NUTRITION AND DIET RESEARCH PROGRESS

NATURE AND NUTRITION

A NEW ERA OF THERAPEUTIC HERBS

NUTRITION AND DIET RESEARCH PROGRESS

Additional books and e-books in this series can be found on Nova's website under the Series tab.

NUTRITION AND DIET RESEARCH PROGRESS

NATURE AND NUTRITION

A NEW ERA OF THERAPEUTIC HERBS

A. K. MOHIUDDIN

nova science publishers
New York

Library of Congress Cataloging-in-Publication Data

ISBN: 978-1-53615-892-2
Library of Congress Control Number:2019944364

Published by Nova Science Publishers, Inc. † New York

CONTENTS

PREFACE

Plants have been well documented for their medicinal uses for thousands of years and traditional medicines are still a major part of habitual treatments of different maladies in different parts of the world. In recent years, there has been growing interest in alternative therapies and the therapeutic use of natural products, especially those derived from plants. Plants are considered as one of the main sources of biologically active materials. Phytochemical screening of medicinal plants has contributed a great deal for the discovery of new drugs. Despite technological developments, herbal drugs still occupy a preferential place in a majority of the population in the Third World and terminal patients in the West. Herbal drugs, in addition to being cost effective and easily accessible, have been used since time immemorial and have passed the test of time without having any side effects. The multitarget effects of herbs (holistic approaches) are the fundamental basis of their utilization. This approach is already used in traditional systems of medicine like Ayurveda, which has become more popular in the West in recent years. However, the integration of modern science with traditional uses of herbal drugs is of the utmost importance if ones wishes to use ancient knowledge for the betterment of humanity.

Chapter 1

PLANT SECONDARY METABOLITES

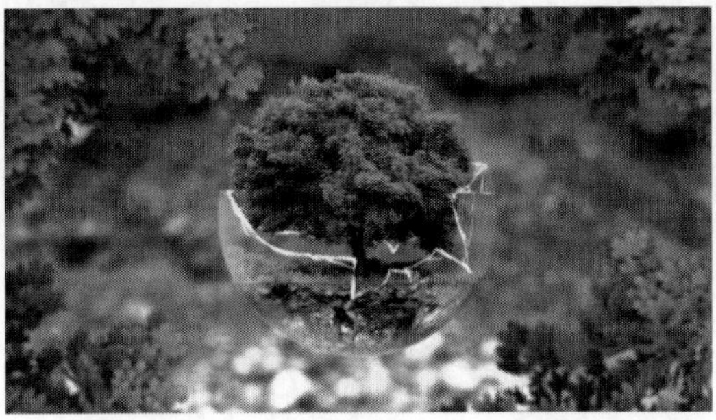

1. INTRODUCTION

Secondary metabolites are organic molecules that are not involved in the normal growth and development of an organism. While primary metabolites have a key role in survival of the species, playing an active function in the photosynthesis and respiration, absence of secondary metabolites does not result in immediate death, but rather in long-term impairment of the organism's survivability, often playing an important role in plant defense. These compounds are an extremely diverse group of natural products synthesized by plants, fungi, bacteria, algae, and animals. Most of secondary metabolites, such as terpenes, phenolic compounds and alkaloids are classified based on their biosynthetic origin. Different classes of these compounds are often associated to a narrow set of species within a phylogenetic group and constitute the bioactive compound in several medicinal, aromatic, colorant, and spice plants and/or functional foods. Secondary metabolites are frequently produced at highest levels during a transition from active growth to stationary phase. The producer organism can grow in the absence of their synthesis, suggesting that secondary metabolism is not essential, at least for short term survival. A second view proposes that the genes involved in secondary metabolism provide a "genetic playing field" that allows mutation and natural selection to fix new beneficial traits via evolution. A third view characterizes secondary metabolism as an integral part of cellular metabolism and biology; it relies on primary metabolism to supply the required enzymes, energy, substrates and cellular machinery and contributes to the long-term survival of the producer. A simple classification of secondary metabolites includes three main groups: terpenes (such as plant volatiles, cardiac glycosides, carotenoids and sterols), phenolics (such as phenolic acids, coumarins, lignans, stilbenes, flavonoids, tannins and lignin) and nitrogen containing compounds (such as alkaloids and glucosinolates). A number of traditional separation techniques with various solvent systems and spray reagents, have been described as having the ability to separate and identify secondary metabolites.

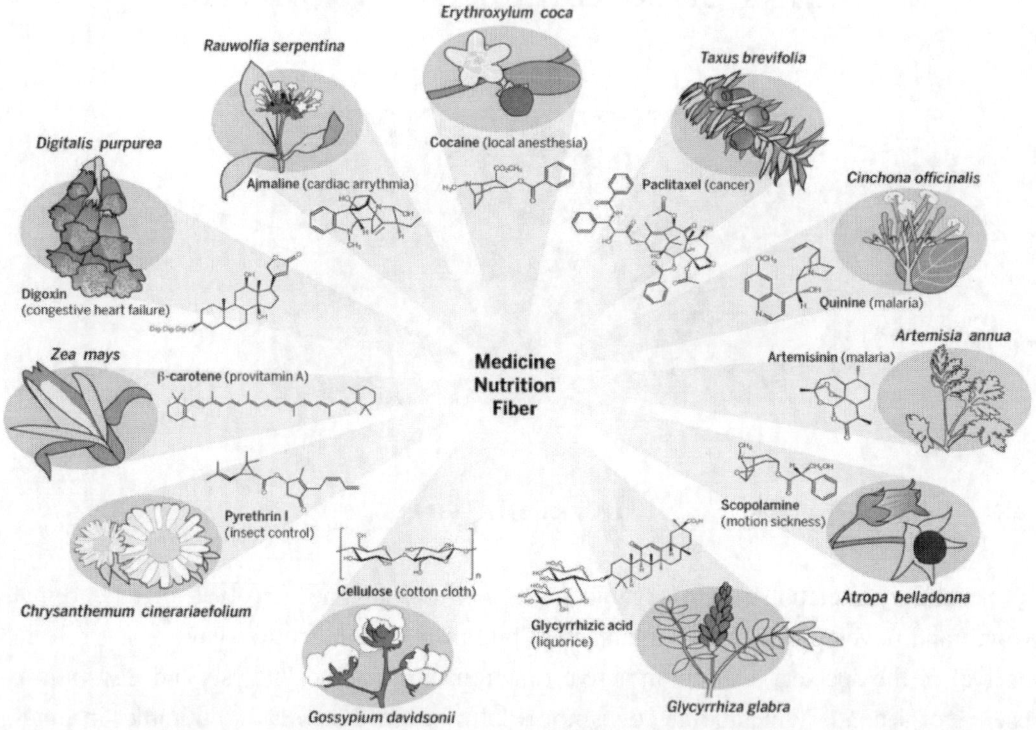

Figure 1. Selected plants and their uses [1]. Throughout history, plants have served as sources of a plethora of chemicals that provide humankind with medicine, fiber, and nutrition. The chemical diversity of plants is enormous. Plants evolved the biosynthesis of a cornucopia of novel chemicals to survive and communicate in a complex ecological environment. Although some plant chemicals are sharp or bitter tasting (glucosinolates and pyrrolizidine alkaloids) to deter herbivory, others such as anthocyanins and carotenoids are brightly colored flower pigments that attract pollinators. Chemicals that are cytotoxic or otherwise physiologically active in mammals are used, for example, as pain-killers, chemotherapeutics, and other drugs. All of these plant chemicals are made through species-specific, specialized biochemical pathways that modify metabolites of primary metabolism. A plethora of new chemicals and metabolic pathways are likely hidden in plant genomes awaiting discovery. Although structures for 200,000 natural products are known, only 15% of the estimated 350,000 plant species have been investigated for their chemical constituents.

2. TERPENOIDS

Terpenoids (isoprenoids) encompass more than 40 000 structures and form the largest class of all known plant metabolites. Some terpenoids have well-characterized physiological functions that are common to most plant species. In addition, many of the structurally diverse plant terpenoids may function in taxonomically more discrete, specialized interactions with other organisms.

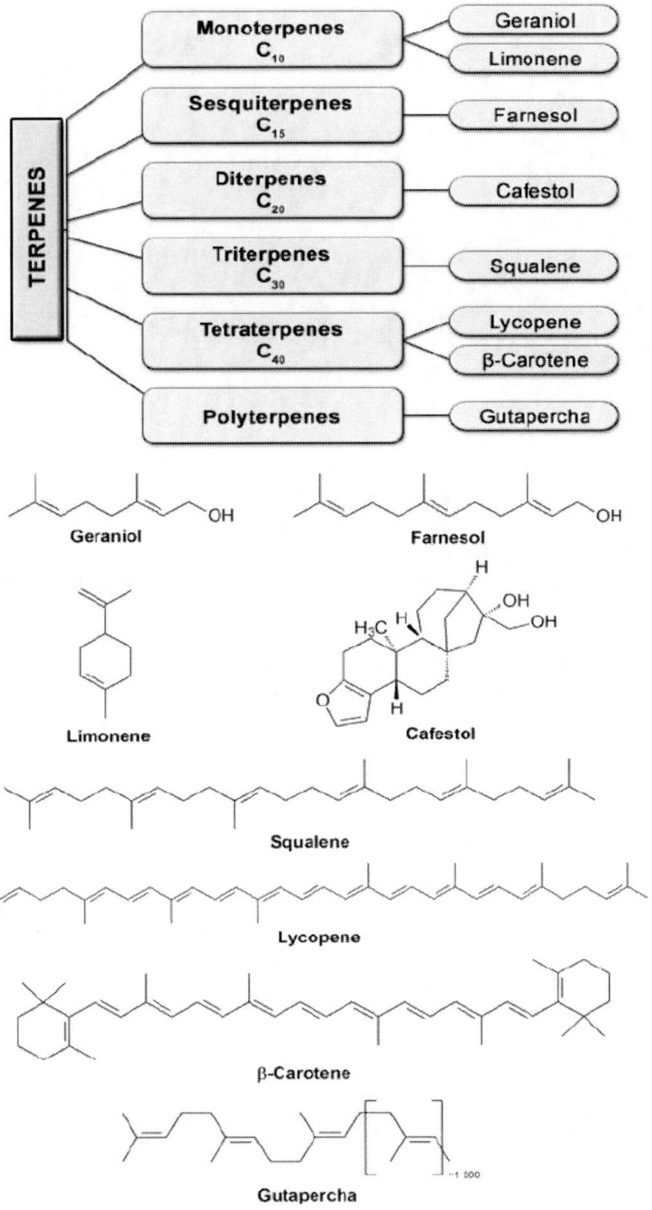

Figure 2. Important carotenoids discovered so far.

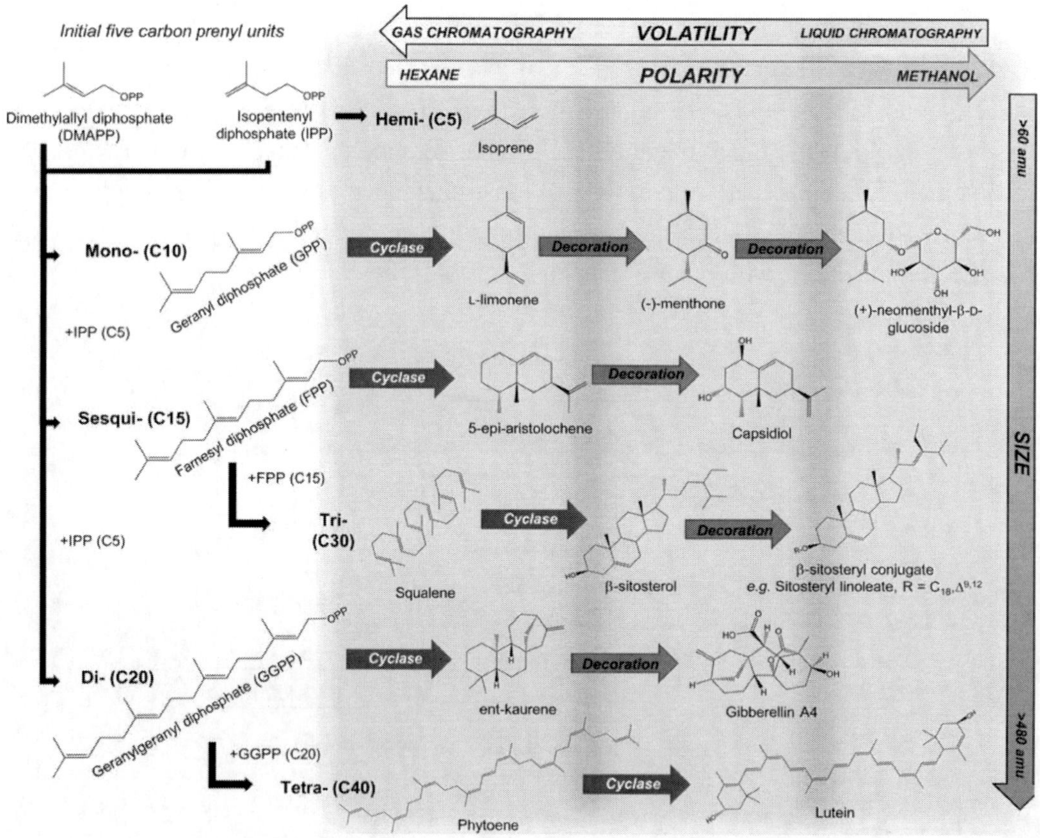

Figure 3. A schematic depiction of terpene metabolism emphasizing the biosynthesis of the different classes of compounds and their physical properties (volatility and polarity) [4]. DMAPP and IPP are the basic building blocks used to generate the allylic diphosphate precursors specific to each terpene class: GPP for monoterpenes; FPP for sesquiterpenes and triterpenes; and GGPP for diterpenes and tetraterpenes. Ionization of the phosphorylated precursors yields linear hydrocarbon forms, while the coupled ionization/cyclization reactions catalyzed by synthases/cyclases yield an incredibly rich array of cyclized hydrocarbons. These linear and cyclized hydrocarbon scaffolds are generally nonpolar or mono-hydroxylated, and their volatility is correlated with their molecular mass. The smaller the compound, the more volatile they will be. But all these terpene scaffolds are also subject to additional layers of modification including hydroxylations, glycosylations, acylations, and aroylations, which alter the physical size and nature of the terpene molecule, and can increase their polarity. This figure is also color coded in reference to the protocols discussed here which might be the most efficient for extraction, quantitation and structural identification of the individual terpene molecules. Protocol 1 is designed for largely nonpolar compounds and is highlighted in green; Protocol 2 is for those molecules having a more polar nature (red); and those terpenes having the greatest polarity are probably best extracted, quantified and qualified by Protocol 3 (blue).

Historically, specialized terpenoids, together with alkaloids and many of the phenolics, have been referred to as secondary metabolites. More recently, these compounds have become widely recognized, conceptually and/or empirically, for their essential ecological functions in plant biology.

Owing to their diverse biological activities and their diverse physical and chemical properties, terpenoid plant chemicals have been exploited by humans as traditional biomaterials in the form of complex mixtures or in the form of more or less pure compounds since ancient times. Plant terpenoids are widely used as industrially relevant chemicals, including many pharmaceuticals, flavors, fragrances, pesticides and disinfectants, and as large-volume feedstocks for chemical industries [2, 3].

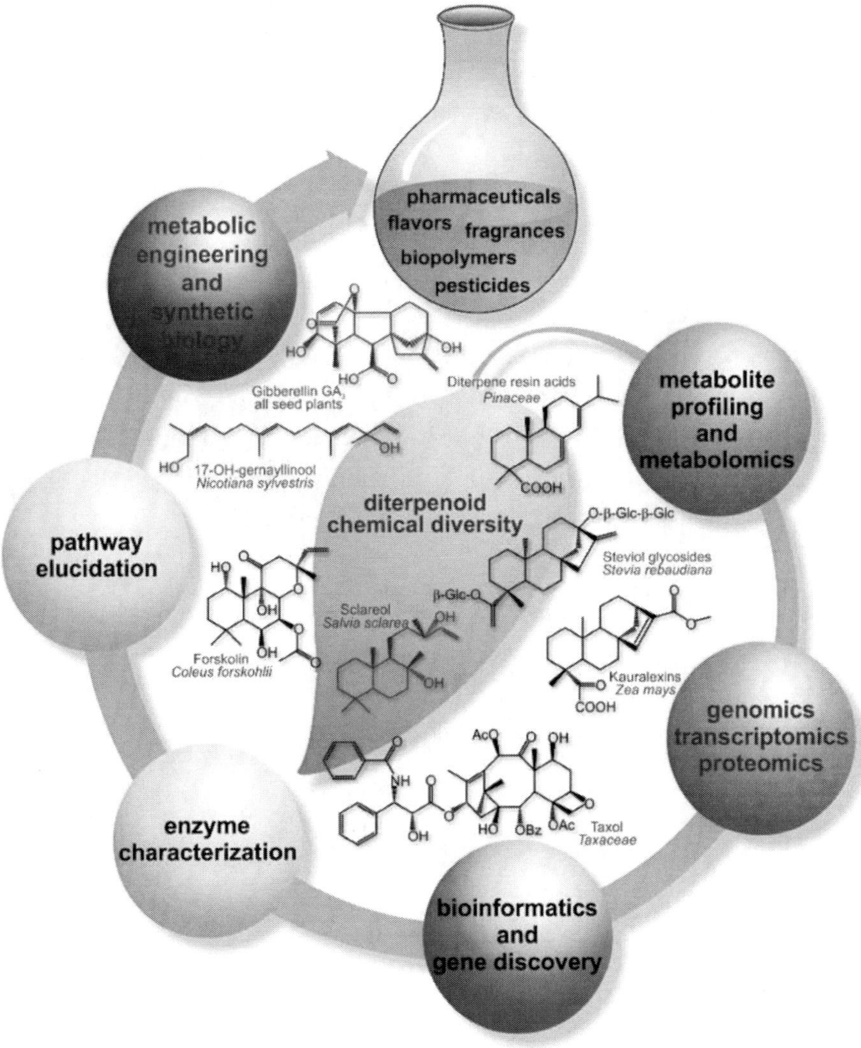

Figure 4. Functional genomics enable efficient discovery of terpenoid metabolic pathways [12]. In order to investigate and ultimately harness the vast chemical repertoire of plant terpenoid metabolism, a core strength of our lab is the efficient identification of terpenoid-metabolic genes, enzymes and pathways by combining genomics-enabled gene discovery using in-house protein databases, rapid enzyme biochemical characterization through microbial and plant co-expression assays, and de novo identification of novel metabolites using mass spectrometry and NMR approaches. Using these tools, we have identified more than 50 functionally distinct TPS and P450 enzymes in over a dozen plant species with relevance for food, bioenergy and medicine. We integrate these biochemical insights with in planta terpenoid profiling via GC- and LC-MS analyses, genetic gene function studies using CRISPR/Cas9-enabled pathway alteration, as well as plant-environment interaction studies using in vitro and in vivo plant-pathogen and plant-microbiome analyses to investigate the bioactivity of teprenoid metabolites and evaluate their potential for agricultural and other biotechnology applications.

2.1. Monoterpenes and Sesquiterpenes (Plant Volatiles)

As nouns the difference between sesquiterpene and monoterpene is that sesquiterpene is (chemistry) any terpene formed from three isoprene units, and having fifteen carbon atoms; includes several plant pigments such as the flavones while monoterpene is (organic chemistry) any terpene formed from two isoprene units, and having ten carbon atoms; either hydrocarbons such as pinene, or compounds with functional groups such as camphor [5]. Monoterpenes evaporate easily and have a low boiling point. Monoterpenes are mostly colorless and odorless, prone to oxidation. Oxidants from monoterpenes could be irritant. Monoterpenes are antiseptic, antiviral and bactericidal [6].

Plant-derived essential oils containing monoterpenoids have been used as antifungal drugs since ancient times, depending both on application method and dose manner. Studies on the antimicrobial activity of essential oils from aromatic species used in Brazil shows that the oils present one or more active fraction, being monoterpenes the major constituents. The monoterpenes citral, citronellal, L-carvone, isopullegol and α-pinene were diluted in ethanol to final concentrations from 0.2 to 1%. All monoterpenes were found to inhibit the growth of the three studies fungi in a dose-dependent manner [8].

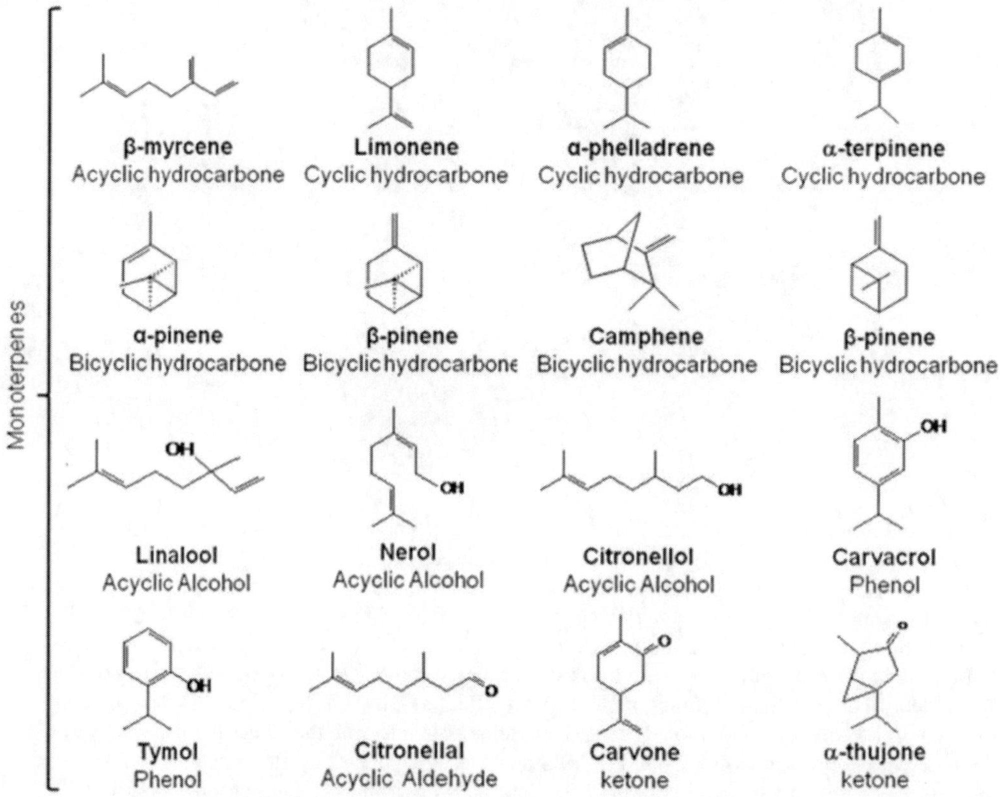

Figure 5. Examples of some mono-terpenes compounds found in essential oils of plants [7].

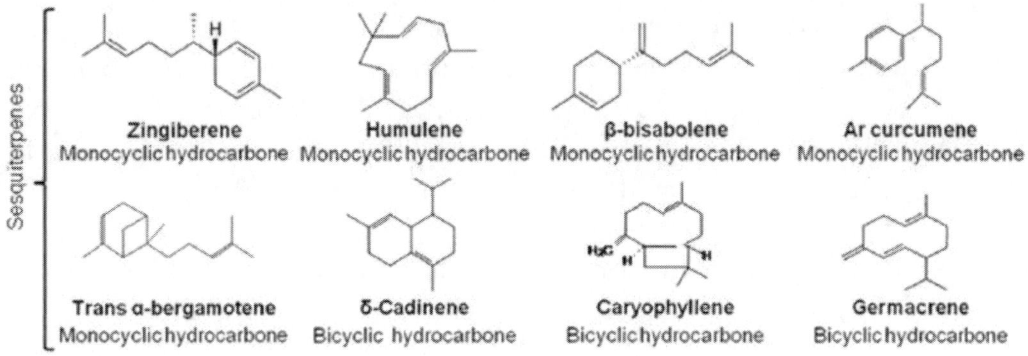

Figure 6. Examples of some sesquiterpenes compounds found in essential oils of plants [7].

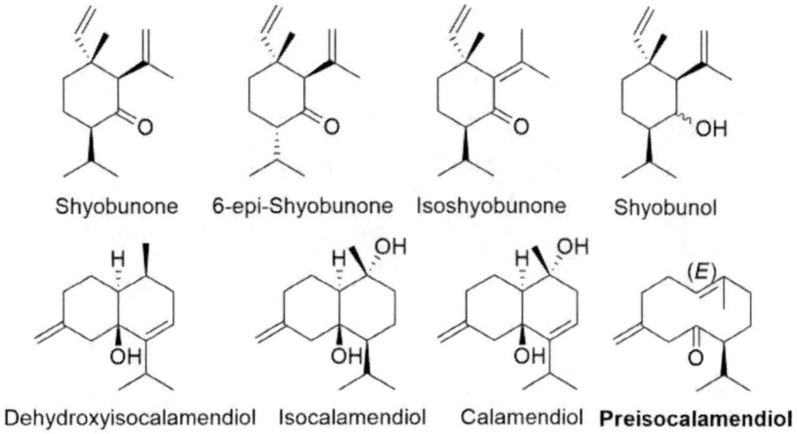

Figure 7. Structures of the uncommon oxygenated sesquiterpenes observed in Bolivian *Schinus molle* essential oils [8].

Sesquiterpenes are less volatile than terpenes, have a greater potential for stereochemical diversity and have stronger odors. They are anti-inflammatory and have bactericidal properties. Sesquiterpenes oxidize over time into sesquiterpenols. In patchouli oil, this oxidation is thought to improve the odor. Sesquiterpenes can be monocyclic, bicyclic or tricyclic and are a very diverse group. When sesquiterpenes occur in essential oils it is mostly in combination with monoterpenes. Sesquiterpenes have a higher melting point than monoterpenes. Sesquiterpenes are anesthetic, antifungal, antiseptic and antibacterial [9-11]. Sesquiterpenes are less volatile than terpenes, have a greater potential for stereochemical diversity and have stronger odors. They are antiinflammatory and have bactericidal properties. Sesquiterpenes oxidize over time into sesquiterpenols. In patchouli oil, this oxidation is thought to improve the odor [10]. Like monoterpenes, sesquiterpenes may be acyclic or contain rings, including many unique combinations. Biochemical modifications such as oxidation or rearrangement produce the related sesquiterpenoids. Sesquiterpenes are found naturally in plants and insects, as semiochemicals, e.g., defensive agents or pheromones [23]. Sesquiterpenes are colorless lipophilic compounds.

Biosynthesis in plants is from three isoprene units, and occurs via farnesyl pyrophosphate (FPP), in the endoplasmic reticulum. Sesquiterpenes consist of a 15-carbon backbone, and whilst diverse in their structure, the majority, and the most functional forms are cyclic, and consequently the focus of this review will rest upon these compounds. The large number of sesquiterpene synthases coupled with the fact that a single synthase may produce numerous products and further modifications after sesquiterpene synthesis, such as oxidation and glycosylation take place result in a vast number of varied structures, many similar synthases may produce the same products, in different ratios which affect the metabolite profile of a plant and can be used to classify closely related species or subspecies [24].

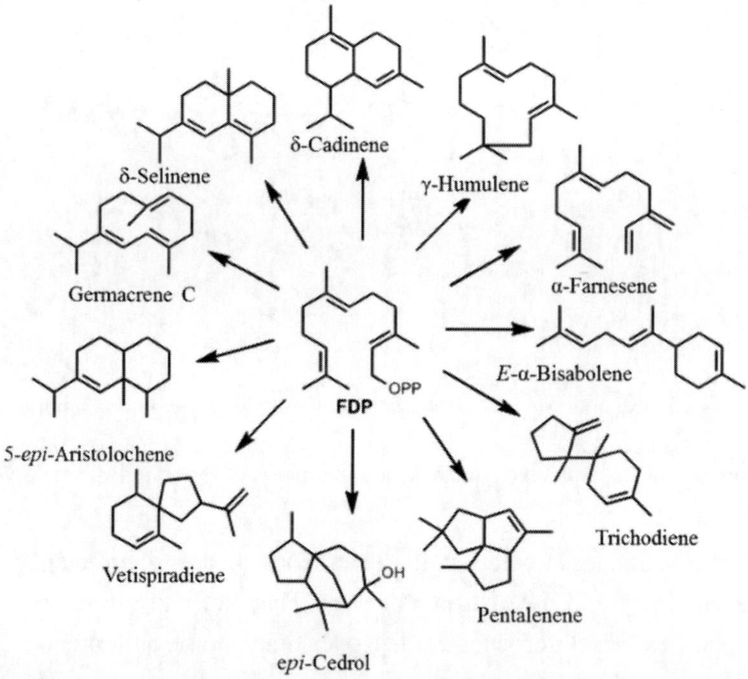

Figure 8. Representative figure of multiproduct terpene synthases converting a single substrate (FDP) into a bouquet of cyclic and acyclic products [13].

Biological Activities

Studies in recent decades have demonstrated that terpenes exert anti-inflammatory effects by inhibiting various proinflammatory pathways in ear edema, bronchitis, chronic obstructive pulmonary disease, skin inflammation, and osteoarthritis. Terpenes have been shown to exert anti-tumorigenic effects against such processes in a number of in vivo and in vitro systems, thus suggesting their potential uses as chemotherapeutic agents for treating tumors. Numerous studies have shown that essential oils derived from various plants have neuroprotective effects against neurodegenerative conditions in vivo and in vitro. Therefore, as a main component of plant essential oils, terpenes may be beneficial to human neuronal health. However, only few studies have focused on the beneficial effects of terpene components of plant essential oils on neuronal health [14, 15]. Antimicrobial and antioxidant properties of essential oils are of great interest in food, cosmetic and pharmaceutical industries since their possible use as natural additives emerged from the tendency to replace synthetic preservatives with natural ones [16]. However, due to the large number of components and synergistic or antagonistic interactions among them, it is possible that essential oils have cellular targets other than cell membranes [17]. Studies into the health benefits of sesquiterpene lactones tend to focus on their anti-tumor potential as some of the SLs have been found to show enough potential to enter clinical trials. Fewer papers look at other applications in disease treatment, and at prospective health benefits. Despite this, work shows that there is much potential for sesquiterpene lactones in the treatment of cardiovascular diseases and their use as antimalarials and are responsible for a range of other effects such as prevention of neurodegeneration, antimigraine activity, analgesic and sedative activities and treatment of ailments such as diarrhea, flu, and burns. The cardiovascular effects are the result of their ability to relax smooth muscle tissue by inhibiting iNOS up-regulation, and consequently increasing levels of NO. The cause of this effect is widely believed to be due to inhibition of NF-κB. In addition, some sesquiterpene lactones protect the gastric lining from ulcer development, another consideration is that parthenolide, the principle component in feverfew and its derived medicines, has been one of the most commonly used sesquiterpenoids, to the exclusion of other compounds [24].

Toxicity Issues

Most of these terpenes easily enter the human body by oral absorption, penetration through the skin, or inhalation leading to measurable blood concentrations. Several studies showed that some monoterpenes (e.g., pulegone, menthofuran, camphor, and limonene) and sesquiterpenes (e.g., zederone, germacrone) exhibited liver toxicity, which is mainly based on reactive metabolites formation, increased concentration of reactive oxygen species and impaired antioxidant defense. There is a high probability that many other terpenes, without sufficiently known metabolism and effects in human liver, could also exert hepatotoxicity. Especially terpenes, that are important components of essential oils with proved hepatotoxicity, should deserve more attention. Intensive research in terpenes metabolism and toxicity represent the only way to reduce the risk of liver injury induced by essential oils and other terpenes-containing products [18]. Sesquiterpene lactones (STLs)-containing plants have long been known to induce a contact dermatitis in exposed farm workers, and also to cause several toxic syndromes in farm animals. More recently, concerns are been raised regarding the genotoxic potential of these compounds and the embryotoxicity of artemisinins. A growing number of STLs are being reported to be mutagenic in different in vitro and in vivo assays [25].

2.2. Diterpenes and Sesterterpenes

Diterpenes are the most important plant metabolites that are derived from geranyl geranyl pyrophosphate (GGPP) and are classified into several categories, namely phytanes, labdanes, halimane, clerodanes, pimaranes, abietanes, cassanes, rosanes, vouacapanes, podocarpanes, trachlobanes, kauranes, aphidicolanes, stemodanes, stemaranes, bayeranes, atisanes, gibberellanes, taxanes, cembranes, daphnanes, tiglianes, and ingenanes classes.

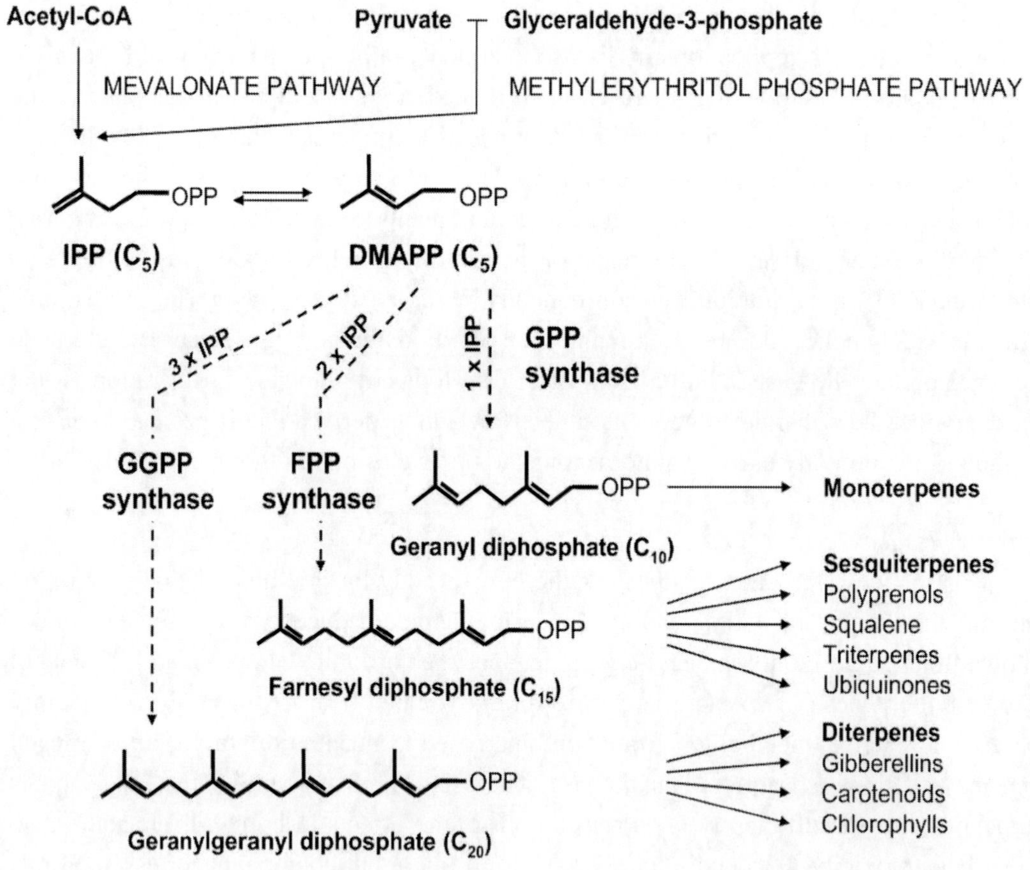

Figure 9. Outline of terpenoid biosynthesis leading to the major conifer oleoresin components, monoterpenes and diterpenes, as well as to other classes of terpenes or compounds with terpene components [19]. In the first phase of terpenoid biosynthesis, IPP and DMAPP are formed via the plastidial methylerythritol phosphate pathway and the cytosolic mevalonate pathway. The next phase consists of the reactions catalyzed by short-chain IDSs, GPP synthase, FPP synthase, and GGPP synthase. GPP synthase condenses one molecule of DMAPP and one molecule of IPP. FPP synthase condenses one molecule of DMAPP with two molecules of IPP in succession. GGPP synthase condenses one molecule of DMAPP with three molecules of IPP in succession. During these repeated condensations, the intermediate prenyl diphosphates are normally bound and not released by the enzymes. The PaIDS1 protein is believed to act like a GGPP synthase, but it releases a significant portion of the GPP formed as an intermediate. The remainder of the GPP is converted directly to GGPP without release of FPP. OPP indicates a diphosphate group.

Diterpenes are derived from a common isoprene precursor, geranylgeranyl diphosphate, via the formation and chemical modification of carbon skeletons. Structural and functional diversity is achieved by the various functions of diterpene cyclases and chemical modification enzymes.

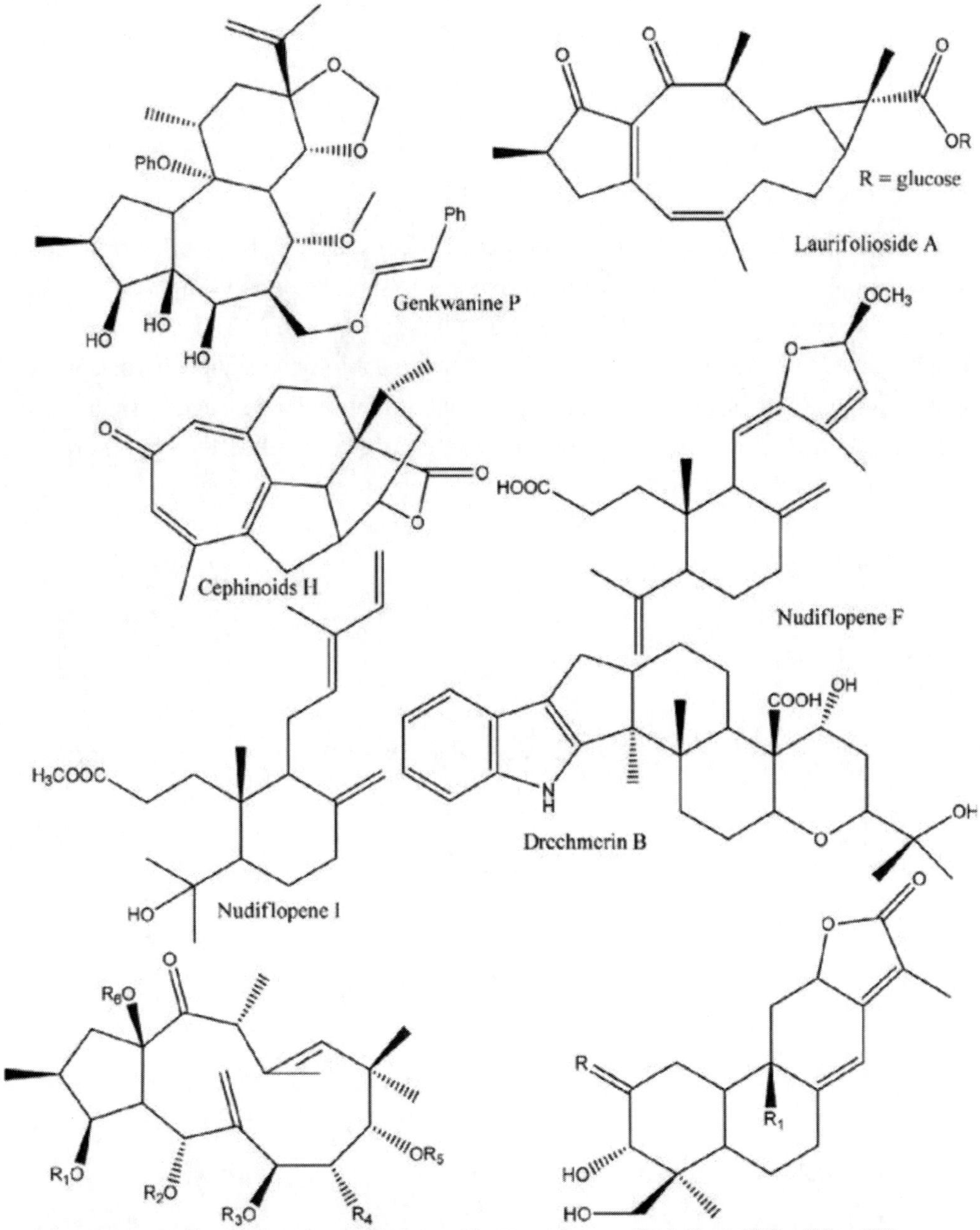

Nicaeenin F R_1 =Ac R_2 =Ac R_3 =*i*Bu R_4 =OAc R_5 =Nic R_6 =Ac
Nicaeenin G R_1 =Pr R_2 =Ac R_3 =*i*Bu R_4 =ONic R_5 =Ac R_6 =H

Eupheliotriol F R =O R_1 =OH
Eupheliotriol L R =H R_1 =H

Figure 10. Structure of diterpenes [20].

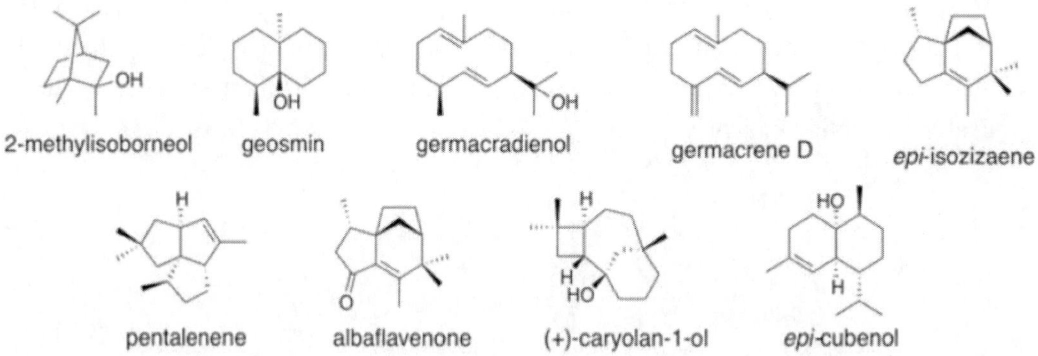

Figure 11. Structure of major known terepenes produced by bacteria.

To date, the cDNAs for a variety of diterpene cyclases responsible for the formation of carbon skeletons or cyclic diphosphate intermediates, such as copalyl diphosphate, have been cloned from higher plants, bryophytes, fungi, and bacteria [21]. Diterpenes have attracted growing attention because of their interesting biological and pharmacological activities. Although thousands of diterpene compounds have been described in nature from terrestrial and marine organisms, only few of them became clinically effective. Overall, the anticancer drug taxol, used in therapy against ovarian, breast, and lung cancer, with its synthetic water-soluble analogue taxotere, is an example of unusual structure discovered from nature and used as medicine.

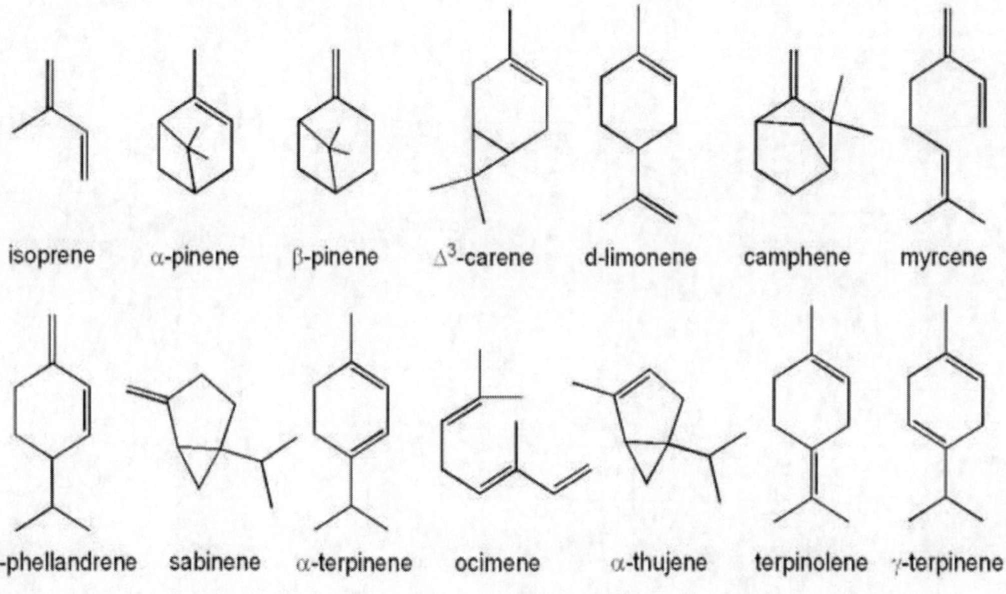

Figure 12. Examples of different terpenes – this diagram shows their chemical structure.

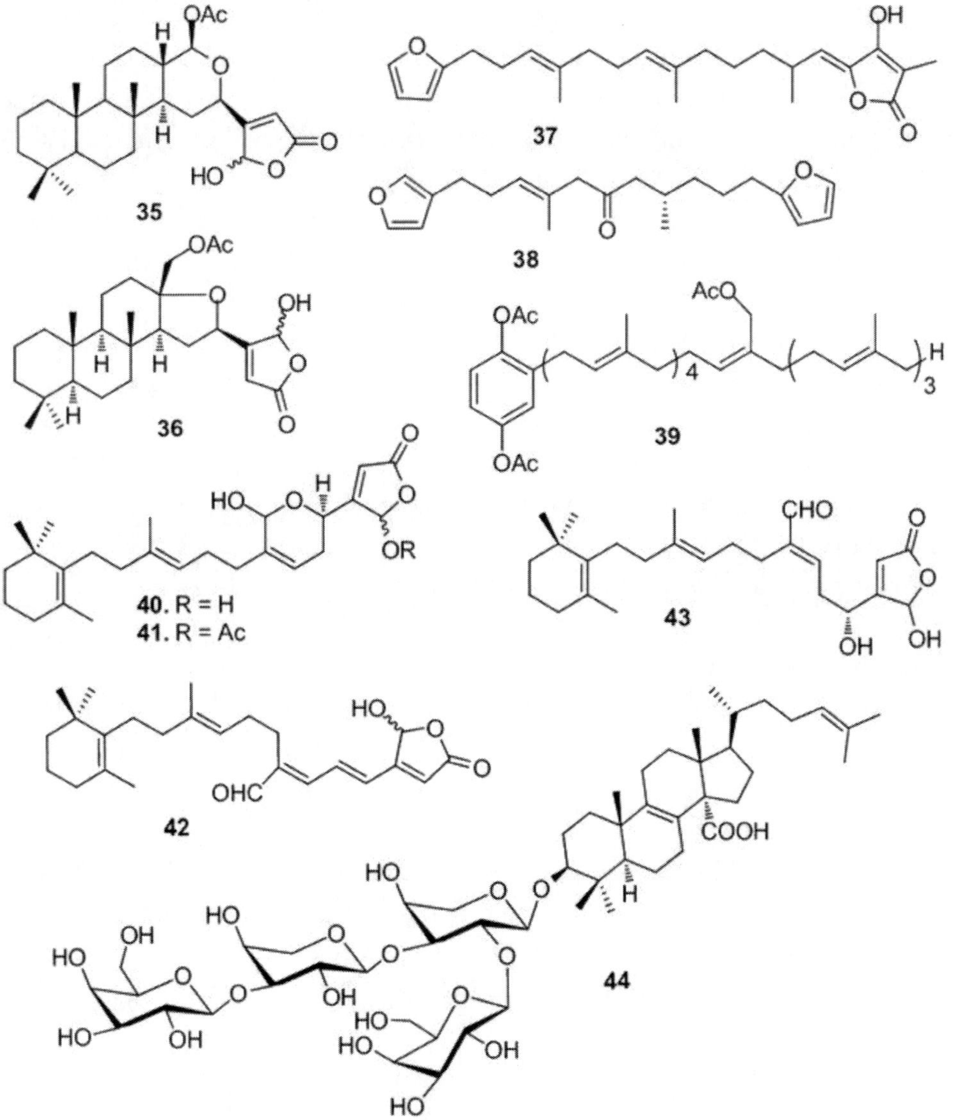

Figure 13. Structures of sesterterpenes and triterpenes from sponges [27]. Sesterterpenes cavernosolide (35), lintenolide A (36) and 7E,12E,20Z-variabilin (37) isolated from the sponge Semitaspongia bactriana, showed strong toxicity against the diatom Nitzschia closterium and against Bugula neritina larvae with EC50 values from 1.22 to 7.41 μM. Two analogues of 37, dihydrofurospongin II (38) and hydroquinone-A acetate (39) obtained from multiple mediterranean sponge extracts showed significant AF activity against B. amphitrite larvae at nontoxic concentrations with EC50 values of about 2.5 and 1.0 μg/mL, respectively. Nortriterpenoids manoalide (40), seco-manoalide (41), manoalide 25-acetate (42) and (4E,6E)-dehydromanoalide (43) from a sponge Smenospongia sp., strongly inhibited the B. amphitrite larval settlement at nontoxic concentrations with EC50 values of 0.24–2.7 μg/mL. Compound 40 could also inhibit bacterial quorum sensing (QS) at low concentrations. Formoside (44), a triterpene glycoside from the sponge Erylus formosus, could strongly deter the biofouling of invertebrates and algae.

Promising diterpenes are the ginkgolides showing potent and selective antagonistic activity toward platelet-activating factor increasing in conditions of shock, burns, ulceration, and inflammation skin diseases. Also used in therapy is the diterpene resiniferatoxin, an ultrapotent vanilloid, isolated from the Euphorbia resinifera latex, in clinical trials for bladder hyperiflexia and diabetic neuropathy. The diterpenes used in therapy will be described together with other promising bioactive diterpenes with particular attention to those isolated from plants [22]. Sesterterpenes are terpene molecules containing a C25 skeleton, which are rare among terpene compounds. Many of them are reported from marine fungi, especially those from mangroves, which include neomangicols A–C and mangicols A–G from the Bahamas mangrove fungus Fusarium sp. In filamentous fungi, genes coding for the enzymes that catalyze secondary metabolites (SM) synthesis, together with those coding for specific regulatory functions and resistance proteins, are usually contiguously aligned in the genome. C25 sesterterpene synthases were discovered only in recent years. Ophiobolin F synthase (AcOS) was found by accident during genome mining for diterpene synthase from *Aspergillus clavatus* [26].

Biological Activities

So far, nearly 1,000 sesterterpenoids have been isolated from terrestrial fungi, lichens, higher plants, insects, and various marine organisms, particularly sponges. Based on the carbocycle numbers contained in their molecular structures, sesterterpenoids can be broadly classified into 6 subgroups: linear, monocarbocyclic, bicarbocyclic, tricarbocyclic, tetracarbocyclic, and miscellaneous sesterterpenoids. All of these six subclasses of sesterterpenoids have been reported to exhibit significant cytotoxicities against tumor cells [31]. Ophiobolins have attracted widespread attention due to their phytotoxic, antimicrobial, nematocidal and cytotoxic bioactivities [32, 33].

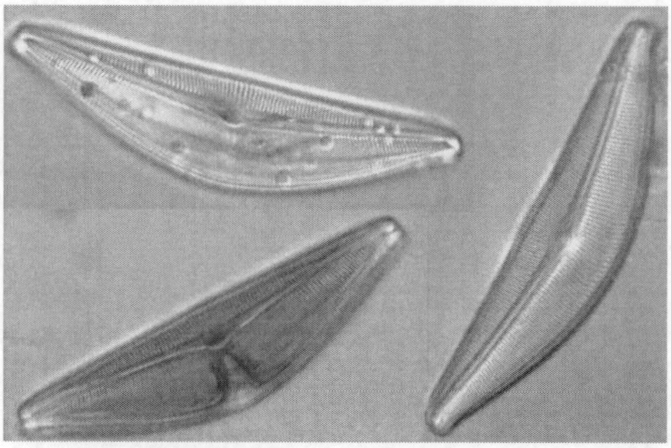

Figure 14. *Nitzschia closterium* [30].

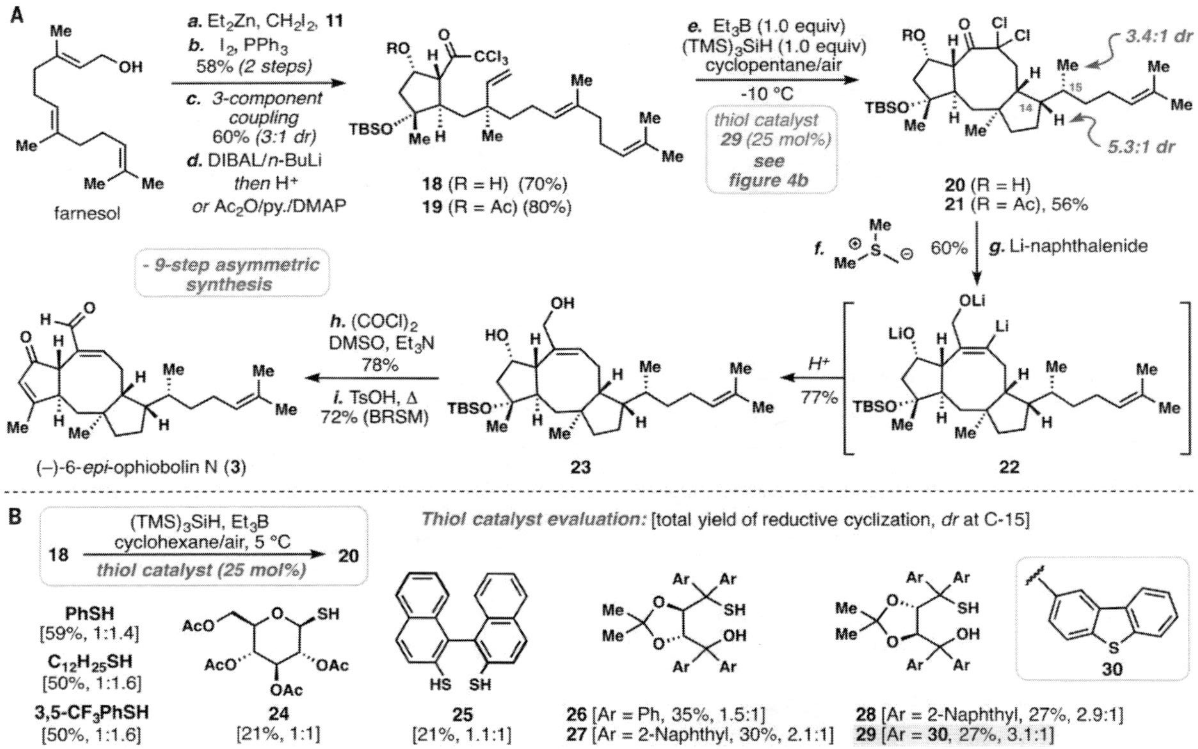

Figure 15. Total synthesis of an ophiobolin sesterterpene [28]. (A) Nine-step asymmetric synthesis of (–)-6-epi-ophiobolin N (3) (yields reported for synthetic steps e to h are for the diastereomeric mixture). (B) Evaluation of thiol catalysts for the transformation of 18→20 (yields and selectivity determined by 1H nuclear magnetic resonance analysis; dr at C-14 was ~4:1). Reagents and conditions: (Steps a to d) See Fig. 3 for analogous conditions. (Step e) 19 (1.0 equiv), TMS3SiH (1.0 equiv), 29 (25 mol %), Et3B (1.0 M solution in THF, 1.25 equiv) added over 12 hours, air, cyclopentane (0.009 M), –10°C, 12 hours, 56% combined yield of reductively cyclized material [the reported dr values at C-14 (5.3:1) and C-15 (3.4:1) were determined after synthetic step h (see supplementary materials)]. (Step f) Me3SI (24.0 equiv), n-BuLi (6.0 equiv), THF, 0°C, 15 min; then add 21 (1.0 equiv), 10 min, 60%. (Step g) Lithium naphthalenide (1.0 M solution in THF, 40 equiv), THF, –78°C, 20 min, 77%. (Step h) (COCl)2 (10.0 equiv), DMSO (15.0 equiv), Et3N (20.0 equiv), CH2Cl2, –78°→0°C, 3 hours, 78%. (Step i) p-TsOH (3.0 equiv), t-BuOH/CH2Cl2, 40°C, 24 hours, 59% plus 19% recovered starting material. p-TsOH, para-toluenesulfonic acid; py, pyridine; DMAP, 4-dimethylaminopyridine; BRSM, based on recovered starting material.

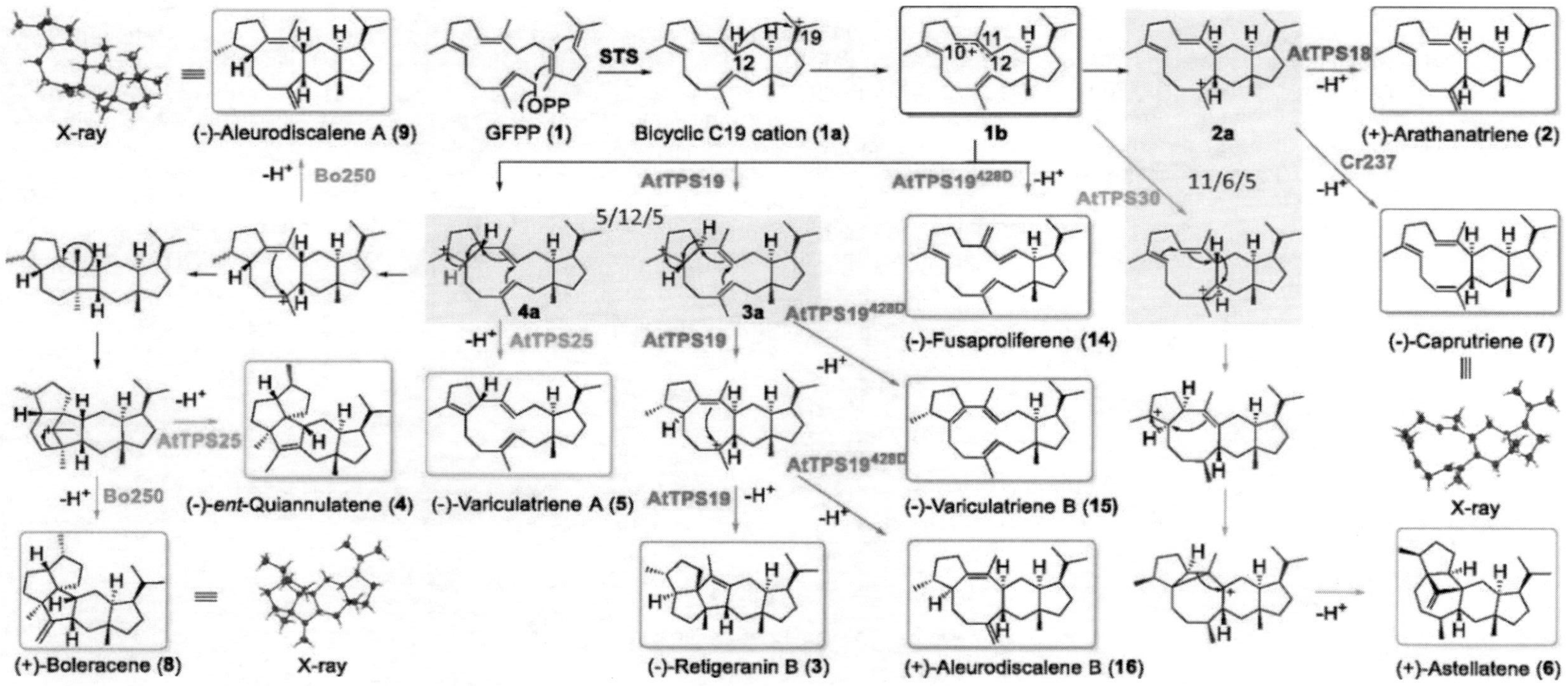

Figure 16. Proposed cyclization paths toward the formation of fungal-type sesterterpenes 2–9 and 14–16 by plant STSs [28]. The universal sesterterpene precursor GFPP is cyclized to form the unified bicyclic C12 cation 1b (black box) following protonation in the active sites of plant STSs and mutated AtTPS19 (AtTPS19428D). Cation 1b diverges to 5/12/5 and 11/6/5 tricyclic carbocations en route to the formation of (+)-arathanatriene (2), (−)-retigeranin B (3), (−)-ent-quiannulatene (4), (−)-variculatriene A (5), (+)-astellatene (6), (−)-caprutriene (7), (+)-boleracene (8), (−)-aleurodiscalene A (9), (−)-fusaproliferene (14), (−)-variculatriene B (15), and (+)-aleurodiscalene B (16). Compounds isolated and characterized are highlighted in colored boxes. Different colors indicate different cyclization paths. Crystal structures 7–9 are presented with displacement ellipsoids shown at 50% probability.

2.3. Triterpenes

Table 1. Examples of neoplastic cell lines sensitive to cytotoxic properties of triterpenes [34]

Triterpene	Type of Neoplasm	Cytotoxicity Evaluation Method
Squalene derivatives	leukemia, melanoma, sarcoma, lung cancer, kidney cancer, cancer of the peripheral nervous system, colon cancer, breast cancer, ovarian carcinoma, cervical carcinoma, prostate cancer	MTT test, evaluation of apoptosis
Dammarane derivatives	glioma, lung cancer, ovarian carcinoma, colorectal carcinoma, colon cancer	MTT test, evaluation of apoptosis
Lanostane and its derivatives	leukemia, melanoma, glioma, gastric carcinoma, pancreatic cancer, colon cancer, hepatic cancer, lung cancer, breast cancer, ovarian carcinoma	MTT test, SRB evaluation of apoptosis
Lupeol	colorectal cancer, gastric cancer	MTT test, LDH evaluation of apoptosis
Oleanolic acid and its derivatives	thyroid carcinoma, ovarian carcinoma, breast cancer, colorectal cancer, glioma, leukemia, gastric adenocarcinoma	MTT test, evaluation of apoptosis
Betulinic acid and its derivatives	lung cancer, prostatic carcinoma, breast cancer, prostate cancer, ovarian carcinoma, cervical carcinoma, lung cancer, colorectal cancer, colon cancer, glioma, melanoma, thyroid tumor, colon adenocarcinoma, leukemia	MTT test, SRB evaluation of apoptosis
Ursolic acid and its derivatives	ovarian carcinoma, pancreatic carcinoma, prostate cancer, cervical carcinoma, hepatic cancer, breast cancer, colorectal cancer, leukemia, neuroma, colon adenocarcinoma	MTT test, SRB evaluation of apoptosis
Vegetal extracts	leukemia, melanoma, glioma, laryngeal cancer, breast cancer, hepatic cancer, gastric cancer, lung cancer, ovarian carcinoma, prostate cancer, colon cancer, epithelial carcinoma	MTT, evaluation of apoptosis
Fungal extracts	melanoma, lymphoma, glioma, breast cancer, ovarian carcinoma, prostate cancer, breast cancer, hepatic cancer, gastric cancer, colon cancer, epidermal nasopharyngeal carcinoma	MTT

*MTT = 3-(4,5-Dimethylthiazol-2-Yl)-2,5-Diphenyltetrazolium Bromide, SRB = Sulforhodamine B, LDH =Lactate dehydrogenase.

Triterpenes are a class of chemical compounds composed of three terpene units with the molecular formula $C_{30}H_{48}$; they may also be thought of as consisting of six isoprene units. Triterpenes are naturally occurring alkenes of vegetable, animal and also fungal origin, classified among an extensive and structurally diverse group of natural substances, referred to as triterpenoids. Their structure includes 30 elements of carbon and they are constituted by isoprene units. Taking into consideration the structure, triterpenes may be divided into linear ones—mainly derivatives of squalene, tetracyclic and pentacyclic, containing respectively four and five cycles, as well as two- and tricyclic ones. Representatives of those show anti-cancer properties as well as anti-inflammatory, anti-oxidative, anti-viral, anti-bacterial and anti-fungal ones. A good example could be the betulinic acid and its derivatives which have been investigated for their strong cytotoxic properties. Other important representatives are the compounds originating from squalene, dammarane, lanostane, oleane (e.g., oleanolic acid), lupane (e.g., lupeol), ursane (e.g., ursolic acid) or triterpenoid sapogenins, for example cycloartane, friedelane, filicane and cucurbitane triterpenoids. Table 1 gives examples of neoplastic cell lines sensitive to cytotoxic properties of triterpenes [34].

Biological Activities

In surgical wounds, the triterpenes induced a reduction in time to closure, and this effect was reported in virtually all wound types. Triterpenes also modulate the production of ROS in the wound microenvironment, accelerating the process of tissue repair [36]. Indeed, this class of compounds presents several biological activities, including anti-inflammatory, antioxidant, anti-viral, anti-diabetic, anti-tumor, hepato-protective and cardio-protective activities [34, 37, 39]. There are many in vitro investigations indicating the ability of various plant-derived triterpenes to inhibit α-glucosidase and α-amylase activity [38]. In the Western world, the individual average human consumption of triterpenes is estimated to be approximately 250 mg per day, and in the Mediterranean countries, the average intake could reach 400 mg per day [39].

2.4. Tetraterpenes (Carotenoids)

Carotenoids are C40-compounds consisting of eight isopentenyl-pyrophosphate units. More than 750 structurally defined carotenoids are found in nature. They are synthesized by oxygenic phototrophs (land plants, algae, and cyanobacteria), anoxygenic phototrophs (purple bacteria, green sulfur bacteria, green filamentous bacteria, and heliobacteria), some eubacteria, some archaea, and some fungi. The yellow, orange, or red fat-soluble plant and animal pigments, known as carotenoids, are classed as tetraterpenes, although they have in general the molecular formula $C_{40}H_{56}$, rather than $C_{40}H_{64}$. The fact that their structures can be built up from isoprene units justifies their classification as terpenes. The carotenoids are isolated from their natural sources by solvent extraction and are purified by chromatography. Lycopene, the red pigment of the ripe tomato, exemplifies the class of acyclic tetraterpenes. The most important and abundant tetraterpene is β-carotene, the principal yellow pigment of the carrot; β-carotene is of nutritional importance because animals are able to cleave the molecule at the point of symmetry with the production of vitamin A [40, 41].

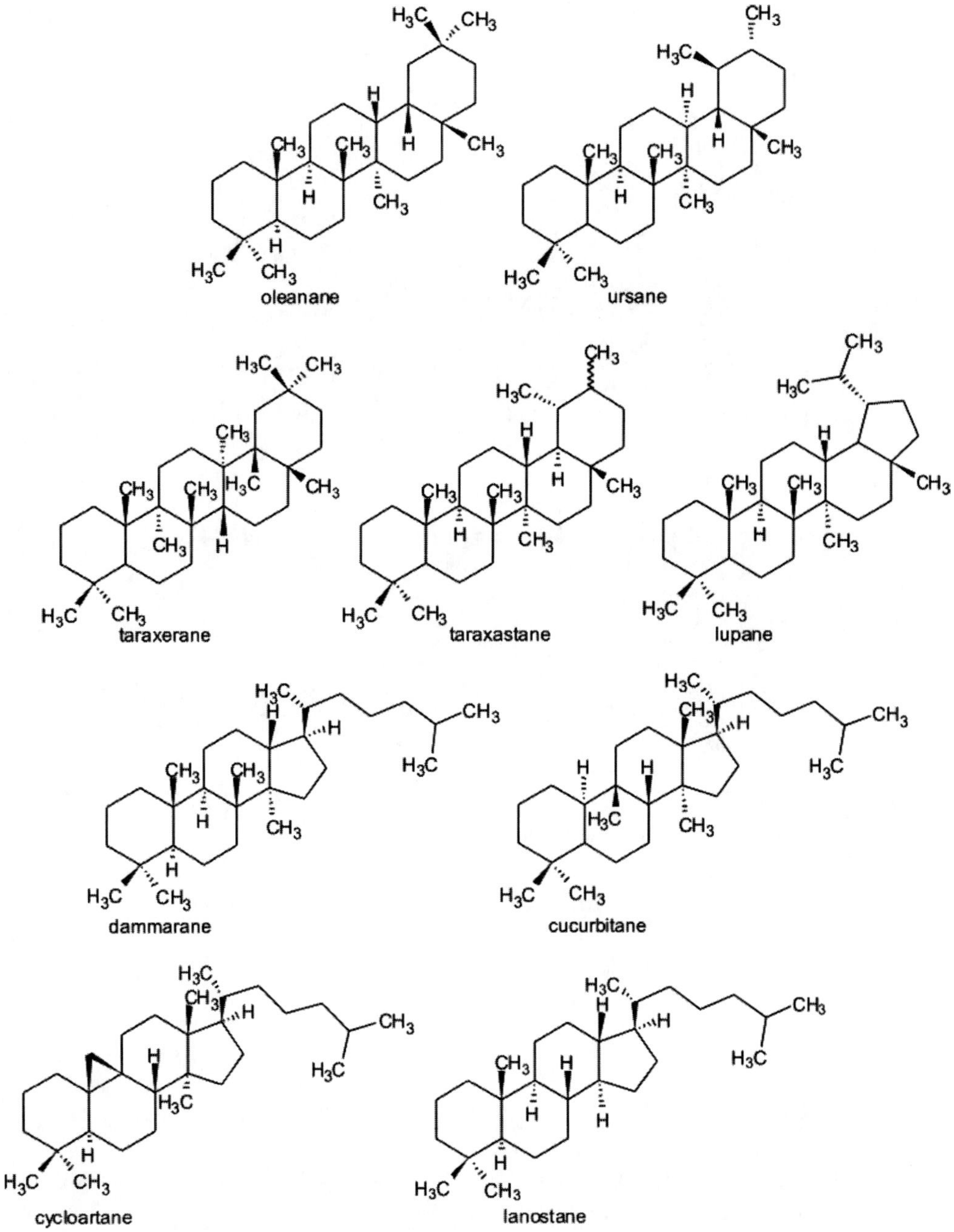

Figure 17. Chemical structures of the main subclasses of triterpenes [38].

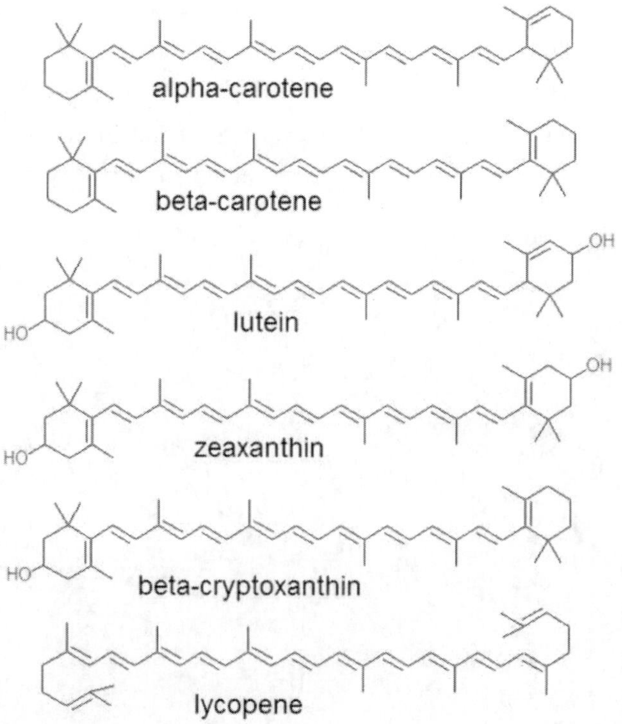

Figure 18. Carotenoids structure.

Table 2. Representative food-derived carotenoids [42]

Carotenoid	Food Source
α-Carotene	Banana, butternut, carrot, pumpkin
β-Carotene	Apricots, banana, broccoli, cantaloupe, carrot, dairy products, honeydew, kale, mango, nectarine, peach, pumpkin, spinach, sweet potato, tomato
Crocetin	Gardenia fruit, saffron stigma
Crocin	Gardenia fruit, saffron stigma
β-Cryptoxanthin	Apple, broccoli, celery, chili, crustaceans, grape, green beans, papaya, pea, peach, peppers, salmonid fish, squashes, tangerine
Lutein	Apple, basil, broccoli, celery, crustaceans, cucumber, dairy products, grapes, green pepper, kale, kiwi, maize, parsley, pea, pumpkin, salmonid fish, spinach, squash
Lycopene	Grapefruit, guava, tomato, watermelon
Zeaxanthin	Basil, crustaceans, cucumber, dairy products, honeydew, kale, maize, mango, orange, parsley, salmonid fish, spinach
Marine	
Astaxanthin	Crustaceans, algae, salmonid fish
Fucoxanthin	Brown seaweeds

The four major carotenoids in terms of their abundance in foods are lutein, zeaxanthin, β-carotene, and lycopene (see Figure 19). Lutein and zeaxanthin belong to the xanthophylls group, while lycopene and β-carotene are hydrocarbon carotenoids. Lycopene has two identical linear 2,6-dimethyl-1,5-heptadiene end-groups, in contrast to β-carotene where the same atoms are arranged into 2,6,6-trimethyl-1-cyclohexene moieties. The two xanthophylls show instead hydroxylated cyclohexene end-groups: two 4-hydroxy-2,6,6-trimethyl-1-cyclohexene for zeaxanthin, while for lutein one end-group is as before and the other is a 4-hydroxy-2,6,6-trimethyl-2-cyclohexene [43].

Biological Activities

Due to their characteristic structure, carotenoids have bioactive properties, such as antioxidant, anti-inflammatory, and autophagy-modulatory activities. Given the protective function of carotenoids, their levels in the human body have been significantly associated with the treatment and prevention of various diseases, including neurodegenerative diseases [44]. Carotenoids protect membranes formed with unsaturated lipids against singlet oxygen through combined activity of different mechanisms: modification of structural properties of the lipid bilayers, physical quenching of singlet oxygen and chemical reactions leading to the pigment oxidation [45]. Carotenoids have a range of functions in human health. They primarily exert antioxidant effects, but individual carotenoids may also act through other mechanisms; for example, β-carotene has a pro-vitamin A function, while lutein/zeaxanthin constitute macular pigment in the eye. The benefit of lutein in reducing progression of age-related macular eye disease and cataracts is strengthening; an intake recommendation would help to generate awareness in the general population to have an adequate intake of lutein rich foods. There is evidence that carotenoids, in addition to beneficial effects on eye health, also produce improvements in cognitive function and cardiovascular health, and may help to prevent some types of cancer [46]. Carotenoids can be associated to fatty acids, sugars, proteins, or other compounds that can change their physical and chemical properties and influence their biological roles. Furthermore, oxidative cleavage of carotenoids produces smaller molecules such as apocarotenoids, some of which are important pigments and volatile (aroma) compounds. Enzymatic breakage of carotenoids can also produce biologically active molecules in both plants (hormones, retrograde signals) and animals (retinoids). Both carotenoids and their enzymatic cleavage products are associated with other processes positively impacting human health. Carotenoids are widely used in the industry as food ingredients, feed additives, and supplements [47].

Toxicity

It is well known that an excess of retinoids induces teratogenic effects and affects xenobiotic metabolism. Although β-carotene is not teratogenic, high doses of β-carotene and vitamin E can be prooxidant and toxic and increase cancer risk. In particular, despite that high intake of β-carotene reduces the risk of many cancers, the effect on breast cancer risk depends on estrogen receptor and progesterone receptor statuses. In general, the relationships between carotenoids and cancer risk depend on type of carotenoids and site of cancer, but the supplementation never confirms the suggestions from intake data. Moreover, the increased risk of lung cancer after β-carotene supplementation had been reported in smokers and people drinking ≥11 g ethanol/d [48].

3. Phenolic Compounds

Phenolics are aromatic benzene ring compounds with one or more hydroxyl groups produced by plants mainly for protection against stress. Phenolics play important roles in plant development, particularly in lignin and pigment biosynthesis. They also provide structural integrity and scaffolding support to plants. Importantly, phenolic phytoalexins, secreted by wounded or otherwise perturbed plants, repel or kill many microorganisms, and some pathogens can counteract or nullify these defenses or even subvert them to their own advantage [49]. Phenolic compounds are secondary metabolites, which are produced in the shikimic acid of plants and pentose phosphate through phenylpropanoid metabolization. They contain benzene rings, with one or more hydroxyl substituents, and range from simple phenolic molecules to highly polymerized compounds. In the synthesis of phenolic compounds, the first procedure is the commitment of glucose to the pentose phosphate pathway (PPP) and transforming glucose-6-phosphate irreversibly to ribulose-5-phosphate. The first committed procedure in the conversion to ribulose-5-phosphate is put into effect by glucose-6-phosphate dehydrogenase (G6PDH). On the one hand, the conversion to ribulose-5-phosphate produces reducing equivalents of nicotinamide adenine dinucleotide phosphate (NADPH) for cellular anabolic reactions. On the other hand, PPP also produces erythrose-4-phosphate along with phosphoenolpyruvate from glycolysis, which is then used through the phenylpropanoid pathway to generate phenolic compounds after being channeled to the shikimic acid pathway to produce phenylalanine. Phenolics are the most pronounced secondary metabolites found in plants, and their distribution is shown throughout the entire metabolic process. These phenolic substances, or polyphenols, contain numerous varieties of compounds: simple flavonoids, phenolic acids, complex flavonoids and colored anthocyanins. (Figure 1). These phenolic compounds are usually related to defense responses in the plant. However, phenolic metabolites play an important part in other processes, for instance incorporating attractive substances to accelerate pollination, coloring for camouflage and defense against herbivores, as well as antibacterial and antifungal activities [50].

Although polyphenols are chemically characterized as compounds with phenolic structural features, this group of natural products is highly diverse and contains several sub-groups of phenolic compounds. Fruits, vegetables, whole grains and other types of foods and beverages such as tea, chocolate and wine are rich sources of polyphenols.

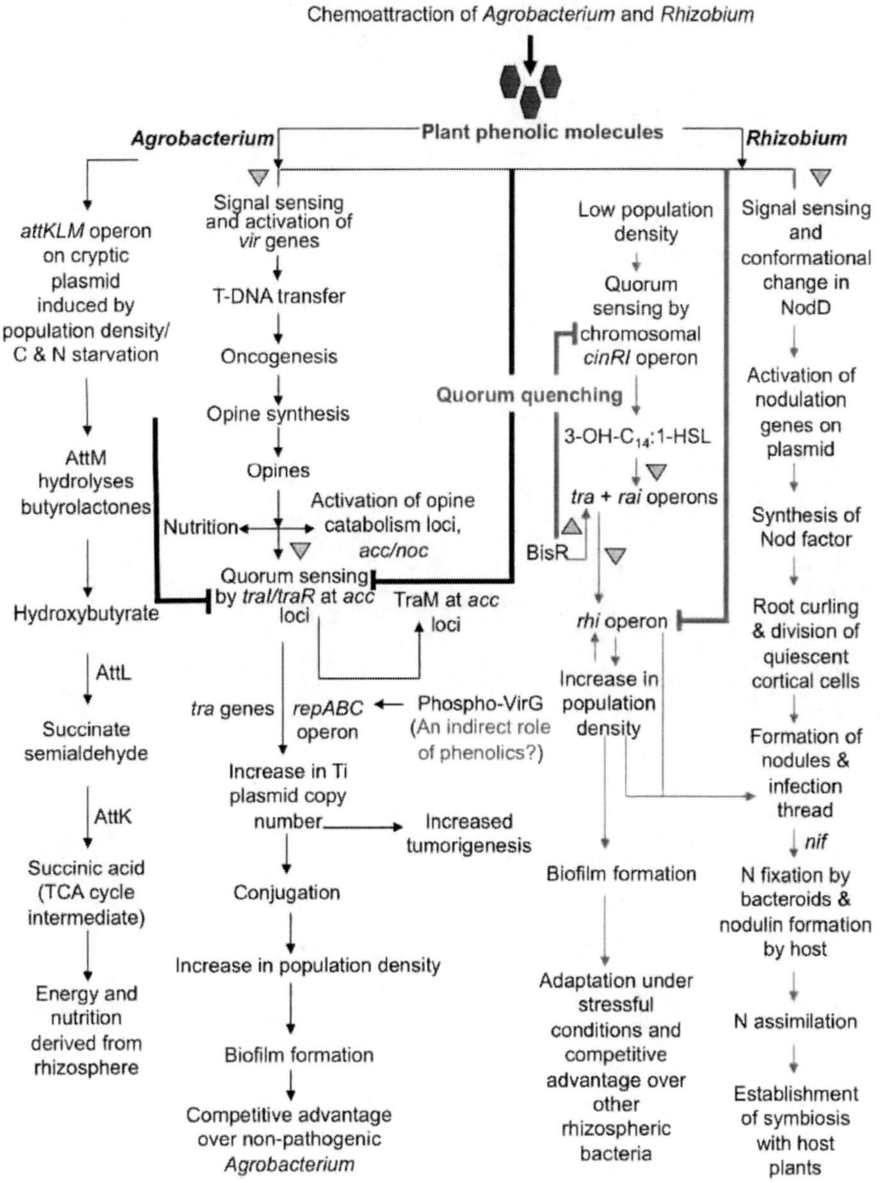

Figure 19. The use of phenolics by Agrobacterium and Rhizobium for survival and infection of the host plant [49]. Black arrows indicate how Agrobacterium uses phenolics to initiate a complex process of pathogenesis, culminating with opine synthesis. In addition to their nutritional value, opines help Agrobacterium's competition with nonpathogenic bacteria, such as A. radiobacter, by increasing its population density and biofilm formation through quorum sensing. Agrobacterium also uses the attKLM operon to regulate its population density during times of nutritional starvation and to synthesize alternative sources of nutrients and energy by degrading g-butyrolactones produced by other rhizospheric bacteria. Green arrows indicate the use of phenolics by Rhizobium leguminosarum bv. viciae for the induction of nod genes followed by the process of symbiosis. Under stress conditions, phenolics also regulate the increase in population density, biofilm formation and effective nodulation by repressing the quorum-sensing rhi operon. An increase in population density as a result of quorum sensing provides a competitive edge to rhizobia over other rhizospheric bacteria. Bold lines indicate the quorum-quenching mechanisms, whereas triangles represent the steps of activation. TCA, tricarboxylic acid.

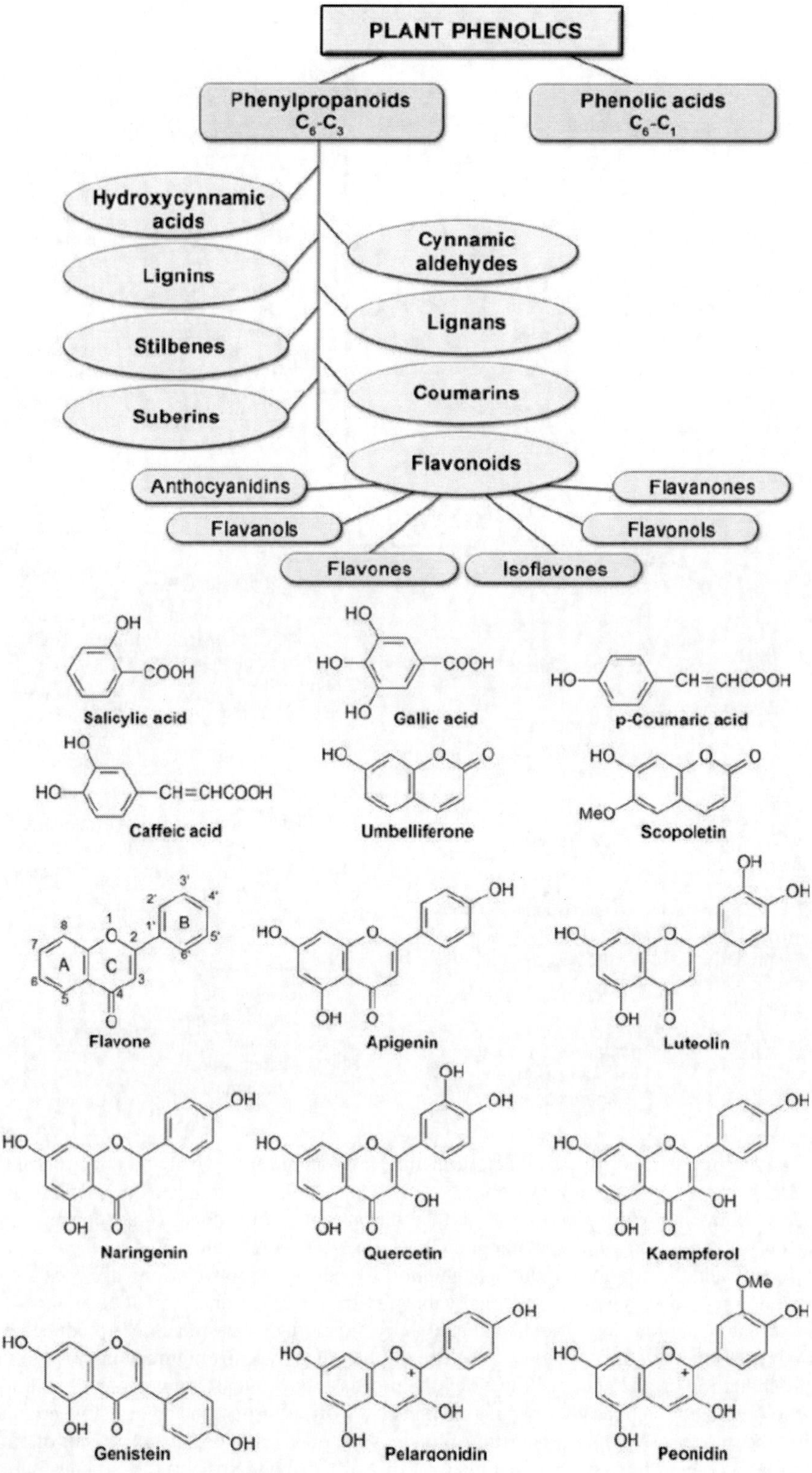

Figure 20. Main phenolic compounds.

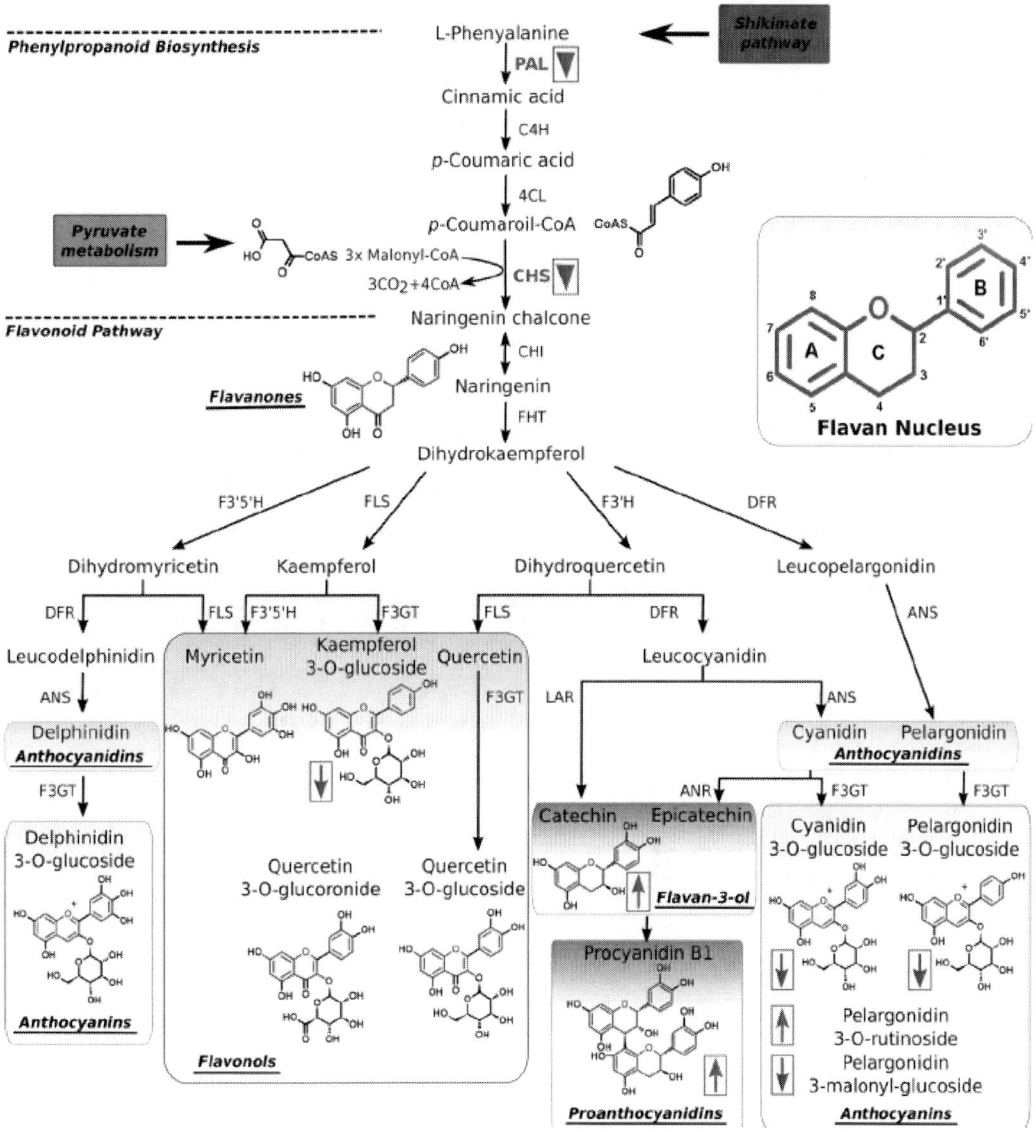

Figure 21. The phenolic compound biosynthesis pathway [52]. A schematic representation of the phenylpropanoid and flavonoid biosynthesis pathway is shown. Major families of flavonoid compounds are highlighted. Flavonoids are characterized by the presence of the flavan nucleus with A, B, and C rings as indicated (inset). Final products of the flavonoid pathway such as pelargonidin 3- O -glucoside, are often glycosylated at the position 3 of the C ring of the flavan nucleus. Suppression of Fra a protein expression affects the expression of phenylalanine ammonia lyase (PAL) and chalcone synthase (CHS) genes (red inverted triangles) and alters phenolic compound accumulation with an increase in the levels of catechin and a decreased accumulation of anthocyanins (as indicated by arrows).

The diversity and wide distribution of polyphenols in plants have led to different ways of categorizing these naturally occurring compounds. Polyphenols have been classified by their source of origin, biological function, and chemical structure. Also, the majority of polyphenols in plants exist as glycosides with different sugar units and acylated sugars at different positions of the polyphenol skeletons [51].

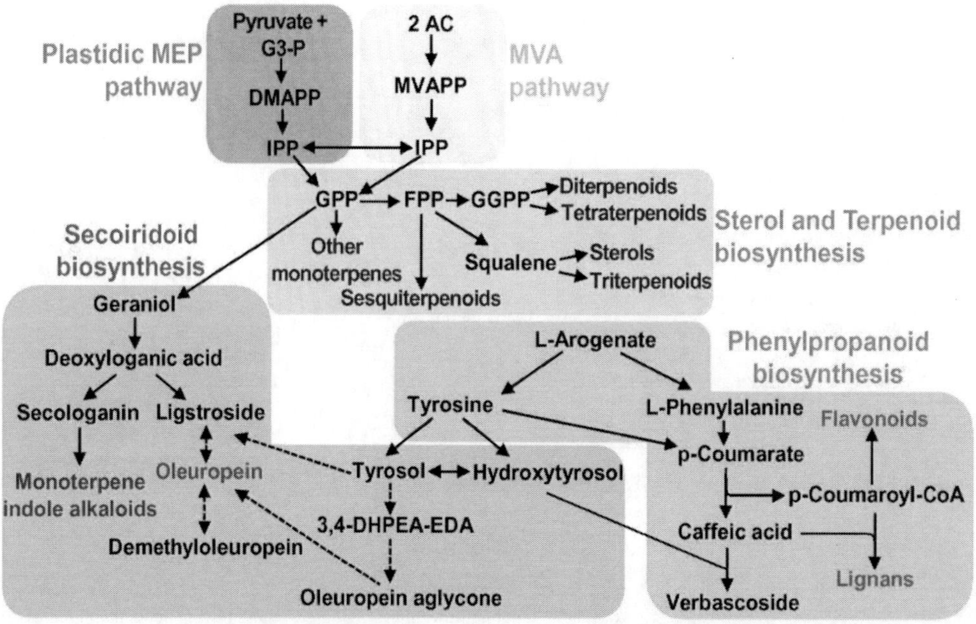

Figure 22. Schematic representation showing the putative biosynthetic pathways of main secondary compounds of olive fruits [61]. G3P: glyceraldehyde 3-phosphate; DMAPP: Dimethylallyl diphosphate; IPP: Isopentenyl diphosphate; AC: Acetyl-CoA; MVAPP: Mevalonate diphosphate; GPP: Geranyl diphosphate; FPP: Farnesyl diphosphate; and GGPP: Geranyl geranyl pyrophosphate. Dotted arrows indicate uncertain biosynthetic steps.

3.1. Phenolic Acids

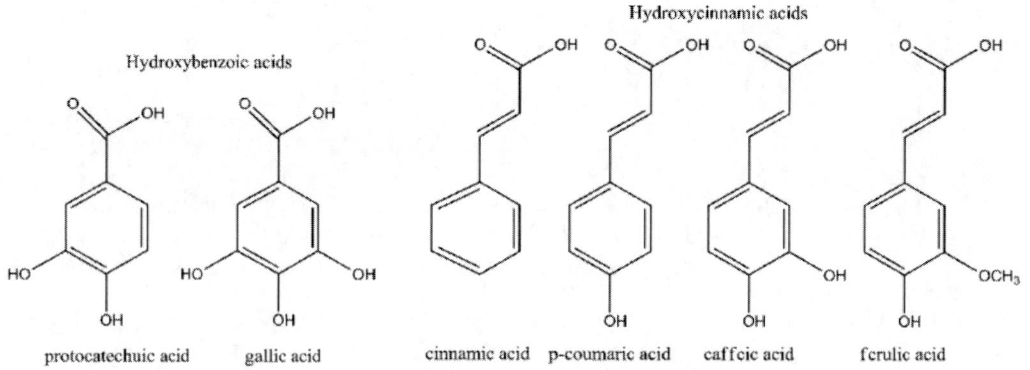

Figure 23. Chemical structure of selected phenolic acids.

Phenolic acids are abundant biomass feedstock that can be derived from the processing of lignin or other byproducts from agro-industrial waste. Although phenolic acids such as p-hydroxybenzoic acid, p-coumaric acid, caffeic acid, vanillic acid, cinnamic acid, gallic acid, syringic acid, and ferulic acid can be used directly in various applications, their value can be significantly increased when they are further modified to high value-added compounds. Thus, biotransformation of phenolic acids provides an economically viable and sustainable means for producing useful materials for society [53]. P-hydroxybenzoic acid used as a raw material for the production of liquid crystal polymers and paraben [54]. Caffeic acid phenethyl ester (CAPE) acts as a specific inhibitor of NF-κB in breast cancer cells [55]. Vanillic acid is a well-known antioxidant and reduce oxidative stress as well Circular Dichroism and FT-IR studies clearly showed efficiency to inhibit collagen fibril formation [56].

3.2. Flavonoids

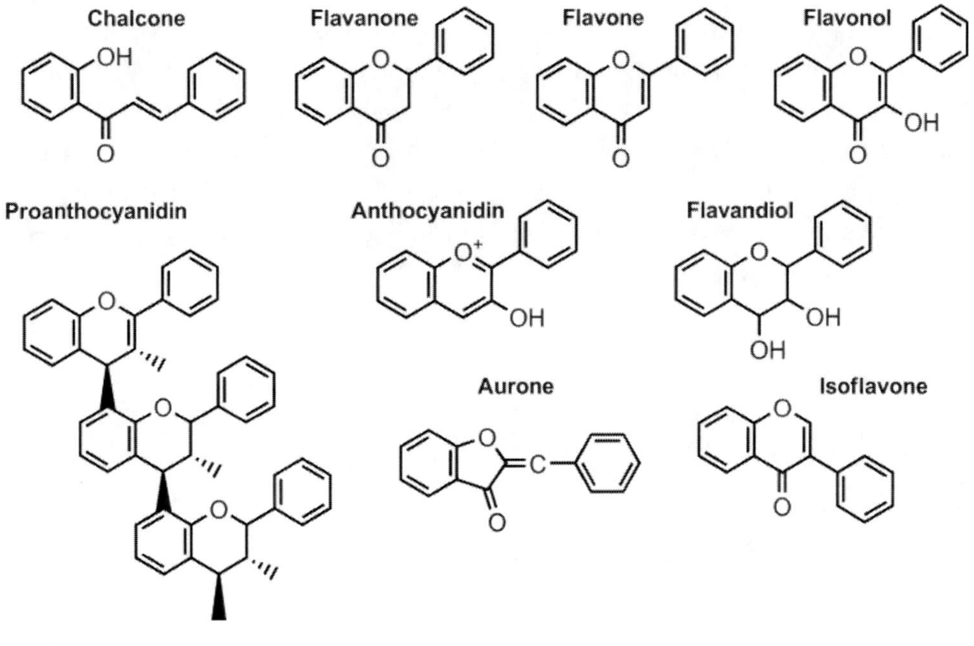

Figure 24. Structure of the main classes of flavonoids.

Flavonoids have the C6–C3–C6 general structural backbone in which the two C6 units (Ring A and Ring B) are of phenolic nature. Due to the hydroxylation pattern and variations in the chromane ring (Ring C), flavonoids can be further divided into different sub-groups such as anthocyanins, flavan-3-ols, flavones, flavanones and flavonols. Some factors influenced flavonoid levels, such as harvest time, shade netting, planting time, development, and using the light transmittance paper bags. Sample processing can influence the quantity and quality of bioactive compounds. For example, the flavonoid content of fresh mulberry leaves was highest and the content in leaves that were oven-dried at 100–105°C was lowest [59]. Due to the reported antioxidant, antibacterial and antiviral effects, presence in normal daily diet and minimal side-effects of flavonoids, they are considered useful resources for drug design. Flavonoids are currently identified not as medicine, but as necessary elements of daily diet that aid functioning of the immune system. The substantial pharmacological properties of flavonoids include antioxidant, anti-inflammatory, antiproliferative, photoprotective, depigmentation, anti-aging which are very promising in the treatment of several skin disorders [57]. Given the putative relationship between inflammation and insulin resistance, the consumption of flavonoids or flavonoid-rich foods has been suggested to reduce the risk of diabetes by targeting inflammatory signals [58].

3.3. Polyphenolic Amides

Some polyphenols may have N-containing functional substituents. Two such groups of polyphenolic amides are of significance for being the major components of common foods: capsaicinoids in chili peppers and avenanthramides in oats. Capsaicinoids such as capsaicin are responsible for the hotness of the chili peppers but have also been found to have strong antioxidant and anti-inflammatory properties, and they modulate the oxidative defense system in cells. Antioxidant activities including inhibition of LDL oxidation by avenanthramides have also been reported.

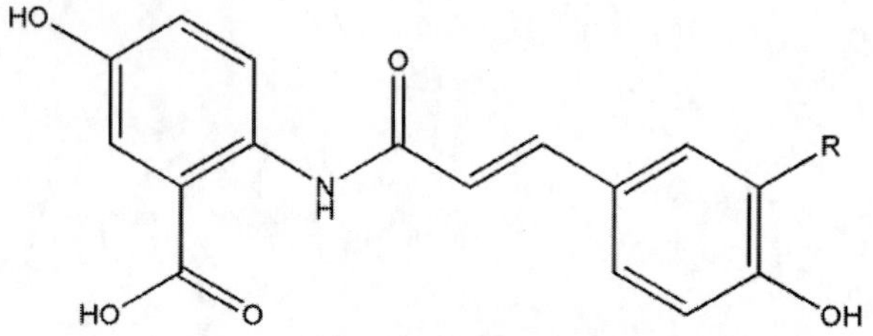

Avenanthramide

Avenanthramide-a R = H
Avenanthramide-b R = OCH_3
Avenanthramide-c R = OH

Figure 25. Structure of avenanthramides. These avenanthramides are now considered to form the active ingredients in oats responsible for their beneficial effects when applied to the skin. They have potent antioxidant properties potentially preventing the oxidation of cholesterol transporting low-density lipoproteins, at least in the lab. Their anti-inflammatory effects may be able to help reduce inflammation in the cells lining our arteries (Another interesting biological effect of avenanthramides is on nitric oxide (NO)-dependent vasodilation, a process that relaxes blood vessels leading to better circulation and reduced blood pressure.

4. ALKALOIDS

Alkaloids are defined as basic compounds synthesized by living organisms containing one or more heterocyclic nitrogen atoms, derived from amino acids (with some exceptions) and pharmacologically active. The class name is directly related to the fact that nearly all alkaloids are basic (alkaline) compounds. Alkaloids constitute a very large group of secondary metabolites, with more than 12,000 substances isolated. A huge variety of structural formulas, coming from different biosynthetic pathways and presenting very diverse pharmacological activities are characteristic of the group. Alkaloid-containing plants are an intrinsic part of the regular Western diet. The present paper summarizes the occurrence of alkaloids in the food chain, their mode of action and possible adverse effects including a safety assessment. Pyrrolizidine alkaloids are a reason for concern because of their bioactivation to reactive alkylating intermediates. Several quinolizidine alkaloids, β-carboline alkaloids, ergot alkaloids and steroid alkaloids are active without bioactivation and mostly act as neurotoxins [63].

4.1. Alkaloid Biosynthesis

The synthesis of the alkaloids is started from the acetate, shikimate, mevalonate and deoxyxylulose pathways. The main criterion for alkaloid precursor determination is the skeleton nucleus of the alkaloid. The following most important alkaloid nuclei exist: piperidine, indolizidine, quinolizidine, pyridon, pyrrolidine, imidazole, manzamine, quinazoline, quinoline, acridine, pyridine, sesquiterpene, phenyl, phenylpropyl, indole, α-β-carboline, pyrroloindole, iboga, corynanthe and aspidosperma. Their synthesis occurs in different pathways, which consist of a series of reactions and compounds as well as enzymes. The sequence of all reactions leading to any alkaloid synthesis is divided into precursor, intermedia, obligatory intermedia, second obligatory intermedia, alkaloid and its post-cursors [65]. For many natural chemicals it is possible to synthesize alternatives from petroleum, coal, or both. The economic limitations of chemical synthesis and the pollution that accompanies this type of chemical synthesis, however, have led to the development of cell culture and molecular engineering of plants for the production of important and commodity chemicals. Plant cell and organ culture offer promising alternatives for the production of chemicals because totipotency enables plant cells and organs to produce useful secondary metabolites in vitro. Cell culture is also advantageous in that useful metabolites are obtained under a controlled environment, independent of climatic changes and soil conditions. In addition, the products are free of microbe and insect contamination. Fermentation technology also can be used to produce desired metabolites and can be optimized to maintain high and stable yields of known quality by cellular and molecular breeding techniques to further improve productivity and quality [66].

4.2. Classification

4.2.1. Non-Heterocyclic Alkaloids or Atypical Alkaloids

These are also sometimes called proto-alkaloids or biological amines. These are less commonly found in nature. These molecules have a nitrogen atom which is not a part of any ring system. Examples of these include ephedrine, colchicine, erythromycin and taxol etc [64].

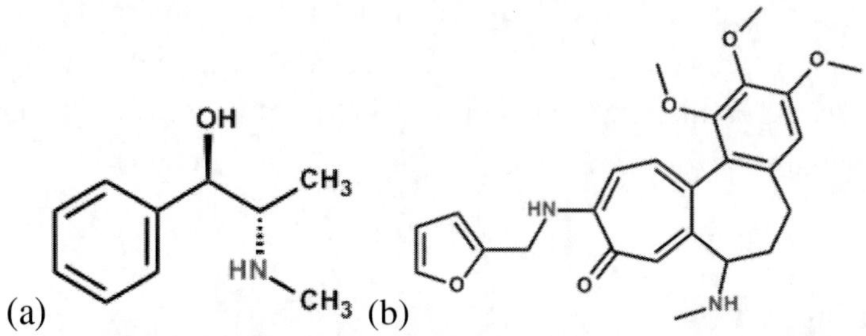

Figure 26. Atypical alkaloids (a) Ephedrine (b) Colchicine.

4.2.2. Heterocyclic Alkaloids or Typical Alkaloids

A large number of specific alkaloids possessing heterocyclic nucleus, preferably true alkaloids. Heterocyclic alkaloids are further subdivided into 14 groups based on the ring structure containing the nitrogen.

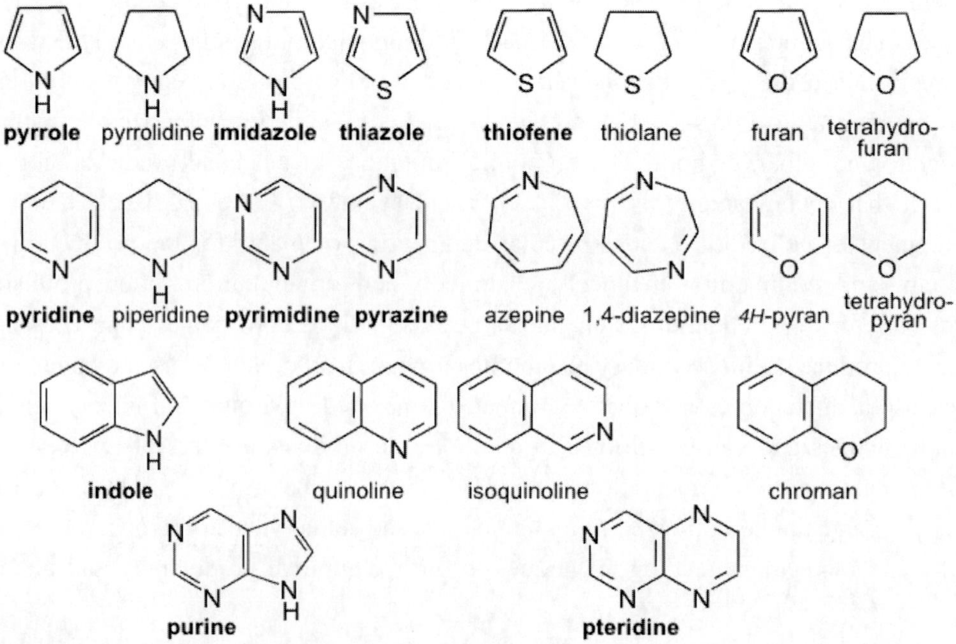

Figure 27. Important chemical classes of heterocyclic alkaloids.

A. Pyrrole

Stachydrine is reported for several pharmacological activities such as anti-inflammatory, anti-cancer, cardioprotective and cerebral ischemia. It was reported that stachydrine has a strong effect on inflammatory pathway [67]. Stachydrine suppresses viability & migration of astrocytoma cells via CXCR4/ERK & CXCR4/Akt pathway activity [68]. Stachydrine protects eNOS uncoupling and ameliorates endothelial dysfunction induced by homocysteine [69]. Stachydrine ameliorates pressure overload-induced diastolic heart failure by suppressing myocardial fibrosis [70]. Hygrine is a pyrrolidine alkaloid, found mainly in coca leaves (0.2%). It was first isolated by Carl Liebermann in 1889 (along with a related compound cuscohygrine) as an alkaloid accompanying cocaine in coca. Hygrine is extracted as a thick yellow oil, having a pungent taste and odor [71]. Hygrine could be considered as markers of coca chewing from cocaine abuse in workplace drug testing [72].

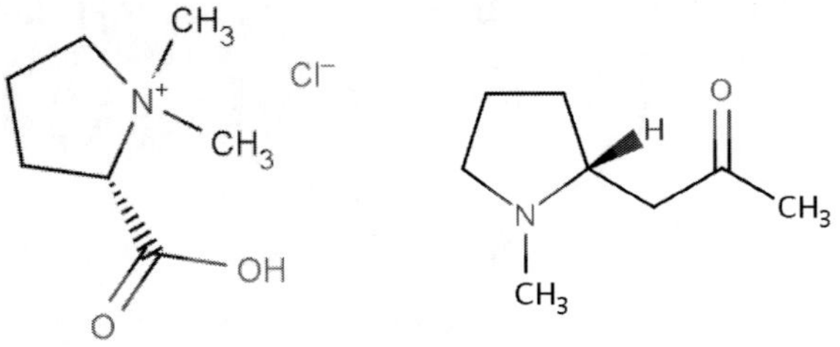

(a) Stachydrine hydrochloride (b) Hygrine

Figure 28. Pyrrole compounds of pharmacological interests.

B. Pyrrolizidine

Pyrrolizidine alkaloids (PA) are widely distributed in plants throughout the world, frequently in species relevant for human consumption. Apart from the toxicity that these molecules can cause in humans and livestock, PA are also known for their wide range of pharmacological properties, which can be exploited in drug discovery programs. In the specific case of PA, the anti-microbial activity of usaramine, monocrotaline and azido-retronecine against some bacteria has been demonstrated. Usaramine was analyzed concerning its ability to inhibit biofilm formation in Staphylococcus epidermidis and Pseudomonas aeruginosa. Crotalaburnine was only efficient against acute edema induced by carrageenin and hyaluronidase, with a dose of 10 mg/kg. In the cotton-pellet granuloma test it was shown that crotalaburnine was two times more potent than hydrocortisone. In a study using different human cancer cell lines (cervical, breast, prostate and cervical squamous) indicine N-oxide from Heliotropium indicum L. inhibited the proliferation of the previous referred cancer cell lines, with IC50 values ranging from 46 to 100 μM. Australine and alexine, isolated from Castanospermum australe A. Cunn. & C. Fraser ex Hook and Alexa Leiopetela Sandwith, are examples of these polyhydroxylated PA that in concentrations between 0.1 and 10 mM inhibited, in distinct degrees, the activity of glycosidases, particularly the nitrogen-linked glycosylation process of HIV. 7-Oangeloyllycopsamine-N-oxide, echimidine-N-oxide, echimidine, and 7-O-angeloylretronecine isolated from Echium confusum Coincy showed the inhibition of AChE, with IC50 values ranging from 0.275 to 0.769 mM [73].

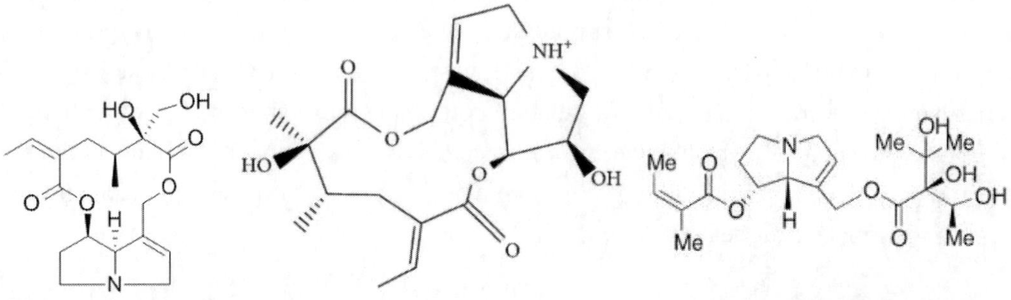

(a) Usaramine (b) Crotalaburnine (c) Echimidine

Figure 29. Pyrrolizidines of pharmacological interests.

C. Pyridine Alkaloids

Nicotine is a pyridine alkaloid belonging to Solanaceae family and majorly found in *Nicotiana tobaccum*. It exhibits extensive pharmacological properties in central nervous system (CNS) as well as the peripheral nervous systems (PNS) mediated by the stimulation of nicotinic acetylcholine receptors (nAChRs). tine elucidates its potential efficacy in promoting the neuroprotection in AD by significantly up regulating the α4 and α7 nAChRs level. Arecoline is a pyridine alkaloid belonging to the family Arecaceae and chiefly found in the fruit of the palm tree *Areca catechu* L. Arecoline possess its efficacy against schizophrenia by directly targeting the OLs and also prevents the demyelination of white matter. It enhances the social and cognitive activity as well as protects the myelin damage in cortex by facilitating oligodendrocyte precursor cells (OPC) differentiation through dephosphorylating the activated protein kinase AMPKα [74].

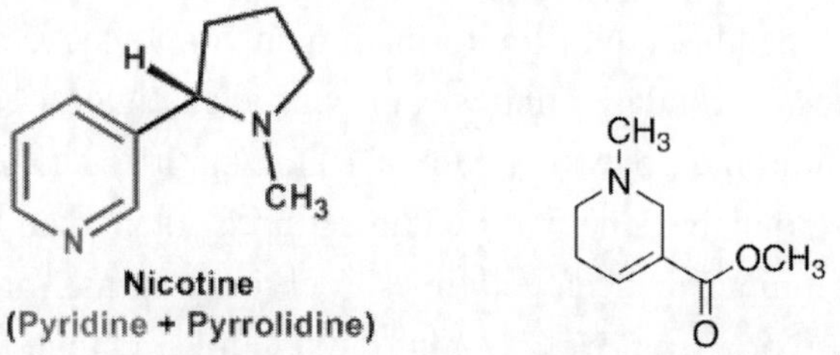

(a) Nicotine (b) Aerecoline

Figure 30. Pyridine alkaloids of pharmacological interests.

D. Piperidine Alkaloids

Lobeline is a piperidine alkaloid isolated from *Lobelia inflata* and exhibits neuroprotective effects. It is a lipophilic alkaloidal component of Indian tobacco. Lobeline protects dopaminergic neurons against 1-methyl-4-phenyl-1,2,3,6-tetrahydropyridine (MPTP) which decreases nigral DA [74]. The consumption of *Prosopis juliflora* as main or sole source of food causes an illness in animals known locally as "cara torta" disease in Brazil due to neurotoxic piperidine compound in P. juliflora leaves and pods [75]. Piperidine alkaloids from *Senna spectabilis* constitute a rare class of natural products with several biological activities [76]. In folk medicine, this plant is indicated for the treatment of constipation, insomnia, anxiety, epilepsy, malaria, dysentery and headache [77]. S. spectabilis is an important source of piperidine alkaloids with leishmanicidal activity [78, 79]. Piperidine is an important pharmacophore, a privileged scaffold and an excellent heterocyclic system in the field of drug discovery which provides numerous opportunities in studying/exploring this moiety as an anticancer agent by acting on various receptors of utmost importance [80].

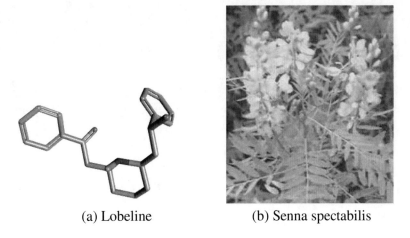

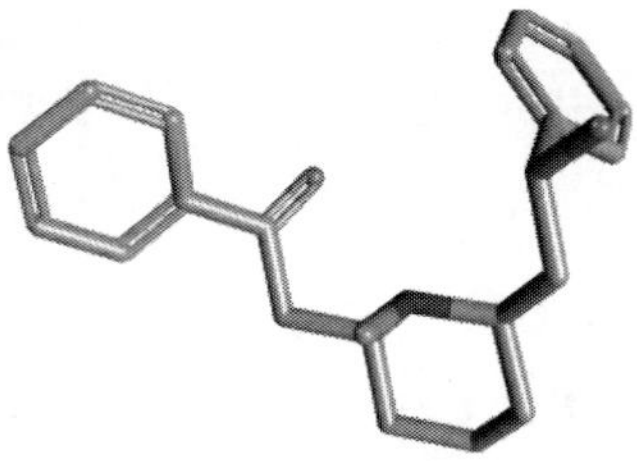

(a) Lobeline

(b) Senna spectabilis

Figure 31. A piperidine alkaloid and an important source.

E. Tropane (Piperidine/N-Methyl-Pyrrolidine)

Tropanes are an important class of alkaloid natural products that are found in plants all over the world. These compounds can exhibit significant biological activity and are among the oldest known medicines. In the early 19th century, tropanes were isolated, characterized, and synthesized by notable chemical researchers. Their significant biological activities have inspired tremendous research efforts toward their synthesis and the elucidation of their pharmacological activity both in academia and in industry [81]. TAs are a class of alkaloids characterized by the presence of a bicyclic nitrogen bridge across a seven-carbon ring. The biosynthesis of hyoscyamine and scopolamine is initiated by decarboxylation of the nonproteinogenic amino acid, ornithine [82]. A closer monitoring of tropane alkaloids in foods is now recommended by the European

Commission, following a series of alerts related to the contamination of buckwheat with weeds of the genus Datura [83]. Homeopathic products prepared from *Atropa belladonna* extracts may present specific problems due to the effects derived from its components [84]. *Scopolia lurida*, also known as Himalayan Scopolia, a native herbal plant species in Tibet, is one of the most effective producers of tropane alkaloids. Some Solanaceae species including *Hyoscyamus niger*, Datura species, *Atropa belladonna* and *S. lurida* are widely used as anticholinergic agents, especially the pharmaceutical tropane alkaloids, such as hyoscyamine and scopolamine that are produced exclusively by the medicinal plant family [85].

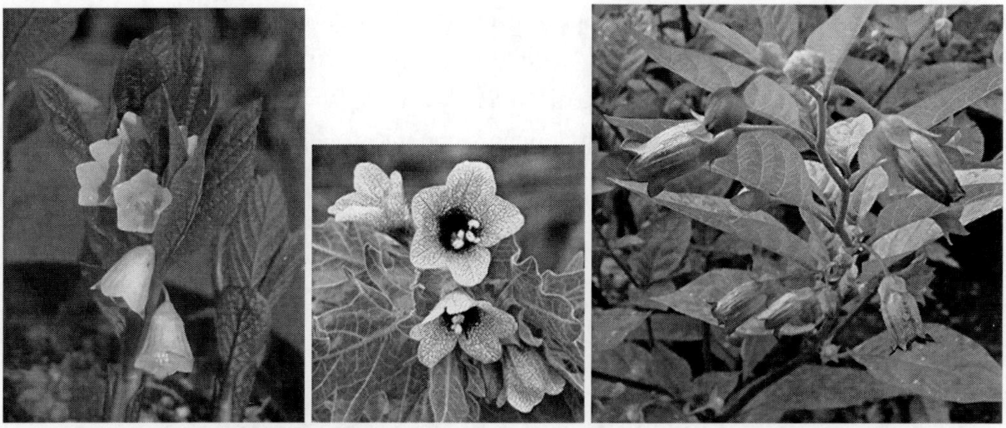

(a) Scopolia lurida (b) Hyoscyamus niger (c) Atropa belladonna

Figure 32. Plants containing tropane alkaloids.

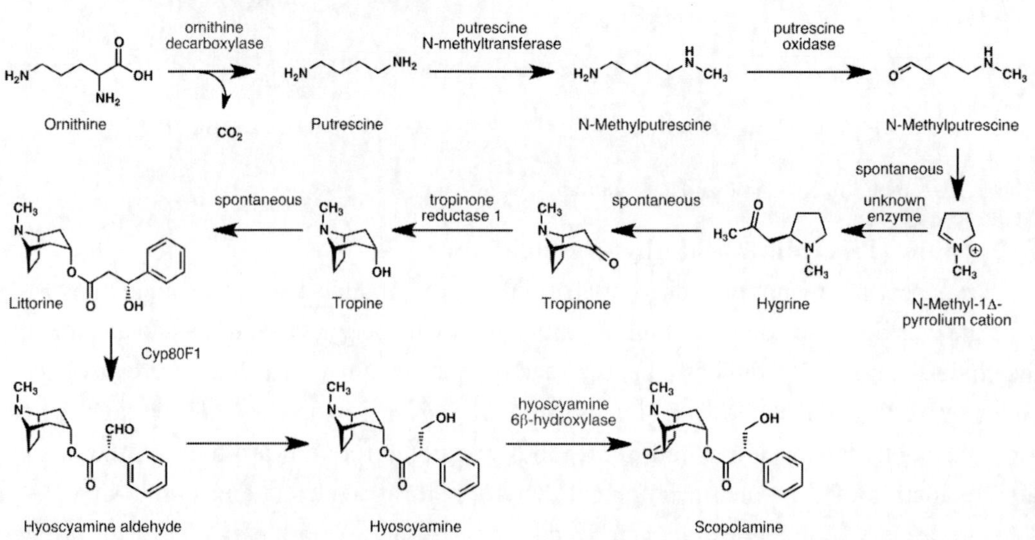

Figure 33. Biosynthesis of scopolamine [86].

F. Quinoline Alkaloids

Quinoline alkaloids are biogenetically derived from anthranilic acid and occur mainly in Rutaceous plants. Quinoline and quinazoline alkaloids, two important classes of N-based heterocyclic compounds, have attracted tremendous attention from researchers worldwide since the 19th century. Over the past 200 years, many compounds from these two classes were isolated from natural sources, and most of them and their modified analogs possess significant bioactivities. Quinine and camptothecin are two of the most famous and important quinoline alkaloids, and their discoveries opened new areas in antimalarial and anticancer drug development, respectively [87]. A reduction in seizures of more than 50% after quinidine treatment was observed in one patient with epilepsy of infancy with migrating focal seizures (EIMFS), whereas two patients with EIMFS and one with focal epilepsy did not achieve apparent seizure reduction [88]. Arrhythmic storm with recurrent polymorphic VT in patients with coronary disease responds to quinidine therapy when other antiarrhythmic drugs (including intravenous amiodarone) fail. There were no recurrent arrhythmias during quinidine therapy [89]. Chloroquine phosphate is the preferred agent if the infection is considered uncomplicated and is caused by chloroquine sensitive P.falciparum. Primaquine phosphate is utilized as an add-on agent to either chloroquine phosphate or hydroxychloroquine when infections are caused by P. vivax or P. ovale with chloroquine sensitivity [90].

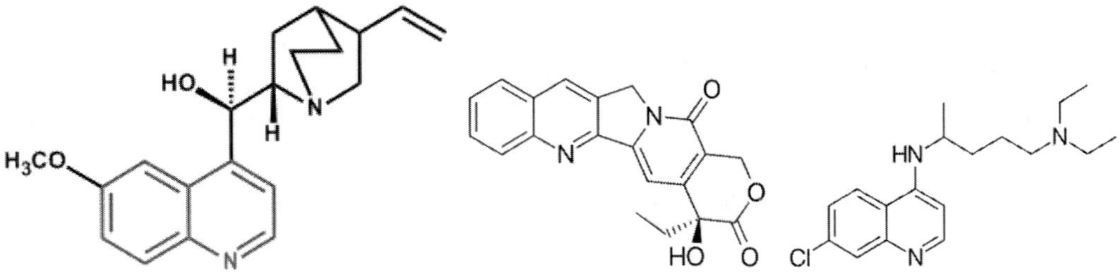

(a) Quinine (b) Camptothecin (c) Chloroquine

Figure 34. Quinoline compounds of pharmacological interests.

G. Isoquinoline Alkaloids

Isoquinoline alkaloids are a large family of natural products which have a broad variety of biological activities. Among the members of this class of compounds, tetrahydroisoquinolines, and the tetrahydroquinoline motif itself, are present in a large group of natural compounds having diverse biological properties. Anti-inflammatory, antimicrobial, antileukemic, and antitumor properties are among the important biological activities that many of these compounds exhibit. Over the years, different methodologies have been reported for the construction of the tetrahydroisoquinoline unit [91]. The isoquinoline alkaloid berberine inhibits human cytomegalovirus replication by interfering with the viral Immediate Early-2 (IE2) protein transactivating activity [92]. Isoquinoline alkaloids and indole alkaloids appear to have a direct anti-atherosclerotic effect in ApoE−/− mice [93]. Berberine is a main component of *Rhizoma Coptidis* (used widely in the field of traditional Chinese medicine for many years). Modern medicine has confirmed that berberine has pharmacological activities, such as anti-inflammatory, analgesic, antimicrobial, hypolipidemic, and blood pressure-lowering effects. Importantly, the active ingredient of berberine has clear inhibitory effects on various cancers, including colorectal cancer, lung cancer, ovarian cancer, prostate cancer, liver cancer, and cervical cancer [94]. In China, *Rhizoma Coptidis* is a common component in traditional medicines used to treat CVD associated problems including obesity, diabetes mellitus, hyperlipidemia, hyperglycemia and disorders of lipid metabolism [95].

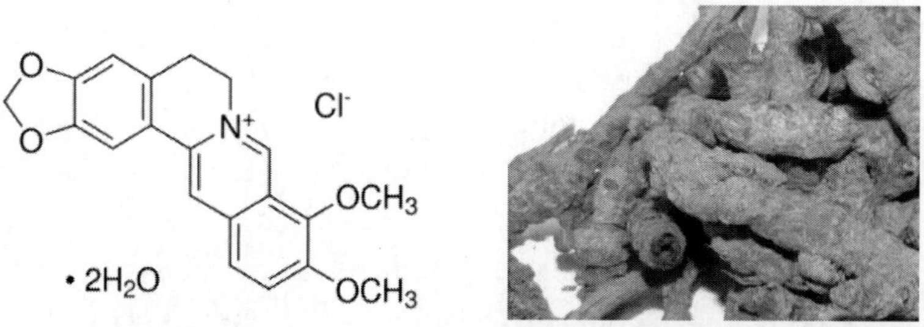

(a) Berberine (b) Huang Lian/*Rhizoma Coptidis*

Figure 35. Barberine and barberine rich rhizome.

H. Aporphine (Reduced Isoquinoline/Naphthalene)

Aporphine alkaloids are natural and synthetic alkaloids that possess a tetracyclic framework. Chemically they incorporate a tetrahydroisoquinoline substructure and belong to the isoquinoline class of alkaloids. More than 500 members of this class of alkaloids have been isolated. Aporphine alkaloids are widely distributed in Annonaceae, Lauraceae, Monimiaceae, Menispermaceae, Hernandiaceae and other plant families [96]. Aporphine Alkaloids from Leaves of *Nelumbo nucifera* Gaertn powerfully enhanced the glucose consumption in adipocytes as rosiglitazone did. These finding may be benefit for the popular use of lotus leaves in blood sugar balance and weight loss in China [97]. Stepharine, an aporphine alkaloid of Stephania glabra plants, exhibits anti-aging, anti-hypertensive, and anti-viral effects [98]. Aporphine alkaloids, characterized by a heterocyclic aromatic basic skeleton, are known from different organisms and exhibit various biological activities: anti-tumor, anti-viral, anti-microbial, anti-inflammatory etc [99]. Crebanine (CN), tetrahydropalmatine (THP), O-methylbulbocapnine (OMBC) and N-methyl tetrahydropalmatine (NMTHP) are isoquinoline derived natural alkaloids isolated from tubers of *Stephania venosa*. Alkaloids obtained from S. venosa could be used as chemo-sensitizers in ovarian cancer to sensitize and minimize the dose related toxicity of platinum-based chemotherapeutic drugs [100].

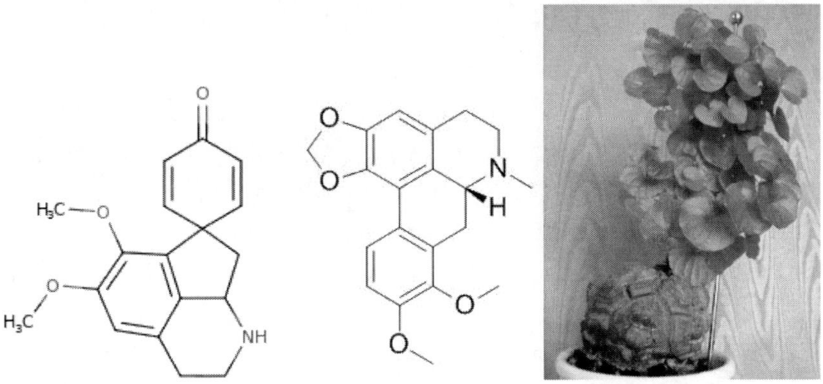

(a) Stepharine (b) Crebanine (c) *Stephania venosa*

Figure 36. Important aporphines and an important source.

I. Quinolizidine Alkaloids

Quinolizidine alkaloids are nontoxic to the legumes that produce them. On the other hand, the quinolizidine alkaloids can be toxic and, in some cases, very toxic to other organisms. The biotoxicity of alkaloids has for some time been considered to be connected with their bitter taste. The quinolizidine alkaloids are certainly bitter in taste to humans. However, not all alkaloids are [101]. 17-Oxo-Sparteine and Lupanine, obtained from *Cytisus scoparius*, exert a neuroprotection against soluble oligomers of amyloid-β toxicity by nicotinic acetylcholine receptors, appears to be an interesting target for the development of new pharmacological tools and strategies against AD [102]. The potential anticonvulsant effect of sparteine may be mediated through the inhibition of acetylcholine release and the subsequent release of GABA in the brain due to the activation of the M2 and M4 subtypes of mAChRs. These effects combined with the systemic effects of decreasing blood pressure and heart rate in addition to the anti-inflammatory and hypoglycemic properties of sparteine, suggest that sparteine promises to be an important anticonvulsant. [103]. Cytisine, a nicotinic acetylcholine receptor partial agonist (like varenicline) found in some plants, is a low-cost, effective smoking cessation medication [104].

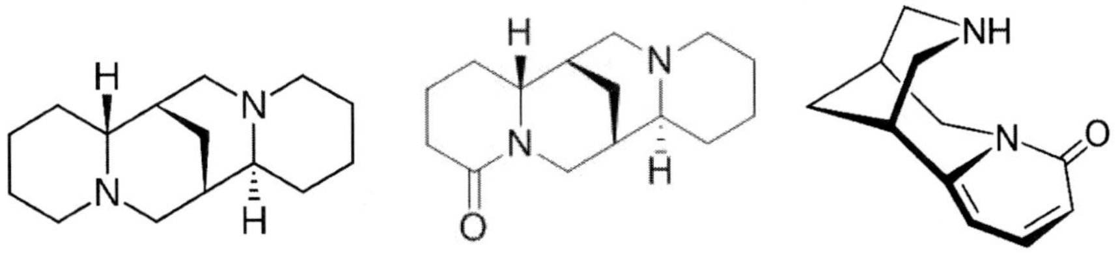

(a) Lupanine (b) Sparteine (c) Sparteine

Figure 37. Important quinolizidine alkaloids.

J. Indole or Benzopyrole Alkaloids

Indole-containing compounds demonstrate an array of biological activities relevant to numerous human diseases. The biological activities of diverse indole-based agents are driven by molecular interactions between indole agent and critical therapeutic target. The chemical inventory of medicinally useful or promising indole compounds spans the entire structural spectrum, from simple synthetic indoles to highly complex indole alkaloids. In an analogous fashion, the chemistry behind the indole heterocycle is unique and provides rich opportunities for extensive synthetic chemistry enabling the construction and development of novel indole compounds to explore chemical space [105]. A survey conducted by the Southmead Hospital Maternity Research Team revealed that 71.4% of UK obstetric units still routinely use oxytocin/ergometrine [106]. Vinblastine is highly active in vitro and demonstrates equivalent antitumoral activity compared to vincristine. Substitution of vincristine with vinblastine in future studies should be considered for all patients with medulloblastoma, particularly those with hereditary neuropathy, severe vincristine toxicity, and adults [107]. Administration of centrally acting physostigmine in cecal ligation and puncture- (CLP-)-induced sepsis in rats has protective effects on polymorphonuclear neutrophils (PMNs) functions and improves survival times, which may be of interest in clinical practice [108].

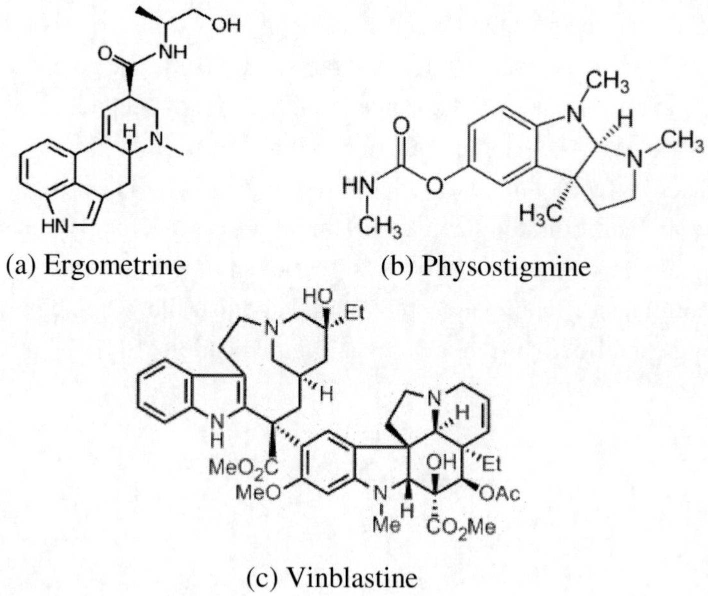

(a) Ergometrine (b) Physostigmine

(c) Vinblastine

Figure 38. Important indole compounds.

K. Purine (Pyrimidine/Imidazole)

Purine is a heterocyclic aromatic organic compound that consists of a pyrimidine ring fused to an imidazole ring. It is water soluble. In order to form DNA and RNA, both purines and pyrimidines are needed by the cell in approximately equal quantities. Both purine and pyrimidine are self-inhibiting and activating. Inborn errors of purine and pyrimidine metabolism are a diverse group of disorders with possible serious or life-threatening symptoms. They may be associated with neurological symptoms, renal stone disease or immunodeficiency. However, the clinical presentation can be nonspecific and mild so that a number of cases may be missed [109]. Caffeine is a naturally occurring, central nervous system (CNS) stimulant of the methylxanthine class and is the most widely taken psychoactive stimulant in the world. The FDA has approved caffeine for the use in the treatment of apnea of prematurity and prevention and treatment of bronchopulmonary dysplasia of premature infants. Caffeine has been linked with decreased all-cause mortality and is also being investigated for its efficacy in the treatment of depression and neurocognitive declines, such as that seen in Alzheimer and Parkinson diseases [110]. Early caffeine therapy is associated with better neurodevelopmental outcomes compared with late caffeine therapy in preterm infants born at <29 weeks' gestation [111]. Both animal and human studies suggested a potential neuroprotective action of long-term assumption of theobromine through a reduction of Aβ amyloid pathology, which is commonly observed in Alzheimer's disease patients' brains [112]. Theobromine and caffeine, in the proportions found in cocoa, are responsible for the liking of the food/beverage. These compounds influence in a positive way our moods and our state of alertness. Theobromine, which is found in higher amounts than caffeine, seems to be behind several effects attributed to cocoa intake. The main mechanisms of action are inhibition of phosphodiesterases and blockade of adenosine receptors [113].

4.3. Alkaloids from Marine Sources

4.3.1. Phenylethylamine (PEA) Alkaloids

These are aromatic amines made up of a benzene ring to which an ethylamine side chain is attached. The PEA alkaloid group includes important alkaloids. It is a precursor of many natural and synthetic compounds. Several substituted PEAs are pharmacologically active compounds found in plants and animals. This group includes simple phenylamine (tyramine, hordenine) and catecholamine (dopamine). Some brown marine algae containing PEA are: *Desmerestia aculeata*, *Desmerestia viridis*; Red: *Ceramium rubrum*, *Cystoclonium purpureum*, *Delesseria sanguine*, *Dumontia incrassata*, *Polysiphonia urceolata*, *Polyides rotundus*. PEA in the human brain acts as a neuromodulator and a neurotransmitter. PEA has been shown to relieve depression in 60% of depressed patients. It has been proposed that a PEA deficit may be the cause of a common form of depressive illness. Substituted PEAs are pharmacologically active compounds as hormones, stimulants, hallucinogens, entactogenes, anorectics, bronchodilators and antidepressants [114].

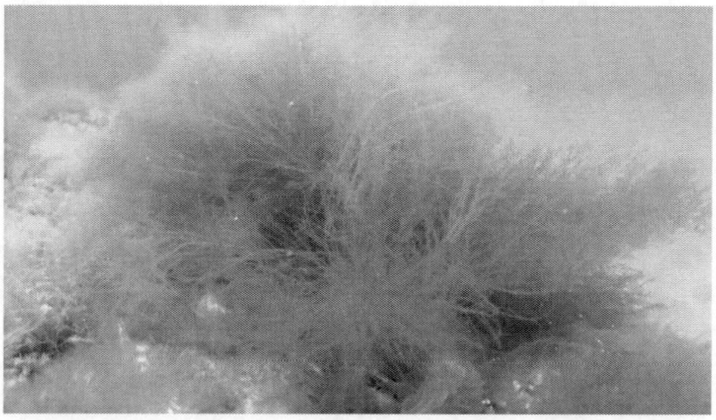

Figure 39. *Desmerestia viridis* [115].

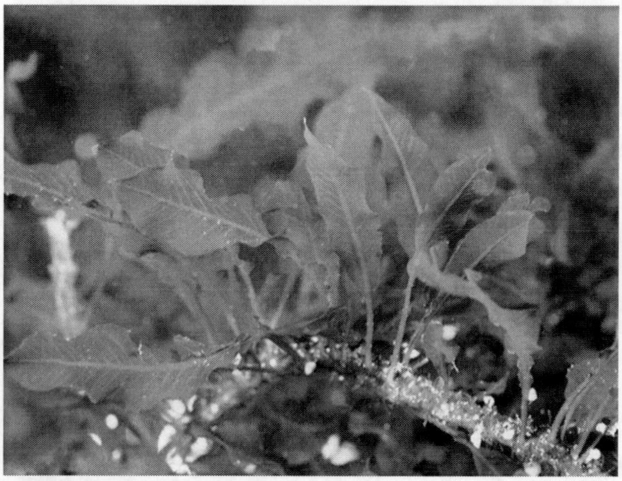

Figure 40. *Delesseria sanguinea* [116].

A. Tyramine (TYR, 4-Hydroxyphenylethylamine)

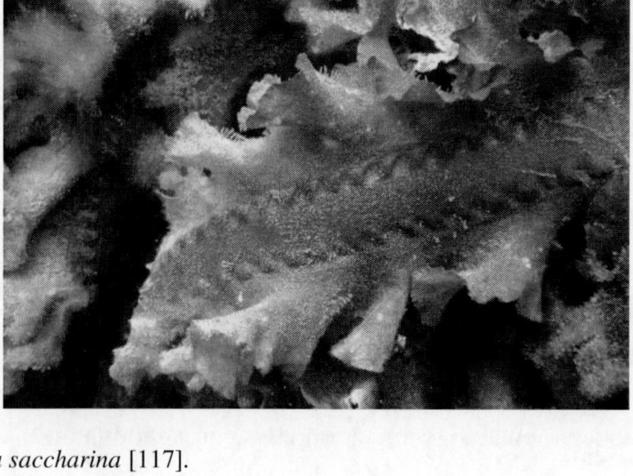

Figure 41. *Laminaria saccharina* [117].

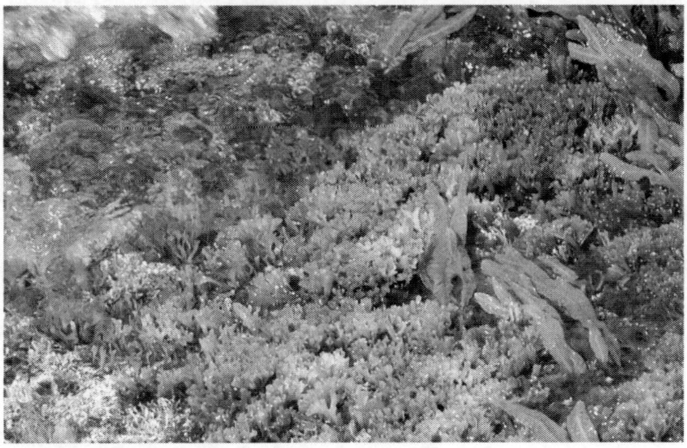

Figure 42. *Chondrus crispus* [118].

A monoamine derivative of the amino acid tyrosine. Tyrosine occurs widely in plants, fungi and animal but is rare in algae. It was detected in the brown alga Laminaria saccharina, and red algae *Chondrus crispus* and *Polysiphonia urceolata* and in the microalgae *Scenedesmus acutus*. Tyrosine is a pharmacologically important compound. It stimulates the CNS, causes vasoconstriction, increases heart rate and blood pressure and is also responsible for migraines [114].

B. Hordenine (Anhaline)

It was first obtained from red algae *Phyllophora nervosa*. Hordenine is a potent phenylethylamine alkaloid with antibacterial and antibiotic properties produced in nature by several varieties of plants in the family Cactacea. The major source of hordenine in humans is beer brewed from barley. Hordenine in urine interferes with tests for morphine, heroin and other opioid drugs. Hordenine is a biomarker for the consumption of beer [119]. Hordenine as an active compound from germinated barley (*Hordeum vulgare* L.). Hordenine inhibited melanogenesis by suppressing cAMP production, which is involved in the expression of melanogenesis-related proteins and suggest that hordenine may be an effective inhibitor of hyperpigmentation [120]. Hordenine treatment inhibited the production of quorum sensing (QS) -related extracellular virulence factors of P. aeruginosa PAO1. Additionally, quantitative real-time polymerase chain reaction analysis demonstrated that the expressions of QS-related genes, lasI, lasR, rhlI, and rhlR, were significantly suppressed. Our results indicated that hordenine can serve as a competitive inhibitor for signaling molecules and act as a novel QS-based agent to defend against foodborne pathogens [121]. The phenethylamine alkaloid hordenine, present in germinated barley, was identified recently as a functionally selective dopamine D2 receptor agonist contributing potentially to the rewarding effects of drinking beer. Hordenine precursor N-methyltyramine binds with a similar affinity to the dopamine D2 receptor as hordenine (Ki 31.3 μM) showing also selectivity towards the G protein-mediated pathway over the βarrestin pathway [122]. Hordenine and insulin function synergistically to play an antioxidant role against oxidative injury in diabetic nephropathy. In conclusion, to the best of our knowledge, we, for the first time, found the anti-diabetic, anti-inflammatory, and anti-fibrotic role of Hordenine in combination with insulin. Hordenine functions synergistically with insulin and prevents diabetic nephropathy [123].

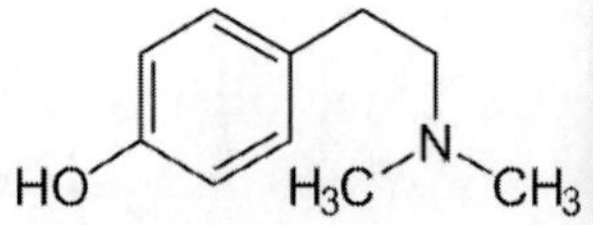

(a) Hordenine

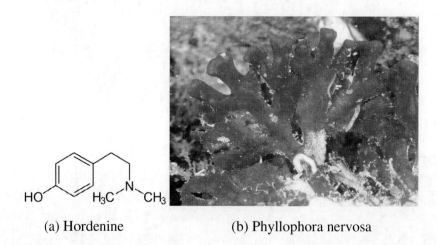

(b) Phyllophora nervosa

Figure 43. Hordenine and an important source.

4.3.2. Marine Indole Alkaloids

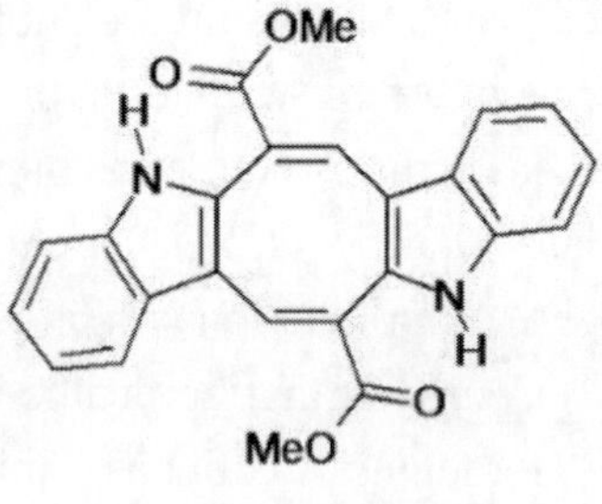

(a) Caulerpin

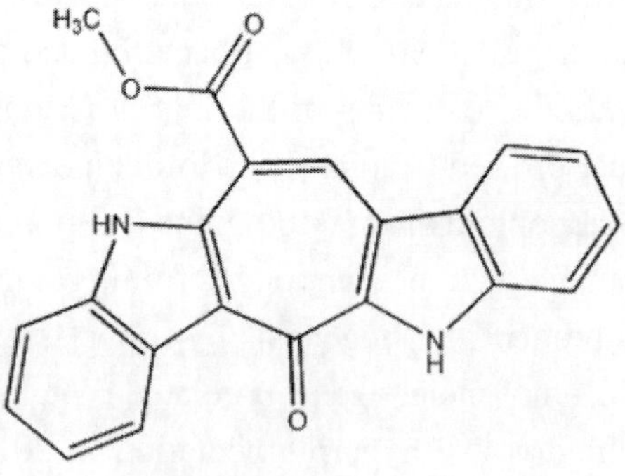

(b) caulersin

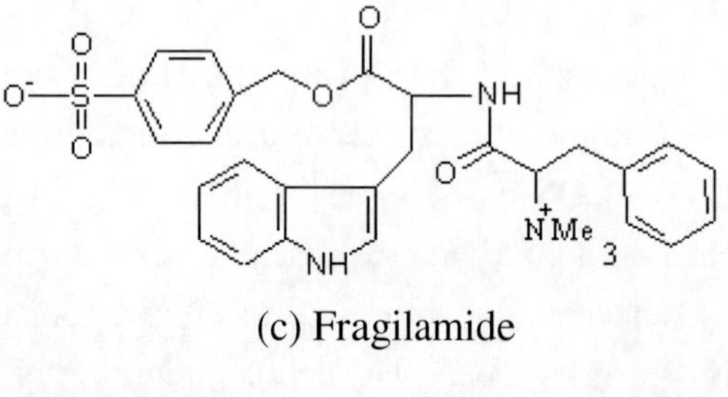

(c) Fragilamide

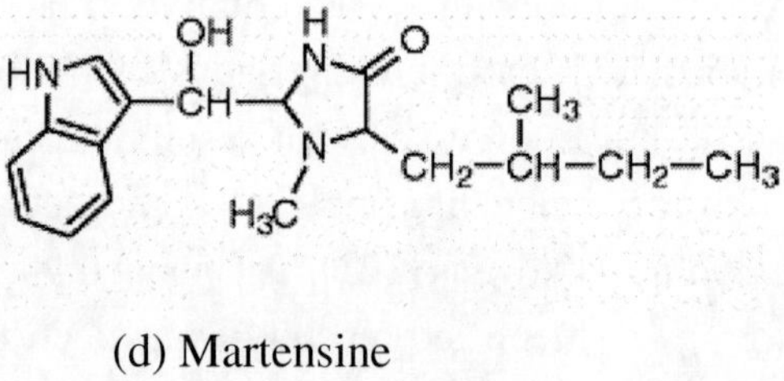

(d) Martensine

Figure 44. Structure of pharmacologically important marine indole alkaloids.

Marine indole alkaloids comprise a large and steadily growing group of secondary metabolites. Their diverse biological activities make many compounds of this class attractive starting points for pharmaceutical development. Several marine-derived indoles were found to possess cytotoxic, antineoplastic, antibacterial and antimicrobial activities, in addition to the action on human enzymes and receptors. Most of the indole group alkaloids are concentrated in red algae. This alkaloid group containing a benzylpyrrole (derived from tryptophan) includes caulerpin, caulersin, fragilamide, martensine, martefragine, denticine and almazolone. The simple indole alkaloids are mostly derived from tryptophan or its direct precursor indole, which itself is formed from chorismate through anthranilate and indole-3-glycerol-phosphate in microorganisms and plants. As the ultimate step of the tryptophan biosynthesis is reversible, free indole can also be formed in this catabolic process [124].

A. Caulerpin

Bis-indole alkaloid caulerpin isolated from marine green algae *Caulerpa* and a red algae *Chondria armata* at various places around the world, and tested against several therapeutic areas such as anti-diabetic, antinociceptive, anti-inflammatory, anti-tumor, anti-larvicidal, anti-herpes, anti-tubercular, anti-microbial and immunostimulating activity as well as means of other chemical agents [125]. Dietary administration of caulerpin decreased aggressiveness *in D. sargus,* suggesting an anxiolytic-like effect of caulerpin possibly mediated by endogenous anxiolytic agents [126]. The Caulerpa Pigment Caulerpin suppressed hypoxic induction of secreted VEGF protein and the ability of hypoxic T47D cell-conditioned media to promote tumor angiogenesis in vitro [130].

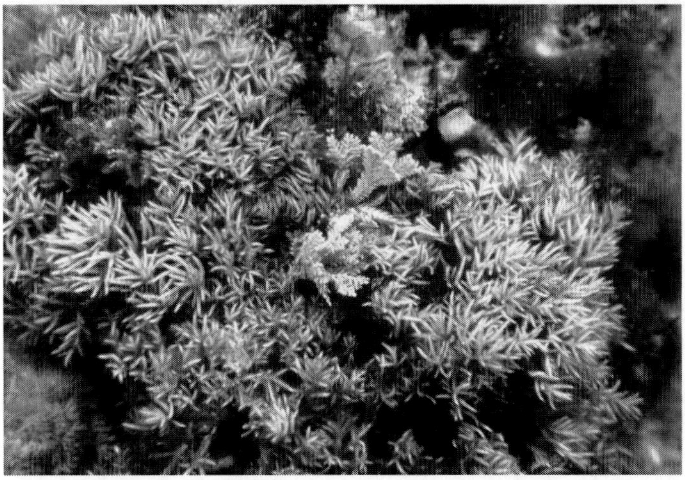

Figure 45. South African seaweeds - *Chondria armata*, typical pink turf [128].

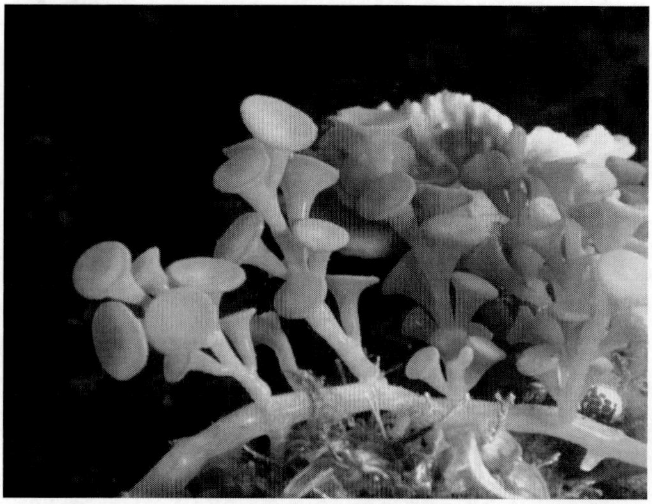

Figure 46. *Caulerpa racemose* [129].

B. Caulersin

Bisindole alkaloid with a 7 members central ring and two ≪anti parallel≫ indole cores, isolated from *Caulerpa serrulata*. The Caulerpa bisindole alkaloids may be considered as a new class of PTP1B inhibitors [127].

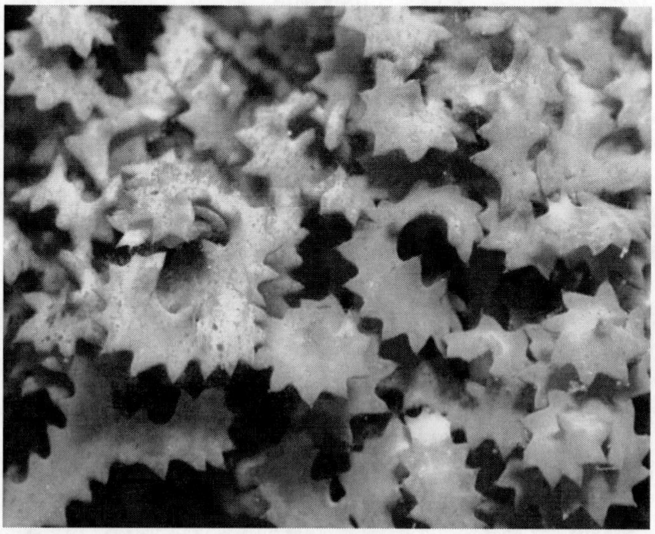

Figure 47. *Caulerpa serrulata* [131].

C. Martensine

Martensines were extracted from the red algae *Martensia fragilis*. Martensine A shows an antibiotic activity against *Bacillus subtilis, Staphylococcus aureus,* and *Mycobacterium smegmatis* [132].

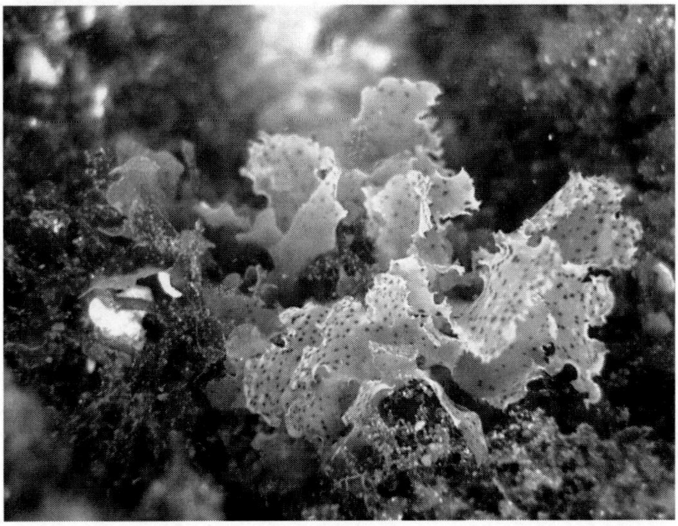

Figure 48. *Martensia fragilis* [133].

4.3.3. Halogenated Indole Alkaloids

The majority of halogenated metabolites contain bromine and they are especially abundant in the marine environment, whereas chlorinated compounds are preferably synthesized by terrestrial organisms. In contrast to brominated and chlorinated metabolites, iodinated and fluorinated compounds are quite rare.

Iodoalkaloids compose a rare group of natural compounds that has been isolated from marine organisms. Antibacterial activities of halogenated alkaloids were examined on terrestrial and some marine bacteria. Meridianins are marine alkaloids which were first isolated from the Ascidian *Aplidium meridianum*. Meridianins have been described as potent inhibitors of various protein kinases and they display antitumor activity. Variolins are rare pyrido-pyrrolo-pyrimidine skeleton has made the variolins an interesting class of alkaloids from both structural and biogenetic viewpoints. This type of compounds exhibits a potent cytotoxic activity against P388 murine leukemia cell line, also being effective against Herpes simplex type I. Variolin B is the most active of this family of natural products. Aplycianins are cytotoxic to the human tumor cell lines MDA-MB-231 (breast adenocarcinoma), A549 (lung carcinoma), and HT-29 (colorectal carcinoma). They also exhibit antimitotic activity. Aplysinopsins exhibit cytoxicity towards tumour cells, as well as some antimalarial and antimicrobial activities. However, properties related to neurotransmission modulation seem to be the most significant pharmacological feature of these compounds. Aplysinopsins have the potential to influence monoaminooxidase (MAO) and nitric oxide synthase (NOS) activities. They have also been found to modulate serotonin receptors [134].

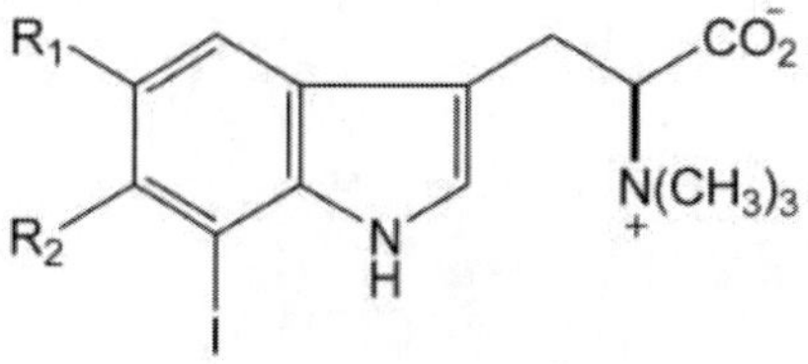

	R_1	R_2
(1) Plakohypaphorine A	H	H
(2) Plakohypaphorine B	H	I
(3) Plakohypaphorine C	I	H

(a) Structures of plakohypaphorines A, B, and C (1–3).

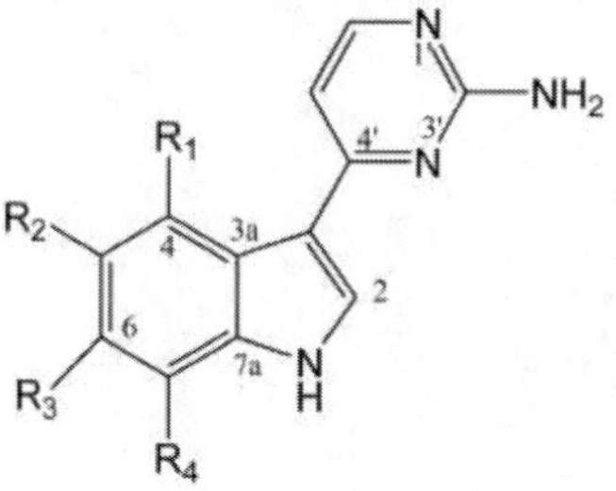

	R_1	R_2	R_3	R_4
(4) Meridianin A	OH	H	H	H
(5) Meridianin B	OH	H	Br	H
(6) Meridianin C	H	Br	H	H
(7) Meridianin D	H	H	Br	H
(8) Meridianin E	OH	H	H	Br
(9) Meridianin F	H	Br	Br	H
(10) Meridianin G	H	H	H	H

(b) Structures of meridianins 4–10

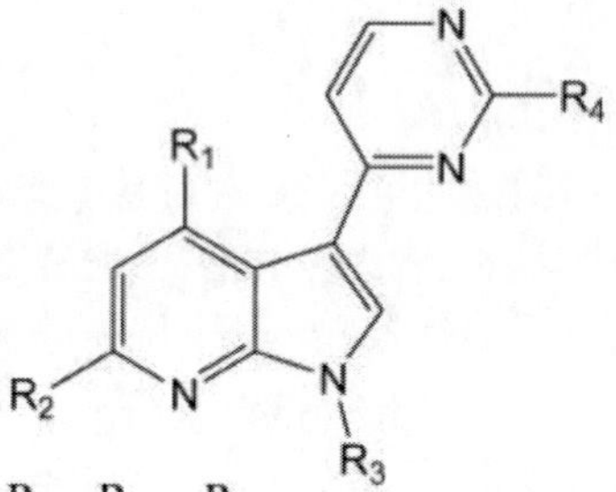

	R_1	R_2	R_3	R_4
(16) Meriolin 1	H	H	H	NH_2
(17) Meriolin 2	OH	H	H	NH_2
(18) Meriolin 3	OMe	H	H	NH_2
(19) Meriolin 4	OEt	H	H	NH_2
(20) Meriolin 5	OPr	H	H	NH_2
(21) Meriolin 6	OiPr	H	H	NH_2
(22) Meriolin 7	$O(CH_2)_2OMe$	H	H	NH_2

	R_1	R_2	R_3	R_4
(23) Meriolin 8	OH	H	Me	NH_2
(24) Meriolin 9	OMe	H	Me	NH_2
(25) Meriolin 10	Cl	H	H	NH_2
(26) Meriolin 11	H	Br	H	NH_2
(27) Meriolin 12	OMe	H	H	SMe
(28) Meriolin 13	OH	H	H	H
(29) Meriolin 14	OMe	H	H	H

(c) Structures of meriolins 16–29

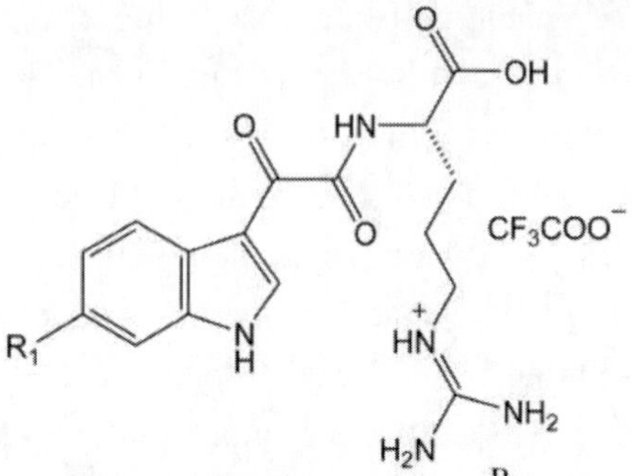

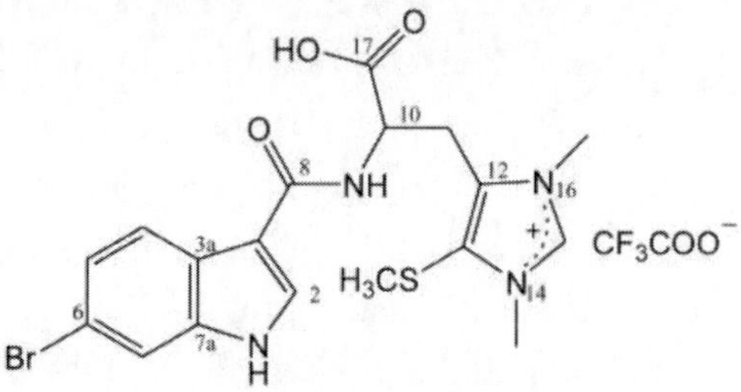

(56) Leptoclinidamine C

	R_1
(54) Leptoclinidamine A	H
(55) Leptoclinidamine B	OH

(d) Structures of leptoclinidamines 54–56.

Figure 49. Halogenated indole alkaloids from marine invertebrates [134].

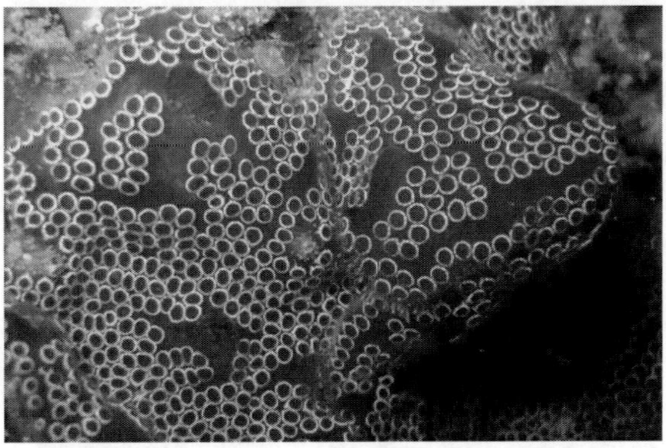

Figure 50. Genus *Aplidium* [135].

4.3.4. Other Marine Alkaloids

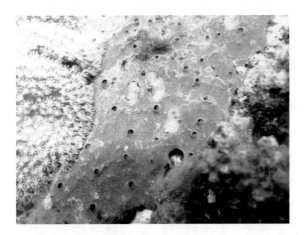

Figure 51. *Suberea molis*—marine sponges [137].

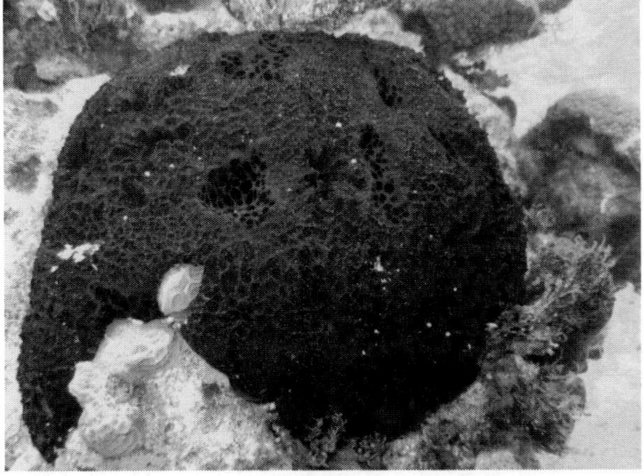

Figure 52. *Asteropus niger*. Location: Bahamas, San Salvador [139].

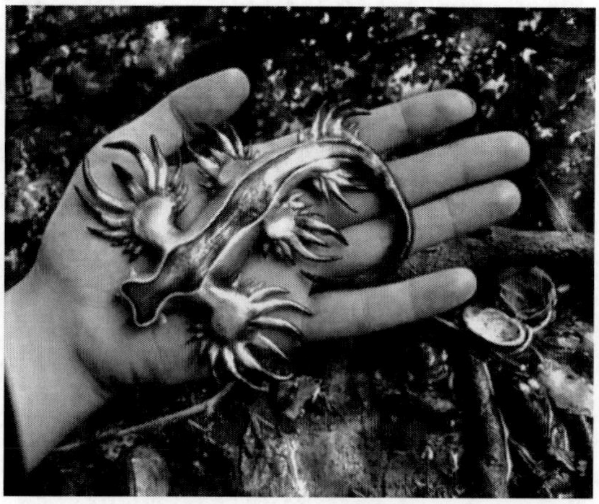

Figure 53. *Glaucus Spp* [140]. "The Blue Fleet" – the siphonophores such as Physalia, Velella, Porpita and the other associated animals including the "Violet snails" of the genus Janthina. All these animals float on the surface of the ocean being carried by the currents and the winds.

A majority of these compounds are found in marine organisms and several recent reviews are available of marine natural products in general, in algae, in sponges, in invertebrates, in gorgonians, in bryophytes, in fungi, in cyanobacteria, in marine bacteria, and those cyano-containing marine triterpenoids [136]. Marine sponges are considered to be a gold mine because of their diversity of secondary vital biological compounds, which are not present in terrestrial organisms. Many worldwide diseases could be treated by drugs extracted from the sponges. They possess an unusual chemical structure due to large amounts of sterols and a lack of terpenes and typical brominated compounds associated with tyrosine. Members of the genus Suberea display diverse bioactivities, including antibacterial, antiviral, enzyme inhibition, and cytotoxic activity. Prenylated toluquinone, hydroquinones, and naphthoquinones are examples of marine-derived natural products with reported antioxidant activities [137]. Antifungal activity was recorded for nakijinamines C and E against *Aspergillus niger* [138]. Eudistomidins were obtained from the Okinawan tunicate Eudistoma glaucus and Eudistomidins G (766) and B (765) showed cytotoxic activity towards murine leukemia cells, whereas eudistomidin J (769) was active against murine leukemia cells P388 (IC50, 0.043 μg/mL) and L1210 (IC50 0.047 μg/mL) and human epidermoid carcinoma cells KB (IC50 0.063 μg/mL) [124].

CONCLUSION

Secondary metabolites are a basic segment to plant survival; in any case, they additionally assume a ground-breaking job in supporting human wellbeing. As opposed to the essential metabolites (sugars, fats, proteins, nutrients and minerals) the secondary metabolites don't have supplement attributes for individuals however have logical demonstrated medicinal impacts. The look for new plant determined chemicals in substitution of engineered medication should along these lines be a need in present and future endeavors towards reasonable protection and objective use of biodiversity. People can profit by devouring secondary metabolites and along these lines, an eating routine wealthy in plants gives heavenly advantages to wellbeing. Significantly, a considerable lot of the secondary metabolites delivered by plants are utilized by pharmaceutical enterprises (since these bioactive compounds trigger a pharmacological or toxicological impact in people and creatures), in beautifying agents, nourishment, for the production of medications, colors, aromas, flavors, dietary enhancements. Consequently, both the logical and mechanical enthusiasm around plant secondary metabolites is gigantic. This audit underlined enormous assortment of atoms of plant secondary metabolism by depicting instances of terpenoids, phenolic compounds and alkaloids that, albeit explicit, can give an outline of the numerous conceivable fields of utilization of these particles. Plant cell and tissue culture systems are being utilized generally for in vitro control and re-vegetation of an extensive number of animal groups for business purposes, including numerous medicinal plants. In plant cell biotechnology, metabolic designing is a rising branch that assumes an essential job in activating explicit pathways for the generation of secondary metabolites (metabolomics). For the generation of explicit secondary metabolite, actuation of a particular way is essential. Event, accessibility, and auxiliary decent variety of these dynamic principals differ as indicated by ecological conditions. Yield of these helpful compounds from various plant sources has been a noteworthy worry over most recent couple of decades.

REFERENCES

[1] Wurtzel ET, Kutchan TM. Plant metabolism, the diverse chemistry set of the future. *Science* 16 Sep 2016: Vol. 353, Issue 6305, pp. 1232-1236. DOI: 10.1126/science.aad2062.

[2] Singh B, Sharma RA. Plant terpenes: defense responses, phylogenetic analysis, regulation and clinical applications. *3 Biotech.* 2014;5(2):129-151.

[3] Bohlmann J, Keeling CI. Terpenoid biomaterials. *Plant J.* 2008 May;54(4):656-69. doi: 10.1111/j.1365-313X.2008.03449.x. PubMed PMID: 18476870.

[4] Jiang Z, Kempinski C, Chappell J. Extraction and Analysis of Terpenes/Terpenoids. *Curr Protoc Plant Biol.* 2016;1:345-358. Epub 2016 Jun 10. PubMed PMID: 27868090; PubMed Central PMCID: PMC5113832.

[5] Web wikidiff.com. *Sesquiterpene vs Monoterpene - What's the difference?*

[6] Web beneforce.com. *Monoterpenes Information.*

[7] Bayala B, Bassole IH, Scifo R, Gnoula C, Morel L, Lobaccaro JM, Simpore J. Anticancer activity of essential oils and their chemical components - a review. *Am J*

Cancer Res. 2014 Nov 19;4(6):591-607. eCollection 2014. Review. PubMed PMID: 25520854; PubMed Central PMCID: PMC4266698.

[8] St-Gelais A. *Published Paper: Interesting and Rare Compounds from Bolivian Molle.* Laboratoire PhytoChemia, 11 July 2015.

[9] Garcia R, Alves ES, Santos MP, Aquije GM, Fernandes AA, Dos Santos RB, Ventura JA, Fernandes PM. Antimicrobial activity and potential use of monoterpenes as tropical fruits preservatives. *Braz J Microbiol.* 2008 Jan;39(1):163-8. doi: 10.1590/S1517-838220080001000032. Epub 2008 Mar 1. PubMed PMID: 24031197; PubMed Central PMCID: PMC3768356.

[10] Buckle J. Chapter 2. Basic Plant Taxonomy, Basic Essential Oil Chemistry, Extraction, Biosynthesis, and Analysis. In: Jane Buckle PhD RN. *Clinical Aromatherapy: Essential Oils in Healthcare* 3rd Edition, published by Churchill Livingstone, December 24, 2014.

[11] Web beneforce.com. *Sesquiterpenes in Oils Information.*

[12] Zerbe P. *Modularity of terpenoid metabolism fuels plant's chemical diversity.* Web Zerbe lab.

[13] Vattekkatte A, Garms S, Brandt W, Boland W. Enhanced structural diversity in terpenoid biosynthesis: enzymes, substrates and cofactors. *Org Biomol Chem.* 2018 Jan 17;16(3):348-362. doi: 10.1039/c7ob02040f. Review. PubMed PMID: 29296983.

[14] Cho KS, Lim YR, Lee K, Lee J, Lee JH, Lee IS. Terpenes from Forests and Human Health. *Toxicol Res.* 2017 Apr;33(2):97-106. doi: 10.5487/TR.2017.33.2.097. Epub 2017 Apr 15. Review. PubMed PMID: 28443180; PubMed Central PMCID: PMC5402865.

[15] Aati H, El-Gamal A, Kayser O. Chemical composition and biological activity of the essential oil from the root of Jatropha pelargoniifolia Courb. native to Saudi Arabia. *Saudi Pharm J.* 2019 Jan;27(1):88-95. doi: 10.1016/j.jsps.2018.09.001. Epub 2018 Sep 11. PubMed PMID: 30662311; PubMed Central PMCID: PMC6323148.

[16] Okoh O., Sadimenko A., Afolayan A. Comparative evaluation of the antibacterial activities of the essential oils of Rosmarinus officinalis L. obtained by hydrodistillation and solvent free microwave extraction methods. *Food Chem.* 2010;120:308–312. doi: 10.1016/j.foodchem.2009.09.084.

[17] Andrade MA, Cardoso Md, Gomes Mde S, de Azeredo CM, Batista LR, Soares MJ, Rodrigues LM, Figueiredo AC. Biological activity of the essential oils from Cinnamodendron dinisii and Siparuna guianensis. *Braz J Microbiol.* 2015 Mar 1;46(1):189-94. doi: 10.1590/S1517-838246120130683. eCollection 2015 Mar. PubMed PMID: 26221107; PubMed Central PMCID: PMC4512063.

[18] Zárybnický T, Boušová I, Ambrož M, Skálová L. Hepatotoxicity of monoterpenes and sesquiterpenes. *Arch Toxicol.* 2018 Jan;92(1):1-13. doi: 10.1007/s00204-017-2062-2. Epub 2017 Sep 13. Review. PubMed PMID: 28905185.

[19] Schmidt A, Wächtler B, Temp U, Krekling T, Séguin A, Gershenzon J. A bifunctional geranyl and geranylgeranyl diphosphate synthase is involved in terpene oleoresin formation in Picea abies. *Plant Physiol.* 2010 Feb;152(2):639-55. doi: 10.1104/pp.109.144691. Epub 2009 Nov 25. PubMed PMID: 19939949; PubMed Central PMCID: PMC2815902.

[20] Toyomasu T, Sassa T. Comprehensive Natural Products II. Chemistry and Biology In: *Reference Module in Chemistry, Molecular Sciences and Chemical Engineering* Volume 1, 2010, Pages 643-672.

[21] Lanzotti V. (2013) Diterpenes for Therapeutic Use. In: Ramawat K., Mérillon JM. (eds) *Natural Products.* Springer, Berlin, Heidelberg DOI https://doi.org/10.1007/978-3-642-22144-6_192. Print ISBN 978-3-642-22143-9, Online ISBN 978-3-642-22144-6.

[22] Perveen S. Introductory Chapter: Terpenes and Terpenoids. In: Shagufta Perveen. *Terpenes and Terpenoids.* Intechopen DOI: 10.5772/intechopen.79683.

[23] *Web Educalingo. Sesquiterpene* (2019). Available hFrom: https://educalingo.com/en/dic-en/sesquiterpene.

[24] Chadwick M, Trewin H, Gawthrop F, Wagstaff C. Sesquiterpenoids lactones: benefits to plants and people. *Int J Mol Sci.* 2013 Jun 19;14(6):12780-805. doi: 10.3390/ijms140612780. Review. PubMed PMID: 23783276; PubMed Central PMCID: PMC3709812.

[25] Amorim MH, Gil da Costa RM, Lopes C, Bastos MM. Sesquiterpene lactones: adverse health effects and toxicity mechanisms. *Crit Rev Toxicol.* 2013 Aug;43(7):559-79. doi: 10.3109/10408444.2013.813905. Review. PubMed PMID: 23875764.

[26] Yan J, Guo J, Yuan W, Mai W, Hong K. Chapter Fifteen - Identification of Enzymes Involved in Sesterterpene Biosynthesis in Marine Fungi. In: *Moore BS. Methods in Enzymology* Volume 604, 2018, Pages 441-498, DOI: https://doi.org/10.1016/bs.mie.2018.04.023.

[27] Qi SH, Ma X. Antifouling Compounds from Marine Invertebrates. *Mar Drugs.* 2017 Aug 28;15(9). pii: E263. doi: 10.3390/md15090263. Review. PubMed PMID: 28846623; PubMed Central PMCID: PMC5618402.

[28] Brill ZG, Grover HK, Maimone TJ. Enantioselective synthesis of an ophiobolin sesterterpene via a programmed radical cascade. *Science.* 2016 May 27;352(6289):1078-82. doi: 10.1126/science.aaf6742. PubMed PMID: 27230373; PubMed Central PMCID: PMC5319821.

[29] Huang AC, Kautsar SA, Hong YJ, Medema MH, Bond AD, Tantillo DJ, Osbourn A. Unearthing a sesterterpene biosynthetic repertoire in the Brassicaceae through genome mining reveals convergent evolution. *Proc Natl Acad Sci U S A.* 2017 Jul 18;114(29):E6005-E6014. doi: 10.1073/pnas.1705567114. Epub 2017 Jul 3. PubMed PMID: 28673978; PubMed Central PMCID: PMC5530694.

[30] *Nitzschia closterium classification essay.* Web http://essaycheap793.web.fc2.com, January 18, 2017.

[31] Zhang C, Liu Y. Targeting cancer with sesterterpenoids: the new potential antitumor drugs. *J Nat Med.* 2015 Jul;69(3):255-66. doi: 10.1007/s11418-015-0911-y. Epub 2015 Apr 19. Review. PubMed PMID: 25894074; PubMed Central PMCID: PMC4506451.

[32] Tian W, Deng Z, Hong K. The Biological Activities of Sesterterpenoid-Type Ophiobolins. *Mar Drugs.* 2017 Jul 18;15(7). pii: E229. doi: 10.3390/md15070229. Review. PubMed PMID: 28718836; PubMed Central PMCID: PMC5532671.

[33] Krisztina Krizsán, Ottó Bencsik, Ildikó Nyilasi, László Galgóczy, Csaba Vágvölgyi, Tamás Papp; Effect of the sesterterpene-type metabolites, ophiobolins A and B, on zygomycetes fungi, *FEMS Microbiology Letters,* Volume 313, Issue 2, 1 December 2010, Pages 135–140, https://doi.org/10.1111/j.1574-6968.2010.02138.x.

[34] Chudzik M, Korzonek-Szlacheta I, Król W. Triterpenes as potentially cytotoxic compounds. *Molecules.* 2015 Jan 19;20(1):1610-25. doi: 10.3390/molecules 20011610. Review. PubMed PMID: 25608043; PubMed Central PMCID: PMC6272502.

[35] Feng L, Liu X, Zhu W, Guo F, Wu Y, Wang R, Chen K, Huang C, Li Y. Inhibition of human neutrophil elastase by pentacyclic triterpenes. *PLoS One.* 2013 Dec 20;8(12):e82794. doi: 10.1371/journal.pone.0082794. eCollection 2013. PubMed PMID: 24376583; PubMed Central PMCID: PMC3869726.

[36] Agra LC, Ferro JN, Barbosa FT, Barreto E. Triterpenes with healing activity: A systematic review. *J Dermatolog Treat.* 2015 Oct;26(5):465-70. doi: 10.3109/09546634.2015.1021663. Epub 2015 Apr 20. Review. PubMed PMID: 25893368.

[37] Ríos JL. Effects of triterpenes on the immune system. *J Ethnopharmacol.* 2010 Mar 2;128(1):1-14. doi: 10.1016/j.jep.2009.12.045. Epub 2010 Jan 14. Review. PubMed PMID: 20079412.

[38] Nazaruk J, Borzym-Kluczyk M. The role of triterpenes in the management of diabetes mellitus and its complications. *Phytochem Rev.* 2015;14(4):675-690. Epub 2014 Jun 24. Review. PubMed PMID: 26213526; PubMed Central PMCID: PMC4513225.

[39] Saleem M. Lupeol, a novel anti-inflammatory and anti-cancer dietary triterpene. *Cancer Lett.* 2009 Nov 28;285(2):109-15. doi: 10.1016/j.canlet.2009.04.033. Epub 2009 May 22. Review. PubMed PMID: 19464787; PubMed Central PMCID: PMC2764818.

[40] Web www.britannica.com. *Isoprenoid chemical compound.*

[41] Takaichi S. (2013) Tetraterpenes: Carotenoids. In: Ramawat K., Mérillon JM. (eds) *Natural Products.* Springer, Berlin, Heidelberg. https://doi.org/10.1007/978-3-642-22144-6_141 Print. ISBN 978-3-642-22143-9. Online ISBN 978-3-642-22144-6.

[42] Cho KS, Shin M, Kim S, Lee SB. Recent Advances in Studies on the Therapeutic Potential of Dietary Carotenoids in Neurodegenerative Diseases. *Oxid Med Cell Longev.* 2018 Apr 16;2018:4120458. doi: 10.1155/2018/4120458. eCollection 2018. Review. PubMed PMID: 29849893; PubMed Central PMCID: PMC5926482.

[43] Marchetti N, Giovannini PP, Catani M, Pasti L, Cavazzini A. Thermodynamic Insights into the Separation of Carotenoids in Reversed-Phase Liquid Chromatography. *Int J Anal Chem.* 2019 Jan 3;2019:7535813. doi: 10.1155/2019/7535813. eCollection 2019. PubMed PMID: 30719042; PubMed Central PMCID: PMC6335859.

[44] Galasso C, Orefice I, Pellone P, Cirino P, Miele R, Ianora A, Brunet C, Sansone C, "On the Neuroprotective Role of Astaxanthin: New Perspectives?," *Marine Drugs,* vol. 16, no. 8, pp. 247, 2018. https://doi.org/10.1155/2018/4120458.

[45] Widomska J, Welc R, Gruszecki WI. The effect of carotenoids on the concentration of singlet oxygen in lipid membranes. *Biochim Biophys Acta Biomembr.* 2019 Apr 1;1861(4):845-851. doi: 10.1016/j.bbamem.2019.01.012. Epub 2019 Jan 26. PubMed PMID: 30689980.

[46] Eggersdorfer M, Wyss A. Carotenoids in human nutrition and health. *Arch Biochem Biophys.* 2018 Aug 15;652:18-26. doi: 10.1016/j.abb.2018.06.001. Epub 2018 Jun 6. Review. PubMed PMID: 29885291.

[47] Rodriguez-Concepcion M, Avalos J, Bonet ML, Boronat A, Gomez-Gomez L, Hornero-Mendez D, Limon MC, Meléndez-Martínez AJ, Olmedilla-Alonso B, Palou A, Ribot J, Rodrigo MJ, Zacarias L, Zhu C. A global perspective on carotenoids: Metabolism, biotechnology, and benefits for nutrition and health. *Prog Lipid Res.* 2018 Apr;70:62-93. doi: 10.1016/j.plipres.2018.04.004. Epub 2018 Apr 19. Review. PubMed PMID: 29679619.

[48] Toti E, Chen CO, Palmery M, Villaño Valencia D, Peluso I. Non-Provitamin A and Provitamin A Carotenoids as Immunomodulators: Recommended Dietary Allowance, Therapeutic Index, or Personalized Nutrition? *Oxid Med Cell Longev.* 2018 May 9;2018:4637861. doi: 10.1155/2018/4637861. eCollection 2018. Review. PubMed PMID: 29861829; PubMed Central PMCID: PMC5971251.

[49] Bhattacharya A, Sood P, Citovsky V. The roles of plant phenolics in defence and communication during Agrobacterium and Rhizobium infection. *Mol Plant Pathol.* 2010 Sep;11(5):705-19. doi: 10.1111/j.1364-3703.2010.00625.x. Review. PubMed PMID: 20696007.

[50] Lin D, Xiao M, Zhao J, Li Z, Xing B, Li X, Kong M, Li L, Zhang Q, Liu Y, Chen H, Qin W, Wu H, Chen S. An Overview of Plant Phenolic Compounds and Their Importance in Human Nutrition and Management of Type 2 Diabetes. *Molecules.* 2016 Oct 15;21(10). pii: E1374. Review. PubMed PMID: 27754463; PubMed Central PMCID: PMC6274266.

[51] Tsao R. Chemistry and biochemistry of dietary polyphenols. *Nutrients.* 2010 Dec;2(12):1231-46. doi: 10.3390/nu2121231. Epub 2010 Dec 10. Review. PubMed PMID: 22254006; PubMed Central PMCID: PMC3257627.

[52] Ulrich AC, Zander ZU. The Strawberry Pathogenesis-related 10 (PR-10) Fra a Proteins Control Flavonoid Biosynthesis by Binding to Metabolic Intermediates. *Journal Of Biological Chemistry* Volume 288, Number 49, December 6, 2013.

[53] Tinikul R, Chenprakhon P, Maenpuen S, Chaiyen P. Biotransformation of Plant-Derived Phenolic Acids. *Biotechnol J.* 2018 Jun;13(6):e1700632. doi: 10.1002/biot.201700632. Epub 2018 Jan 30. Review. PubMed PMID: 29278307.

[54] Kitade Y, Hashimoto R, Suda M, Hiraga K, Inui M. Production of 4-Hydroxybenzoic Acid by an Aerobic Growth-Arrested Bioprocess Using Metabolically Engineered Corynebacterium glutamicum. *Appl Environ Microbiol.* 2018 Mar 1;84(6). pii: e02587-17. doi: 10.1128/AEM.02587-17. Print 2018 Mar 15. PubMed PMID: 29305513; PubMed Central PMCID: PMC5835730.

[55] Kabała-Dzik A, Rzepecka-Stojko A, Kubina R, Wojtyczka RD, Buszman E, Stojko J. Caffeic Acid Versus Caffeic Acid Phenethyl Ester in the Treatment of Breast Cancer MCF-7 Cells: Migration Rate Inhibition. *Integr Cancer Ther.* 2018 Dec;17(4):1247-1259. doi: 10.1177/1534735418801521. Epub 2018 Sep 24. PubMed PMID: 30246565; PubMed Central PMCID: PMC6247537.

[56] Rasheeda K, Bharathy H, Nishad Fathima N. Vanillic acid and syringic acid: Exceptionally robust aromatic moieties for inhibiting in vitro self-assembly of type I collagen. *Int J Biol Macromol.* 2018 Jul 1;113:952-960. doi: 10.1016/j.ijbiomac.2018.03.015. Epub 2018 Mar 6. PubMed PMID: 29522822.

[57] Sadati SM, Gheibi N, Ranjbar S, Hashemzadeh MS. Docking study of flavonoid derivatives as potent inhibitors of influenza H1N1 virus neuraminidase. *Biomed Rep.* 2019 Jan;10(1):33-38. doi: 10.3892/br.2018.1173. Epub 2018 Nov 23. PubMed PMID: 30588301; PubMed Central PMCID: PMC6299203.

[58] Ren N, Kim E, Li B, Pan H, Tong T, Yang CS, Tu Y. Flavonoids alleviating insulin resistance through inhibition of inflammatory signaling. *J Agric Food Chem.* 2019 Jan 5. doi: 10.1021/acs.jafc.8b05348. [Epub ahead of print] PubMed PMID: 30612424.

[59] Nagula RL, Wairkar S. Recent advances in topical delivery of flavonoids: A review. *Journal of Controlled Release* Volume 296, 28 February 2019, Pages 190-201. https://doi.org/10.1016/j.jconrel.2019.01.029. PMID 30682442.

[60] Zhang X, Wang X, Wang M, Cao J, Xiao J, Wang Q. Effects of different pretreatments on flavonoids and antioxidant activity of Dryopteris erythrosora leave. *PLoS One.* 2019 Jan 2;14(1):e0200174. doi: 10.1371/journal.pone.0200174. eCollection 2019. PubMed PMID: 30601805; PubMed Central PMCID: PMC6314590.

[61] Alagna F, Mariotti R, Panara F, et al. Olive phenolic compounds: metabolic and transcriptional profiling during fruit development. *BMC Plant Biol.* 2012;12:162. Published 2012 Sep 10. doi:10.1186/1471-2229-12-162.

[62] *Oat Avenanthramides.* Web honey-guide.com, June 20 2015.

[63] Koleva II, van Beek TA, Soffers AE, Dusemund B, Rietjens IM. Alkaloids in the human food chain--natural occurrence and possible adverse effects. *Mol Nutr Food Res.* 2012 Jan;56(1):30-52. doi: 10.1002/mnfr.201100165. Epub 2011 Aug 8. Review. PubMed PMID: 21823220.

[64] Mehta S. Classification of Alkaloids. Web pharmaxchange.info July 28, 2012.

[65] Aniszewski T. Alkaloids - *Secrets of Life Alkaloid Chemistry, Biological Significance, Applications and Ecological Role.* Elsevier Science, 2007. https://doi.org/10.1016/B978-0-444-52736-3.X5000-4. ISBN 978-0-444-52736-3.

[66] Sato F, Hashimoto T, Hachiya A, Tamura K, Choi KB, Morishige T, Fujimoto H, Yamada Y. Metabolic engineering of plant alkaloid biosynthesis. *Proc Natl Acad Sci U S A.* 2001 Jan 2;98(1):367-72. PubMed PMID: 11134522; PubMed Central PMCID: PMC14596.

[67] Yu N, Hu S, Hao Z. Benificial Effect of Stachydrine on the Traumatic Brain Injury Induced Neurodegeneration by Attenuating the Expressions of Akt/mTOR/PI3K and TLR4/NFκ-B Pathway. *Transl Neurosci.* 2018 Dec 31;9:175-182. doi: 10.1515/tnsci-2018-0026. eCollection 2018. PubMed PMID: 30687544; PubMed Central PMCID: PMC6341910.

[68] Liu Y, Wei S, Zou Q, Luo Y. Stachydrine suppresses viability & migration of astrocytoma cells via CXCR4/ERK & CXCR4/Akt pathway activity. *Future Oncol.* 2018 Jun;14(15):1443-1459. doi: 10.2217/fon-2017-0562. Epub 2018 Jun 6. PubMed PMID: 29873242.

[69] Xie X, Zhang Z, Wang X, Luo Z, Lai B, Xiao L, Wang N. Stachydrine protects eNOS uncoupling and ameliorates endothelial dysfunction induced by homocysteine. *Mol Med.* 2018 Mar 19;24(1):10. doi: 10.1186/s10020-018-0010-0. PubMed PMID: 30134790; PubMed Central PMCID: PMC6016886.

[70] Chen HH, Zhao P, Zhao WX, Tian J, Guo W, Xu M, Zhang C, Lu R. Stachydrine ameliorates pressure overload-induced diastolic heart failure by suppressing myocardial fibrosis. *Am J Transl Res.* 2017 Sep 15;9(9):4250-4260. eCollection 2017. PubMed PMID: 28979698; PubMed Central PMCID: PMC5622267.

[71] CHEBI:46750 – *hygrine.* Available From: https://www.ebi.ac.uk/chebi/searchId.do?chebiId=CHEBI:46750.

[72] Rubio C, Strano-Rossi S, Tabernero MJ, Anzillotti L, Chiarotti M, Bermejo AM. Hygrine and cuscohygrine as possible markers to distinguish coca chewing from cocaine abuse in workplace drug testing. *Forensic Sci Int.* 2013 Apr 10;227(1-3):60-3. doi: 10.1016/j.forsciint.2012.09.005. Epub 2012 Oct 11. PubMed PMID: 23063180.

[73] Moreira R, Pereira DM, Valentão P, Andrade PB. Pyrrolizidine Alkaloids: Chemistry, Pharmacology, Toxicology and Food Safety. *Int J Mol Sci.* 2018 Jun 5;19(6). pii: E1668. doi: 10.3390/ijms19061668. Review. PubMed PMID: 29874826; PubMed Central PMCID: PMC6032134.

[74] Hussain G, Rasul A, Anwar H, Aziz N, Razzaq A, Wei W, Ali M, Li J, Li X. Role of Plant Derived Alkaloids and Their Mechanism in Neurodegenerative Disorders. *Int J Biol Sci.* 2018 Mar 9;14(3):341-357. doi: 10.7150/ijbs.23247. eCollection 2018. Review. PubMed PMID: 29559851; PubMed Central PMCID: PMC5859479.

[75] da Silva VDA, da Silva AMM, E Silva JHC, Costa SL. Neurotoxicity of Prosopis juliflora: from Natural Poisoning to Mechanism of Action of Its Piperidine Alkaloids. *Neurotox Res.* 2018 Nov;34(4):878-888. doi: 10.1007/s12640-017-9862-2. Epub 2018 Jan 16. Review. PubMed PMID: 29340871.

[76] Freitas TR, Danuello A, Viegas Júnior C, Bolzani VS, Pivatto M. Mass spectrometry for characterization of homologous piperidine alkaloids and their activity as acetylcholinesterase inhibitors. *Rapid Commun Mass Spectrom.* 2018 Aug 15;32(15):1303-1310. doi: 10.1002/rcm.8172. PubMed PMID: 29785738.

[77] de Albuquerque Melo GM, Silva MC, Guimarães TP, Pinheiro KM, da Matta CB, de Queiroz AC, Pivatto M, Bolzani Vda S, Alexandre-Moreira MS, Viegas C Jr. Leishmanicidal activity of the crude extract, fractions and major piperidine alkaloids from the flowers of Senna spectabilis. *Phytomedicine.* 2014 Feb 15;21(3):277-81. doi: 10.1016/j.phymed.2013.09.024. Epub 2013 Nov 1. PubMed PMID: 24188737.

[78] Fernandes ÍA, de Almeida L, Ferreira PE, Marques MJ, Rocha RP, Coelho LF, Carvalho DT, Viegas C Jr. Synthesis and biological evaluation of novel piperidine-benzodioxole derivatives designed as potential leishmanicidal drug candidates. *Bioorg Med Chem Lett.* 2015 Aug 15;25(16):3346-9. doi: 10.1016/j.bmcl.2015. 05.068. Epub 2015 Jun 4. PubMed PMID: 26094119.

[79] Lacerda RBM, Freitas TR, Martins MM, Teixeira TL, da Silva CV, Candido PA, Oliveira RJ, Júnior CV, Bolzani VDS, Danuello A, Pivatto M. Isolation, leishmanicidal evaluation and molecular docking simulations of piperidine alkaloids from Senna spectabilis. *Bioorg Med Chem.* 2018 Dec 1;26(22):5816-5823. doi: 10.1016/j.bmc.2018.10.032. Epub 2018 Nov 2. PubMed PMID: 30413343.

[80] Goel P, Alam O, Naim MJ, Nawaz F, Iqbal M, Alam MI. Recent advancement of piperidine moiety in treatment of cancer- A review. *Eur J Med Chem.* 2018 Sep 5;157:480-502. doi: 10.1016/j.ejmech.2018.08.017. Epub 2018 Aug 8. Review. PubMed PMID: 30114660.

[81] Afewerki S, Wang JX, Liao WW, Córdova A. The Chemical Synthesis and Applications of Tropane Alkaloids. *Alkaloids Chem Biol.* 2019;81:151-233. doi: 10.1016/bs.alkal.2018.06.001. Epub 2018 Sep 7. PubMed PMID: 30685050.

[82] Guo Z, Tan H, Lv Z, Ji Q, Huang Y, Liu J, Chen D, Diao Y, Si J, Zhang L. Targeted expression of Vitreoscilla hemoglobin improves the production of tropane alkaloids

in Hyoscyamus niger hairy roots. *Sci Rep.* 2018 Dec 19;8(1):17969. doi: 10.1038/s41598-018-36156-y. PubMed PMID: 30568179; PubMed Central PMCID: PMC6299274.

[83] Cirlini M, Demuth TM, Biancardi A, Rychlik M, Dall'Asta C, Bruni R. Are tropane alkaloids present in organic foods? Detection of scopolamine and atropine in organic buckwheat (Fagopyron esculentum L.) products by UHPLC-MS/MS. *Food Chem.* 2018 Jan 15;239:141-147. doi: 10.1016/j.foodchem.2017.06.028. Epub 2017 Jun 23. PubMed PMID: 28873551.

[84] Marín-Sáez J, Romero-González R, Garrido Frenich A, Egea-González FJ. Screening of drugs and homeopathic products from Atropa belladonna seed extracts: Tropane alkaloids determination and untargeted analysis. *Drug Test Anal.* 2018 Oct;10(10):1579-1589. doi: 10.1002/dta.2416. Epub 2018 Jun 29. PubMed PMID: 29808589.

[85] Zhao K, Zeng J, Zhao T, Zhang H, Qiu F, Yang C, Zeng L, Liu X, Chen M, Lan X, Liao Z. Enhancing Tropane Alkaloid Production Based on the Functional Identification of Tropine-Forming Reductase in Scopolia lurida, a Tibetan Medicinal Plant. *Front Plant Sci.* 2017 Oct 16;8:1745. doi: 10.3389/fpls.2017. 01745. eCollection 2017. PubMed PMID: 29085381; PubMed Central PMCID: PMC5650612.

[86] Biosynthesis of scopolamine. Adapted from Ziegler J, Facchini PJ (2008). "Alkaloid biosynthesis: metabolism and trafficking." *Annual Review of Plant Biology* 59 (1): 735–69. DOI:10.1146/annurev.arplant.59.032607.092730. PMID 18251710.

[87] Shang XF, Morris-Natschke SL, Liu YQ, Guo X, Xu XS, Goto M, Li JC, Yang GZ, Lee KH. Biologically active quinoline and quinazoline alkaloids part I. *Med Res Rev.* 2018 May;38(3):775-828. doi: 10.1002/med.21466. Epub 2017 Sep 13. Review. PubMed PMID: 28902434.

[88] Yoshitomi S, Takahashi Y, Yamaguchi T, Oboshi T, Horino A, Ikeda H, Imai K, Okanishi T, Nakashima M, Saitsu H, Matsumoto N, Yoshimoto J, Fujita T, Ishii A, Hirose S, Inoue Y. Quinidine therapy and therapeutic drug monitoring in four patients with KCNT1 mutations. *Epileptic Disord.* 2019 Feb 1;21(1):48-54. doi: 10.1684/epd.2019.1026. PubMed PMID: 30782581.

[89] Viskin S, Chorin E, Viskin D, Hochstadt A, Halkin A, Tovia-Brodie O, Lee JK, Asher E, Laish-Farkash A, Amit G, Havakuk O, Belhassen B, Rosso R. Quinidine-Responsive Polymorphic Ventricular Tachycardia in Patients with Coronary Heart Disease. *Circulation*. 2019 Jan 30. doi: 10.1161/CIRCULATIONAHA. 118.038036. [Epub ahead of print] PubMed PMID: 30696267.

[90] Hill SR, Sharma GK. Antimalarial Medications. [Updated 2018 Dec 2]. In: *StatPearls* [Internet]. Treasure Island (FL): StatPearls Publishing; 2019 Jan-. Available from: https://www.ncbi.nlm.nih.gov/books/NBK470158/

[91] Gunatilaka AAL. Chapter 1 - Alkaloids from Sri Lankan Flora. In: Geoffrey A. Cordell. *The Alkaloids: Chemistry and Biology* Volume 52, 1999, Pages 1-101. Gulf Professional Publishing, Aug 23, 2005 https://doi.org/10.1016/S0099-9598(08)60025-5.

[92] Luganini A, Mercorelli B, Messa L, Palù G, Gribaudo G, Loregian A. The isoquinoline alkaloid berberine inhibits human cytomegalovirus replication by interfering with the viral Immediate Early-2 (IE2) protein transactivating activity. *Antiviral Res.* 2019 Feb 8;164:52-60. doi: 10.1016/j.antiviral.2019.02.006. [Epub ahead of print] PubMed PMID: 30738836.

[93] Zhang Y, Li M, Li X, Zhang T, Qin M, Ren L. Isoquinoline Alkaloids and Indole Alkaloids Attenuate Aortic Atherosclerosis in Apolipoprotein E Deficient Mice: A Systematic Review and Meta-Analysis. *Front Pharmacol.* 2018 Jun 5;9:602. doi: 10.3389/fphar.2018.00602. eCollection 2018. PubMed PMID: 29922166; PubMed Central PMCID: PMC5996168.

[94] Liu D, Meng X, Wu D, Qiu Z, Luo H. A Natural Isoquinoline Alkaloid With Antitumor Activity: Studies of the Biological Activities of Berberine. *Front Pharmacol.* 2019 Feb 14;10:9. doi: 10.3389/fphar.2019.00009. eCollection 2019. Review. PubMed PMID: 30837865; PubMed Central PMCID: PMC6382680.

[95] Tan HL, Chan KG, Pusparajah P, Duangjai A, Saokaew S, Mehmood Khan T, Lee LH, Goh BH. Rhizoma Coptidis: A Potential Cardiovascular Protective Agent. *Front Pharmacol.* 2016 Oct 7;7:362. eCollection 2016. Review. PubMed PMID: 27774066; PubMed Central PMCID: PMC5054023.

[96] Kapadia N, Harding W. Aporphine Alkaloids as Ligands for Serotonin Receptors. *Med chem (Los Angeles)* 6:241-249. doi:10.4172/2161-0444.1000353.

[97] Ma C, Wang J, Chu H, Zhang X, Wang Z, Wang H, Li G. Purification and characterization of aporphine alkaloids from leaves of Nelumbo nucifera Gaertn and their effects on glucose consumption in 3T3-L1 adipocytes. *Int J Mol Sci.* 2014 Feb 26;15(3):3481-94. doi: 10.3390/ijms15033481. PubMed PMID: 24577311; PubMed Central PMCID: PMC3975348.

[98] Gorpenchenko TY, Grigorchuk VP, Bulgakov DV, Tchernoded GK, Bulgakov VP. Tempo-Spatial Pattern of Stepharine Accumulation in Stephania Glabra Morphogenic Tissues. *Int J Mol Sci.* 2019 Feb 13;20(4). pii: E808. doi: 10.3390/ijms20040808. PMID 30781887.

[99] Ge YC, Wang KW. New Analogues of Aporphine Alkaloids. *Mini Rev Med Chem.* 2018;18(19):1590-1602. doi: 10.2174/1389557518666180423151426.

[100] Mon MT, Yodkeeree S, Punfa W, Pompimon W, Limtrakul P. Alkaloids from Stephania venosa as Chemo-Sensitizers in SKOV3 Ovarian Cancer Cells via Akt/NF-κB Signaling. *Chem Pharm Bull* (Tokyo). 2018;66(2):162-169. doi: 10.1248/cpb.c17-00687. PubMed PMID: 29386467.

[101] Aniszewski T. Chapter 2 - *Alkaloid chemistry Alkaloids: Chemistry, Biology, Ecology, and Applications*. Elsevier Science, Apr 25, 2015. https://doi.org/10.1016/C2011-0-04166-2. ISBN 978-0-444-59433-4.

[102] Gavilan J, Mennickent D, Ramirez-Molina O, Triviño S, Perez C, Silva-Grecchi T, Godoy PA, Becerra J, Aguayo LG, Moraga-Cid G, Martin VS, Yevenes GE, Castro PA, Guzman L, Fuentealba J. 17 Oxo Sparteine and Lupanine, Obtained from Cytisus scoparius, Exert a Neuroprotection against Soluble Oligomers of Amyloid-β Toxicity by Nicotinic Acetylcholine Receptors. *J Alzheimers Dis*. 2019;67(1):343-356. doi: 10.3233/JAD-180945. PubMed PMID: 30584148.

[103] Villalpando-Vargas F, Medina-Ceja L. Sparteine as an anticonvulsant drug: Evidence and possible mechanism of action. *Seizure* Volume 39, July 2016, Pages 49-55. https://doi.org/10.1016/j.seizure.2016.05.010.

[104] Walker N, Smith B, Barnes J, Verbiest M, Kurdziel T, Parag V, Pokhrel S, Bullen C. Cytisine versus varenicline for smoking cessation for Māori (the indigenous people of New Zealand) and their extended family: protocol for a randomized non-inferiority trial. *Addiction*. 2019 Feb;114(2):344-352. doi: 10.1111/add.14449. Epub 2018 Nov 9. PubMed PMID: 30276931.

[105] Norwood Iv VM, Huigens Iii RW. Harnessing the Chemistry of the Indole Heterocycle to Drive Discoveries in Biology and Medicine. *Chembiochem*. 2019 Jan 4. doi: 10.1002/cbic.201800768. [Epub ahead of print] PubMed PMID: 30609199.

[106] van der Nelson H, O'Brien S, Lenguerrand E, Marques E, Alvarez M, Mayer M, Burnard S, Siassakos D, Draycott T. Intramuscular oxytocin versus oxytocin/ergometrine versus carbetocin for prevention of primary postpartum haemorrhage after vaginal birth: study protocol for a randomised controlled trial (the IMox study). *Trials*. 2019 Jan 3;20(1):4. doi: 10.1186/s13063-018-3109-2. PubMed PMID: 30606246; PubMed Central PMCID: PMC6319006.

[107] Nobre L, Pauck D, Golbourn B, Maue M, Bouffet E, Remke M, Ramaswamy V. Effective and safe tumor inhibition using vinblastine in medulloblastoma. *Pediatr Blood Cancer*. 2019 Mar 8:e27694. doi: 10.1002/pbc.27694. [Epub ahead of print] PubMed PMID: 30848061.

[108] Bitzinger DI, Gruber M, Tümmler S, Malsy M, Seyfried T, Weber F, Redel A, Graf BM, Zausig YA. In Vivo Effects of Neostigmine and Physostigmine on Neutrophil Functions and Evaluation of Acetylcholinesterase and Butyrylcholinesterase as Inflammatory Markers during Experimental Sepsis in Rats. *Mediators Inflamm*. 2019 Jan 20;2019:8274903. doi: 10.1155/2019/8274903. eCollection 2019. PubMed PMID: 30804708; PubMed Central PMCID: PMC6360579.

[109] Monostori P, Klinke G, Hauke J, Richter S, Bierau J, Garbade SF, Hoffmann GF, Langhans CD, Haas D, Okun JG. Extended diagnosis of purine and pyrimidine disorders from urine: LC MS/MS assay development and clinical validation. *PLoS*

One. 2019 Feb 28;14(2):e0212458. doi: 10.1371/journal.pone.0212458. eCollection 2019. PubMed PMID: 30817767; PubMed Central PMCID: PMC6394934.

[110] Evans J, Battisti AS. Caffeine. [Updated 2019 Jan 16]. In: *StatPearls [Internet].* Treasure Island (FL): StatPearls Publishing; 2019 Jan-. Available from: https://www.ncbi.nlm.nih.gov/books/NBK519490/

[111] Lodha A, Entz R, Synnes A, Creighton D, Yusuf K, Lapointe A, Yang J, Shah PS; investigators of the Canadian Neonatal Network (CNN) and the Canadian Neonatal Follow-up Network (CNFUN). Early Caffeine Administration and Neurodevelopmental Outcomes in Preterm Infants. *Pediatrics.* 2019 Jan;143(1). pii: e20181348. doi: 10.1542/peds.2018-1348. Epub 2018 Dec 5. PubMed PMID: 30518670.

[112] Cova I, Leta V, Mariani C, Pantoni L, Pomati S. Exploring cocoa properties: is theobromine a cognitive modulator? *Psychopharmacology (Berl).* 2019 Feb;236(2):561-572. doi: 10.1007/s00213-019-5172-0. Epub 2019 Jan 31. Review. PubMed PMID: 30706099.

[113] Martínez-Pinilla E, Oñatibia-Astibia A, Franco R. The relevance of theobromine for the beneficial effects of cocoa consumption. *Front Pharmacol.* 2015 Feb 20;6:30. doi: 10.3389/fphar.2015.00030. eCollection 2015. PubMed PMID: 25750625; PubMed Central PMCID: PMC4335269.

[114] Güven KC, Percot A, Sezik E. Alkaloids in marine algae. *Mar Drugs.* 2010 Feb 4;8(2):269-84. doi: 10.3390/md8020269. Review. PubMed PMID: 20390105; PubMed Central PMCID: PMC2852838.

[115] Web shutterstock.com. *Brown (Phaeophita) algae (Desmarestia viridis) on rocks in March in the Black Sea.*

[116] Web european-marine-life.org. *Delesseria sanguinea* (Hudson) J.V. Lamouroux, 1813.

[117] *Web A few seaweeds of Newfoundland* (part 4) (2011). Available From: http://micksmarinebiology.blogspot.com.

[118] Between the Tides of Nova Scotia. Available From: http://intertidal-novascotia.blogspot.com/

[119] *Showing metabocard for Hordenine* (HMDB0004366). Available From: http://www.hmdb.ca/metabolites/HMDB0004366.

[120] Kim SC, Lee JH, Kim MH, Lee JA, Kim YB, Jung E, Kim YS, Lee J, Park D. Hordenine, a single compound produced during barley germination, inhibits melanogenesis in human melanocytes. *Food Chem.* 2013 Nov 1;141(1):174-81. doi: 10.1016/j.foodchem.2013.03.017. Epub 2013 Mar 14. PubMed PMID: 23768344.

[121] Zhou JW, Luo HZ, Jiang H, Jian TK, Chen ZQ, Jia AQ. Hordenine: A Novel Quorum Sensing Inhibitor and Antibiofilm Agent against Pseudomonas aeruginosa. *J Agric Food Chem.* 2018 Feb 21;66(7):1620-1628. doi: 10.1021/acs.jafc.7b05035. Epub 2018 Feb 8. PubMed PMID: 29353476.

[122] Sommer T, Dlugash G, Hübner H, Gmeiner P, Pischetsrieder M. Monitoring of the dopamine D2 receptor agonists hordenine and N-methyltyramine during the brewing process and in commercial beer samples. *Food Chem.* 2019 Mar 15;276:745-753. doi: 10.1016/j.foodchem.2018.10.067. Epub 2018 Oct 13. PubMed PMID: 30409657.

[123] Su S, Cao M, Wu G, Long Z, Cheng X, Fan J, Xu Z, Su H, Hao Y, Li G, Peng J, Li S, Wang X. Hordenine protects against hyperglycemia-associated renal complications in streptozotocin-induced diabetic mice. *Biomed Pharmacother.* 2018 Aug;104:315-324. doi: 10.1016/j.biopha.2018.05.036. Epub 2018 May 15. PubMed PMID: 29775900.

[124] Netz N, Opatz T. Marine Indole Alkaloids. *Mar Drugs.* 2015 Aug 6;13(8):4814-914. doi: 10.3390/md13084814. Review. PubMed PMID: 26287214; PubMed Central PMCID: PMC4557006.

[125] Lunagariya J, Bhadja P, Zhong S, Vekariya R, Xu S. Marine Natural Product Bis-indole Alkaloid Caulerpin: Chemistry and Biology. *Mini Rev Med Chem.* 2017 Sep 27. doi: 10.2174/1389557517666170927154231. [Epub ahead of print] PubMed PMID: 28971770.

[126] Magliozzi L, Maselli V, Almada F, Di Cosmo A, Mollo E, Polese G. Effect of the algal alkaloid caulerpin on neuropeptide Y (NPY) expression in the central nervous system (CNS) of Diplodus sargus. *J Comp Physiol A Neuroethol Sens Neural Behav Physiol.* 2019 Mar 9. doi: 10.1007/s00359-019-01322-8. [Epub ahead of print] PubMed PMID: 30852662.

[127] Yang H, Liu DQ, Liang TJ, Li J, Liu AH, Yang P, Lin K, Yu XQ, Guo YW, Mao SC, Wang B. Racemosin C, a novel minor bisindole alkaloid with protein tyrosine phosphatase-1B inhibitory activity from the green alga Caulerpa racemosa. *J Asian Nat Prod Res.* 2014 Dec;16(12):1158-65. doi: 10.1080/10286020.2014.965162. Epub 2014 Oct 8. PubMed PMID: 25296343.

[128] Web http://southafrseaweeds.uct.ac.za. *Seaweeds of the South African South Coast.*

[129] Web en.wikipedia.org. Caulerpa racemosa.

[130] Liu Y, Morgan B, Coothankandaswamy V et al. *The Caulerpa Pigment Caulerpin Inhibits HIF-1 Activation and Mitochondrial Respiration.* November 2009Journal of Natural Products 72(12):2104-9 DOI: 10.1021/np9005794.

[131] Web poppe-images.com. *CAULERPACEAE - Caulerpa serrulate.*

[132] Kirkup MP, Moore RE. Indole alkaloids from the marine red alga Martensia fragilis. *Tetrahedron Lett.* 1983;24:2087–2090.

[133] Expat I. Limu of the Day | Turtle Bay, Oahu. In: Hawaiian Time Machine Views Of Hawaii Through The Distorting Lens Of Time. *Blog hawaiiantimemachine,* 21st July 2012. Available From: http://hawaiiantimemachine.blogspot.com/

[134] Pauletti PM, Cintra LS, Braguine CG, da Silva Filho AA, Silva ML, Cunha WR, Januário AH. Halogenated indole alkaloids from marine invertebrates. *Mar Drugs.*

2010 Apr 28;8(5):1526-49. doi: 10.3390/md8051526. Review. PubMed PMID: 20559487; PubMed Central PMCID: PMC2885079.

[135] *Photos by Susana Martins.* Available From: http://skaphandrus.com/en/underwater-photography/photo/23840.

[136] Gribble GW. Biological Activity of Recently Discovered Halogenated Marine Natural Products. *Mar Drugs.* 2015 Jun 30;13(7):4044-136. doi: 10.3390/md13074044. Review. PubMed PMID: 26133553; PubMed Central PMCID: PMC4515607.

[137] Abbas AT, El-Shitany NA, Shaala LA, et al. Red Sea Suberea mollis Sponge Extract Protects against CCl4-Induced Acute Liver Injury in Rats via an Antioxidant Mechanism. *Evid Based Complement Alternat Med.* 2014; 2014:745606.

[138] Agostini-Costa TS, Vieira RF, Bizzo HR, Silveira D, Gimenes MA (2012) Chromatography and its applications. In: Dhanarasu S (ed) *Plant secondary metabolites*, pp. 131-164. InTech Publisher, Rijeka, Croatia.

[139] Sven Zea (Photographer). *Asteropus niger,* Web spongeguide.

[140] Welsh Blogging at its Very Best Info. *Ten Amazing Sea Slugs You Simply Won't Believe Are Real.*

Chapter 2

ENVIRONMENTAL FACTORS ON SECONDARY METABOLISM OF MEDICINAL PLANTS

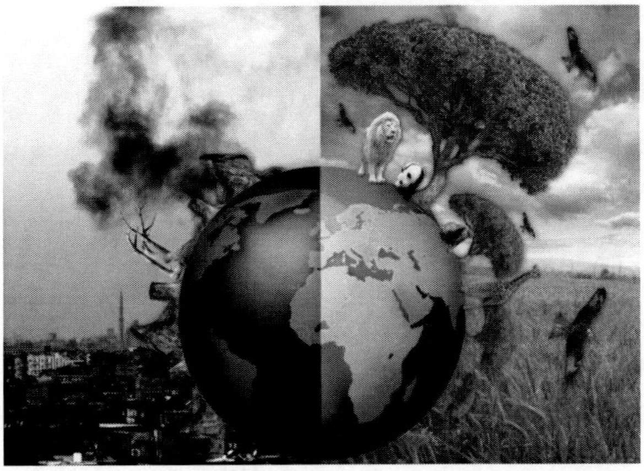

1. ABSTRACT

Plants are unrivaled in the natural world in both the number and complexity of secondary metabolites they produce, and the ubiquitous phenylpropanoids and the lineage-specific glucosinolates represent two such large and chemically diverse groups. Advances in genome-enabled biochemistry and metabolomic technologies have greatly increased the understanding of their metabolic networks in diverse plant species. There also has been some progress in elucidating the gene regulatory networks that are key to their synthesis, accumulation and function. Secondary metabolites have important defense and signaling roles, and they contribute to the overall quality of developing and ripening fruits. Especially, light conditions and temperature are demonstrated to have a prominent role on the composition of phenolic compounds. The present review focuses on the studies on mechanisms associated with the regulation of key secondary metabolites, mainly phenolic compounds, in various plants. are not only a useful array of natural products but also an important part of plant defense system against pathogenic attacks and environmental stresses. With remarkable biological activities, plant SMs are increasingly used as medicine ingredients and food additives for therapeutic, aromatic and culinary purposes. Various genetic, ontogenic, morphogenetic and environmental factors can influence the biosynthesis and accumulation of SMs. According to the literature reports, for example, SMs accumulation is strongly dependent on a variety of environmental factors such as light, temperature, soil water, soil fertility and salinity, and for most plants, a change in an individual factor may alter the content of SMs even if other factors remain constant. Here, we review with emphasis how each of single factors to affect the accumulation of plant secondary metabolites, and conduct a comparative analysis of relevant natural products in the stressed and unstressed plants. Expectantly, this documentary review will outline a general picture of environmental factors responsible for fluctuation in plant SMs, provide a practical way to obtain consistent quality and high quantity of bioactive compounds in vegetation, and present some suggestions for future research and development.

Keywords: medicinal plants, organic compounds, secondary metabolite, biosynthesis

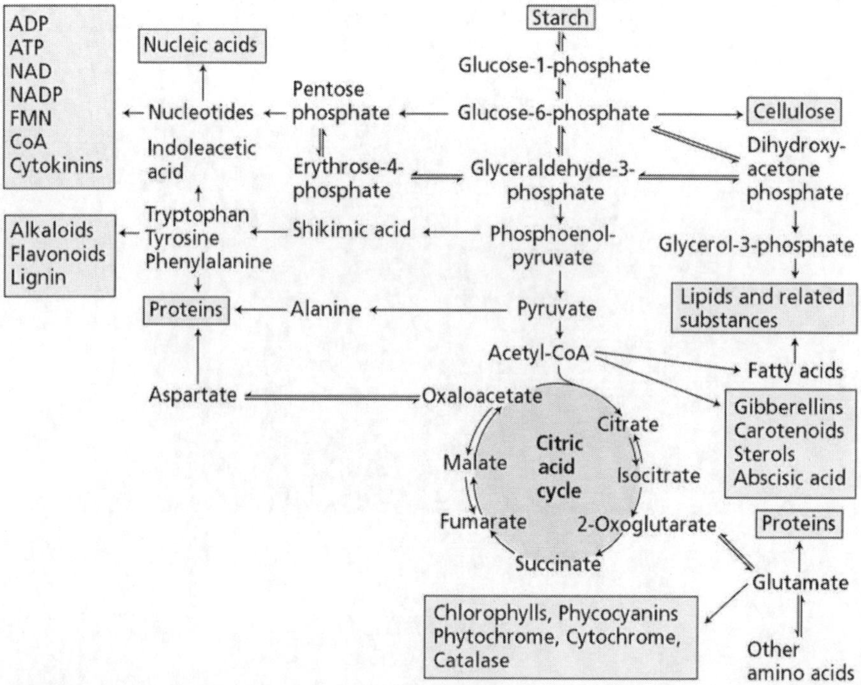

Figure 1. Cell Metabolic Cycle and Production of Secondary metabolites. Plants are sessile organisms and, in order to defend themselves against exogenous (a) biotic constraints, they synthesize an array of secondary metabolites which have important physiological and ecological effects. Plant secondary metabolites can be classified into four major classes: terpenoids, phenolic compounds, alkaloids and sulphur-containing compounds. These phytochemicals can be antimicrobial, act as attractants/repellents, or as deterrents against herbivores. The synthesis of such a rich variety of phytochemicals is also observed in undifferentiated plant cells under laboratory conditions and can be further induced with elicitors or by feeding precursors. (Source: Guerriero G, Berni R, Muñoz-Sanchez JA, et al. Production of Plant Secondary Metabolites: Examples, Tips and Suggestions for Biotechnologists. Genes (Basel). 2018;9(6):309. Published 2018 Jun 20. doi:10.3390/genes9060309.)

2. Introduction

While in food plants our main interest is the carbohydrate/ sugars, proteins, fats and other vitamins, in medicinal plants we look for therapeutically useful chemicals which are generally termed as secondary metabolites which are not that essential for the normal growth and development of the plants/organisms. Plants synthesize these compounds to protect themselves, i.e., to adjust, adapt or defend/ offend, from the hostile organisms or diseases or the environment. SMs that are useful in medicine are mostly polyphenols, alkaloids, glycosides, terpenes, flavonoids, coumarins, tannins etc. The production of secondary metabolites although controlled by genes but their specific expression is greatly influenced by various factors including biotic and abiotic environments such as climate and edaphic factors or other associated living organisms. During the course of evolution plants have evolved various physical and chemical mechanisms to protect themselves from the vagaries of nature (drought, heat, rain, flood, etc.) and also to defend or offend the predators or to protect from predators and pathogens. The most successful adaptation of plants while developing various physiological mechanisms is through the production of a variety of phytochemicals by which they were able to face both biotic and abiotic stresses and threats. In this process of defense/ offence from abiotic stress or the invading diseases causing organisms or the predators (animals, birds, insects and herbivorous animals), the plant synthesize a variety of chemical compounds. Apparently, plants produce many antioxidants for protecting themselves from the oxidative stress. These compounds are in general stored in the leaves or other parts such as, bark, hardwood, fruits, etc., so that the predators or the disease-causing organisms can be either knocked down or paralyzed or even get killed. In many cases, the production of the secondary metabolites in plant also depends on the association of other living organisms, more particularly, the plant or soil microbes. Such differential expressions of therapeutically active principles in plant on account of the above said factors appears to have known and well understood by the ancient scholars, when they gave specific instructions in the procurement of medicinal plants.

3. Biosynthesis

The pathways of biosynthesis are responsible for the occurrence of both primary and secondary metabolites illustrated in Figure 1. Biosynthetic reactions are energy consuming, fueled by the energy released by glycolysis of carbohydrates and through the citric acid cycle. Oxidation of glucose, fatty acids and amino acids results in ATP formation, which is a high-energy molecule formed by catabolism of primary compounds. ATP is recycled in fuel anabolic reactions involving intermediate molecules on the pathways. Whereas, catabolism involves oxidation of starting molecules, biosynthesis or anabolism involves reduction reaction. Hence, the need of reducing agent or hydrogen donor, which is usually the NADP. These catalysts are known as coenzymes and the most widely occurring is CoA made up of ADP and pantetheine phosphate. The most common pathways taken for biosynthesis are performed through the pentose for glycosides, polysaccharides; shikimic acid for phenols, tannins, aromatic alkaloids; acetate-malonate for phenols and alkaloids and mevalonic acid for terpenes, steroids and alkaloids. As showed in the Fig. 1, the scheme outlines how metabolites from the process of photosynthesis, glycolysis and Krebs cycle are tapped off from energy-generating process to provide biosynthetic intermediates. By far, the important building blocks employed in the biosynthesis of secondary metabolites are derived from Acetyl-CoA, shikimic acid, mevalonic acid and 1-deoxylulose 5-phosphate [1-7].

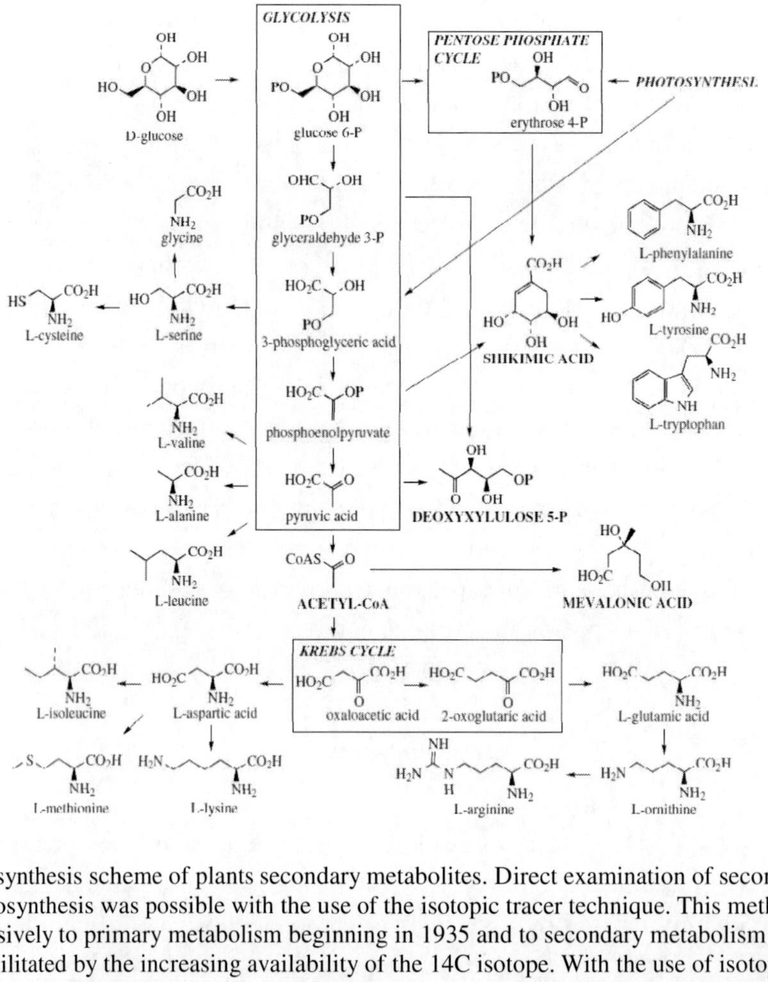

Figure 2. Biosynthesis scheme of plants secondary metabolites. Direct examination of secondary metabolite biosynthesis was possible with the use of the isotopic tracer technique. This methodology, applied extensively to primary metabolism beginning in 1935 and to secondary metabolism from about 1950, was facilitated by the increasing availability of the 14C isotope. With the use of isotopes as tracers, the broad outlines of secondary metabolite biosynthesis, reviewed here, were established in the period 1950 to 1965. (Source: Ronald Bentley. Secondary Metabolite Biosynthesis: The First Century. *Critical Reviews in Biotechnology* Volume 19, 1999 - Issue 1. https://doi.org/10.1080/0738-859991229189.)

4. Expression of Secondary Metabolites

The presence of or absence of certain secondary metabolites in medicinal plants are influenced by a variety of factors, which include climate/ season, edaphic conditions or the association of other plants and other living organisms [8, 9]. Another factor that influenced the production of secondary metabolites in plants are the inter relationship between plants and the insect flora. It is now generally accepted that the flora and the insect flora in a tropical ecosystem have been co-evolving and co-adapting. Many of the medicinal plants are cross-pollinated and they need the help of pollinators. In an open area the wind could do the function, but in a canopied forest many of the shrubs and herbs growing under the big trees cannot get wind to pollinate. These plants are thus heavily depending upon the insects or even the birds to pollinate them. To attract the insects or birds the plants develop pleasant aroma (essential oils) and provide honey and pollen as food to these pollinators. Many flowers contain honey or pollen, which are the normal food of many insects and birds [10, 11]. The insects like bees and butterflies visit flowers after flowers, and take honey or pollen or both. During this process they also carry pollen on their body part, which then help in pollinating while visiting other plants. Many flowers have structurally evolved flower parts to affect such pollinations by insects. These insects also multiply on plants. They lay millions of eggs and the larvae that emerge from these eggs then feed on leaves of the plants, sometimes destroying the plants altogether by over feeding. During the course of evolution, the plants began to synthesize certain toxic substance so that a good percentage of the feeding larvae could be killed [12, 13, 14]. The insect on the other hand began to develop resistance so that many of the larvae could survive. The plants on the other hand again counteracted. It synthesizing more and more toxic compounds. This was something like the love and hate relationship between plants and the insects, which during the course of millions of years of evolutions have resulted in the synthesis of innumerable chemical compounds, mostly the secondary metabolites in plants as well as in insects [15, 16]. The variability in living organisms is indeed the insurance for survival. The evolutionary origin of cross breeding was indeed a nature's device for reshuffling of genes so that new variants could be produced. Similarly, the abiotic conditions also exerted certain influence in the plants and the plants responded by developing various chemicals [17]. In extreme drought conditions the desert exerts a kind of stress on the plants and the plants evolve by synthesizing chemicals that would help them to protect from stress induced by the desert conditions. An excellent example for this is the plant *Commiphora wightii*; an important medicinal plant used extensively as complimentary medicine named 'Guggul'. The medicinal part of the plant is the gum exudates from the stem bark of living plants. This gum is traditionally collected from the desert regions of Rajasthan, Gujarat and even Afghanistan. To everyone's surprise the chemical data of this gum revealed that it does not contain most of the active compounds. A logical explanation may be that this plant growing in a warm humid tropical forest region. It has no desert like conditions and therefore there is no question of any drought induced stress. The same plant when growing in desert has to confront drought induced stress and the plant synthesizes the stress beating chemicals. There are many similar cases that demonstrate that certain specific climatic conditions and edaphic situations are extremely important in the production of therapeutically desirable medicinal compounds. Sandalwood is another classical example. The specific aroma of sandalwood is due to the presence of certain essential oil chemicals, mostly monoterpenes and sesquiterpenes. The production of the specific aroma chemicals is fully expressed only in those sandalwood trees that grow in certain forest regions of Karnataka. The sandalwood growing in other places in India or elsewhere in the world do not have the same kind of aroma with the corresponding chemical constituents [18-20].

5. Importance of Secondary Metabolites

Secondary metabolites, which are a characteristic feature of plants, are especially important and can protect plants against a wide variety of microorganisms (viruses, bacteria, fungi) and herbivores (arthropods, vertebrates). As is the situation with all defense systems of plants and animals, a few specialized pathogens have evolved in plants and have overcome the chemical defense barrier. Secondary metabolites, including antibiotics, are produced in nature and serve survival functions for the organisms producing them. Secondary metabolites serve:

i. As competitive weapons used against other bacteria, fungi, amoebae, plants, insects, and large animals;
ii. As metal transporting agents;
iii. As agents of symbiosis between microbes and plants, nematodes, insects, and higher animals;
iv. As sexual hormones; and
v. As differentiation effectors.

Although antibiotics are not obligatory for sporulation, some secondary metabolites (including antibiotics) stimulate spore formation and inhibit or stimulate germination. Formation of secondary metabolites and spores are regulated by similar factors. Thus, the secondary metabolite can:

i. Slow down germination of spores until a less competitive environment and more favorable conditions for growth exist;
ii. Protect the dormant or initiated spore from consumption by amoebae; or
iii. Cleanse the immediate environment of competing microorganisms during germination [21- 24].

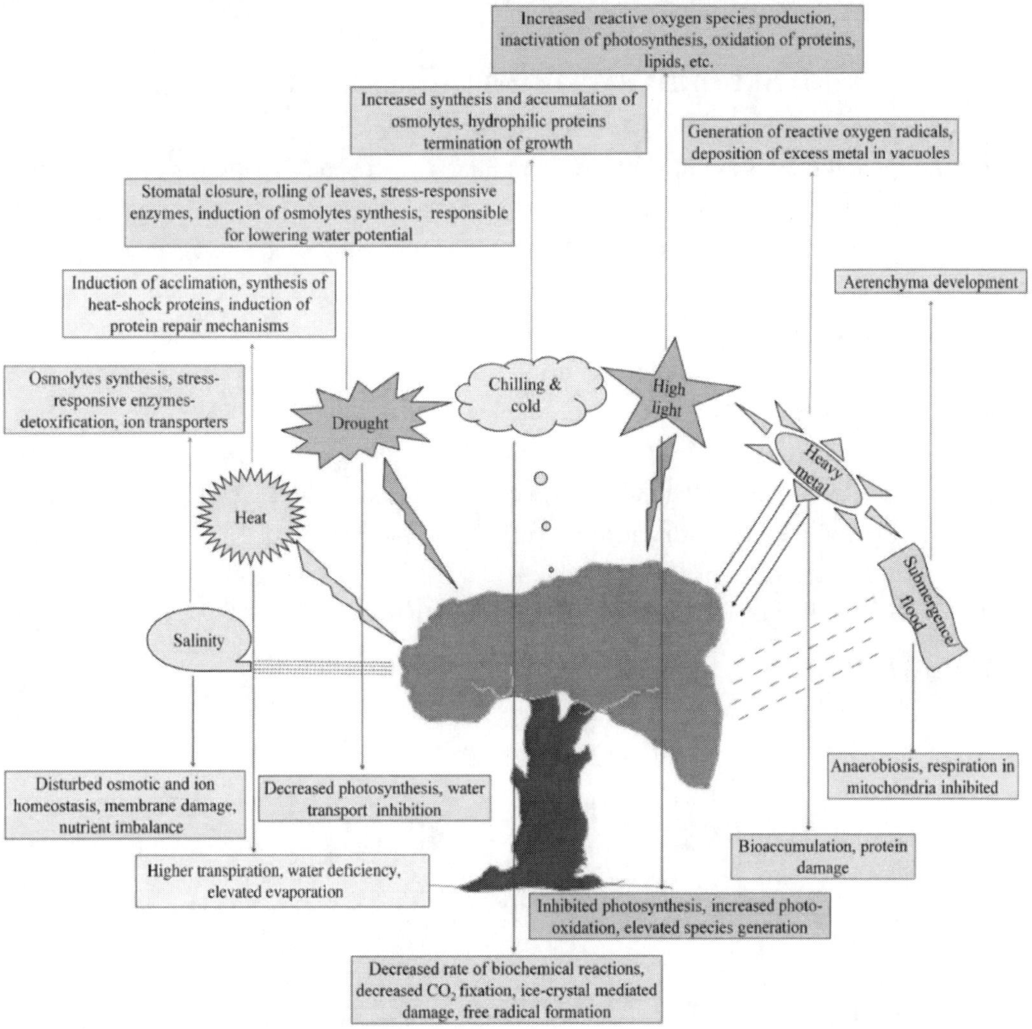

Figure 3. Diverse abiotic stresses and the strategic defense mechanisms adopted by the plants. Extreme conditions (below or above the optimal levels) limit plant growth and development. An unfavorable environment comprising extreme high or low of temperature, salinity and drought pose a complex set of stress conditions. Plants can sense and react to stresses in many ways that favor their sustenance. They remember past exposure to abiotic stresses and even mechanisms to overcome them in such a way that responses to repeated stresses can be modified accordingly. Though the consequences of heat, drought, salinity and chilling are different, the biochemical responses seem more or less similar. High light intensity and heavy metal toxicity also generate similar impact but submergence/flood situation leads to degenerative responses in plants where aerenchyma are developed to cope with anaerobiosis.
It is therefore, clear that adaptive strategies of plants against variety of abiotic stresses are analogous in nature. It may provide an important key for mounting strategic tolerance to combined abiotic stresses in crop plants (Meena KK, Sorty AM et al. Abiotic Stress Responses and Microbe-Mediated Mitigation in Plants: The Omics Strategies. *Front. Plant Sci*., 09 February 2017 | https://doi.org/10.3389/fpls.2017.00172).

6. ENVIRONMENTAL STRESS AND SECONDARY METABOLITES IN PLANTS

Environmental factors significantly affect plant growth and biosynthesis of SMs. Plant growth and productivity is negatively affected by temperature extremes, salinity, and drought stress. Plant SMs are compounds that play an essential part in the interaction of plants with abiotic stresses [25]. In addition, plant growth and development are also largely mediated by the endogenous levels of these SMs. A wide range of SMs are produced from primary metabolites such as amino acids, lipids, and carbohydrates in higher plants. Particular colors, tastes, and odors of plants are associated with SMs. Plant SMs also serve as essential sources of industrially important chemicals, flavors, food additives, and pharmaceuticals [26]. Plants accumulate such compounds in response to different signaling molecules. SM production is influenced by various environmental stresses. Environmental factors determine the synthesis and subsequent accumulation of SM. Alteration in any one factor triggers perturbations in the biosynthesis of plant SMs [27].

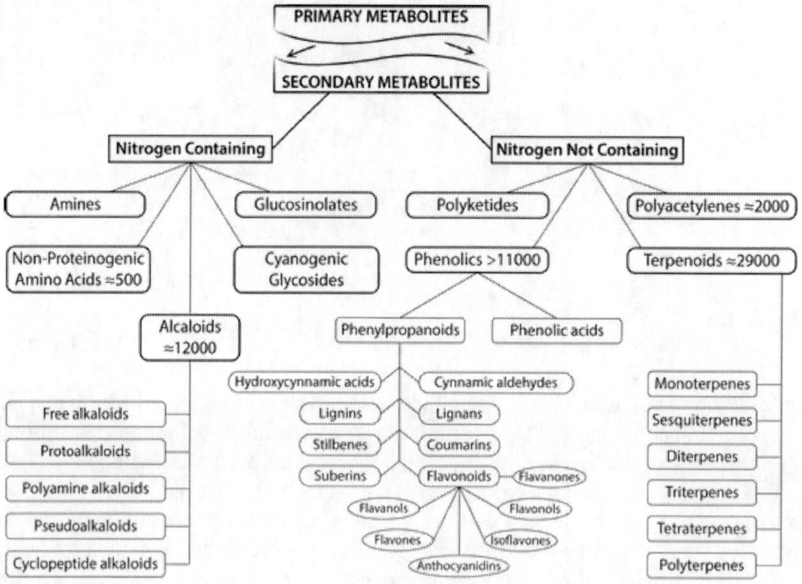

Figure 4. Secondary Metabolites and Plant Growth Regulators. As the plants require oxygen, water, sunlight, and nutrition to grow and develop, they do require certain chemical substances to manage their growth and development. These chemicals substances are called Plant Growth Regulators and are produced naturally by the plants itself. The plant growth regulators are simple organic molecules having several chemical compositions. They are also described as phytohormones, plant growth substances, or plant hormones. Based on their action, plant growth regulators are broadly classified into two major groups: Plant growth promoters and Plant growth inhibitors. (Source: Katerova Z., Todorova D., Sergiev I. (2017) Plant Secondary Metabolites and Some Plant Growth Regulators Elicited by UV Irradiation, Light And/Or Shade. In: Ghorbanpour M., Varma A. (eds) *Medicinal Plants and Environmental Challenges*. Springer, Cham DOI https://doi.org/10.1007/978-3-319-68717-9_6.)

7. Differential Responses of Plants to Biotic Stress

Plants contribute a lot to this universe but they have to face many stresses of biotic or abiotic nature. Biotic stress is a severe environmental constraint to the plant's productivity. Biotic stress induces loss in crop yield probably more than the cumulative losses from all other factors. In any stress, the type and duration are critical for plant growth [28]. Plants use various defensive strategies to tolerate these adverse factors. Of the various defensive mechanisms, one is the production of reactive oxygen species. These defensive mechanisms against biotic stress are generated as a result of the continuous interaction between plant and pathogen [29]. Plants' responses to biotic stress are not only the alteration in anatomical features, such as formation of a waxy cuticle, trichrome, setae, and spines, but also the production of various secondary metabolites. Such types of plant responses have been observed against bacteria, fungi, and pests. These secondary metabolites trigger different plant defense mechanisms in the form of ascorbic acid, antioxidative enzymes (peroxidase, polyphenol oxidase, lipoxygenases), salicylic acid, jasmonic acid, and Ca2+ against biotic stress and also act as toxins (terpenes, alkaloids, and phenolic compounds) against plant pathogens [30].

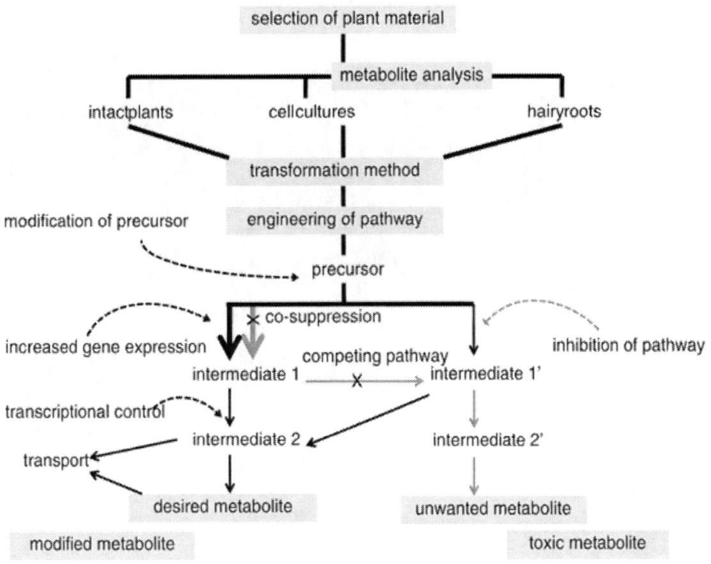

Figure 5. Metabolic Engineering of Selected Secondary Metabolites. The demand for the production of valuable secondary metabolites is increasing rapidly. While many metabolites can be directly extracted from intact plants, others are routinely produced using cell or organ cultures. The latter, also called Hairy roots when generated through the transformation with the bacterium Agrobacterium rhizogenes, are also amenable to molecular modifications. Similar to intact plants metabolic pathways can be altered by introducing homologous or foreign genes. The better the knowledge of a given pathway, the more efficient will be the genetic alteration. (Source: Ludwig-Müller J. (2014) Metabolic Engineering of Selected Secondary Metabolites. In: Paek KY., Murthy H., Zhong JJ. (eds) *Production of Biomass and Bioactive Compounds Using Bioreactor Technology*. Springer, Dordrechthttps://doi.org/10.1007/978-94-017-9223-3_21.)

8. Engineering of Biomass Accumulation and Secondary Metabolite Production

Plants are the source of valuable secondary metabolites that are commonly used in pharmaceutical, food, agricultural, cosmetic, and textile industries [31]. Plant cell and tissue culture technologies can be established routinely under sterile conditions from explants, such as plant leaves, stems, roots, and meristems for both the ways for multiplication and extraction of secondary metabolites. In vitro production of secondary metabolite in plant cell suspension cultures has been reported from various medicinal plants, and bioreactors are the key step for their commercial production. Based on this lime light, the present review is aimed to cover phytotherapeutic application and recent advancement for the production of some important plant pharmaceuticals [32]. The increasing commercial importance of secondary metabolites has resulted in a great interest in research focusing on secondary metabolism and finding alternative ways for secondary metabolite production. Plant cell and tissue cultures are branches of plant biotechnology and they have been introduced as alternative ways for the production of valuable secondary metabolites. Plant technology provides a continuous and reliable source for pharmaceutical phytochemicals and can easily be scaled up [33]. Therefore, plant cell and tissue cultures have a great potential to be used as an alternative to traditional agriculture for the industrial production of secondary metabolites [34, 35].

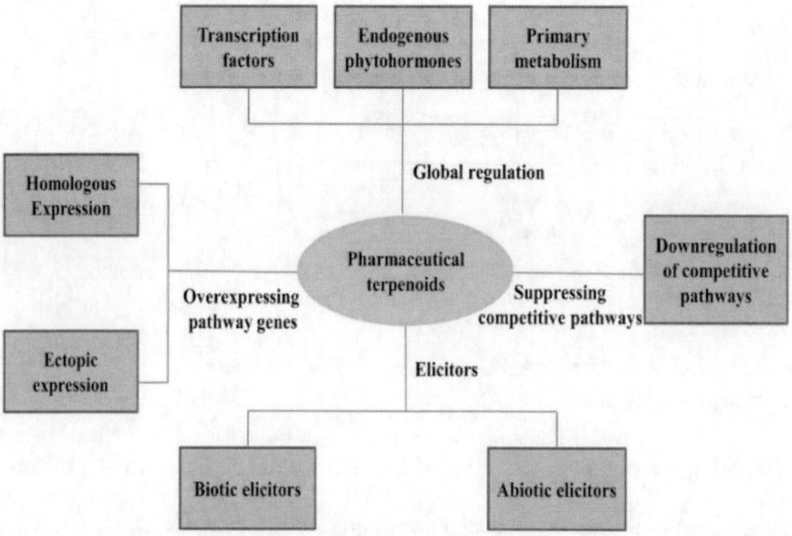

Figure 6. Plant metabolic engineering strategies to regulate pharmaceutical terpenoids. Pharmaceutical terpenoids of medicinal plants are often natural defense metabolites against pathogen attacks. Elicitors, including biotic and abiotic elicitors, can be used to activate the pathway of secondary metabolism and enhance the production of target terpenoids. (Xu Lu, Kexuan Tang, Ping Li1. Plant Metabolic Engineering Strategies for the Production of Pharmaceutical Terpenoids. *Front. Plant Sci.*, 08 November 2016 | https://doi.org/10.3389/fpls.2016.01647.)

9. Response to Secondary Metabolism to Light Irradiation

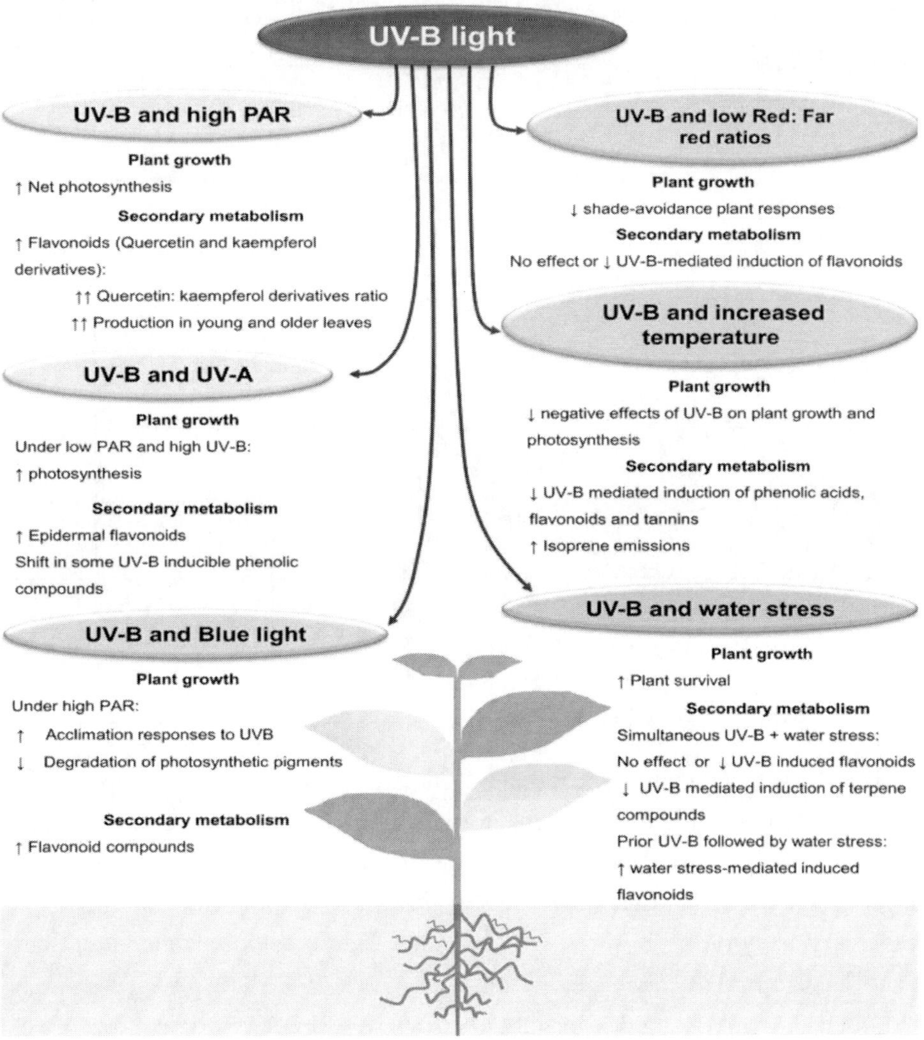

Figure 7. Interactive effects of UV-B light with other abiotic factors on plant growth and production of plant secondary metabolites. Under high Photosynthetic active radiation. UV-B light increases the net plant photosynthesis in several plant species. Higher production of flavonoids can be induced under both UV-B and high PAR in young and old plant leaves. UV-A radiation has a positive effect on the photosynthesis when plants are exposed to UV-B. Higher epidermal flavonoids are detected in plants under both UV-A and B radiations in some plant species. Exposition of plants to blue light prior or subsequent to UV-B also increases the acclimation responses to UV-B by reducing the degradation of photosynthetic pigments. Antagonistic responses between UV-B radiation and low-Red:far-red ratios have been reported. UV-B can inhibit the shade avoidance associated responses under low-Red:far-red ratios. Likewise, a low-Red:far red ratio can reduce the UV-B-mediated induction of plant flavonoids. Increased temperature increases acclimation of plants to UV-B, though it can reduce the UV-B-mediated induction of plant phenolics. Under combined UV-B radiation and increased temperature, however, higher emission of the plant volatile isoprene can be detected in some plant species. Similarly, under UV-B and water stress conditions, a positive effect on plant survival is reported. Production of UV-B-induced flavonoids can be modulated by the application of UV-B prior or subsequent to water stress.

Table 1. Photoperiod change on the content of various plant SMs [37-41]

Metabolite Class	Metabolite Name	Structural Image	Environment Factor	Concentration Change	Plant Species
Phenols	Caffeoyl-quinic acids	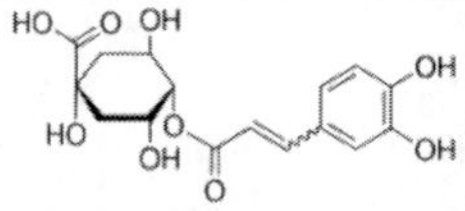	Short day of light	Decrease	*X. pensylva-nicuim*
Phenols	Pelargonidin	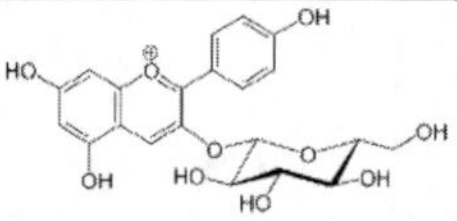	Short day of light	Decrease	*P. contorta*
Phenols	Catechins	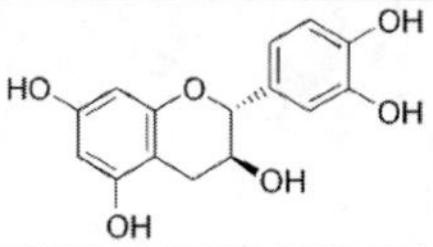	Long day of light	Increase	*I. batatas*
Phenols	Hydroxy-benzoic acids	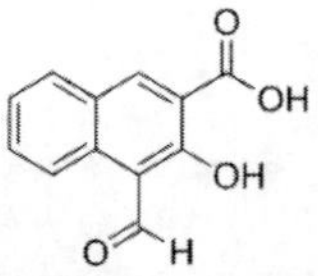	Long day of light	Increase	*I. batatas*
Phenols	Chlorogenic acid	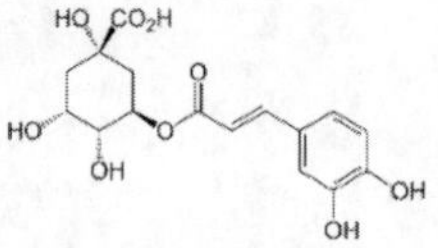	Long day of light	Increase	*V. myrtillus*

The key factors related light radiation include photoperiod (duration), intensity (quantity), direction and quality (frequency or wavelength). In response to light radiation, plants are able to adapt to the changes of circumstances by the release and accumulation of various secondary metabolites including phenolic compounds, triterpenoids and flavonoids, and many of them, have high economic and utilization value due to the well-known antioxidant property [36].

In comparison with a long day of light exposure, a short day of light exposure caused a decrease of, caffeoylquinic acids by about 40% and even an approximately double reduction in the content of flavonoid aglycones.

Camptothecin (CPT) class of compounds has been demonstrated to be effective against a broad spectrum of tumors. Their molecular target has been firmly established to be human DNA topoisomerase I (topo I). The medicinal plant Centella asiatica (L.) Urban contains mainly ursane-type triterpene saponins, the most prominent one is asiaticoside. It is now firmly established that the major bioactivities of C. asiatica leaf extracts are due to these saponins, including memory improvement, wound and vein healing, antihistaminic, antiulcer and antilepsory treatments, as an antidepressant, and as antibacterial, antifungal, and antioxidant agents. As a familiar indole alkaloid, the SM camptothecin can respond to environmental stresses and its accumulation rate can change with light irradiation conditions. It is known that overshadowing can induce biochemical changes in plants, particularly in leaves, and heavy shading of only 27% full sunlight, for example, can elevate the concentration of camptothecin in leaves of Camptotheca acuminata, whereas substantially reduce that in the lateral roots of this tree.

Table 2. Light intensity changes on the content of various plant SMs [42-45]

Metabolite Class	Metabolite Name	Structural Image	Environment Factor	Concentration Change	Plant Species
Alkaloids	Camptothecin	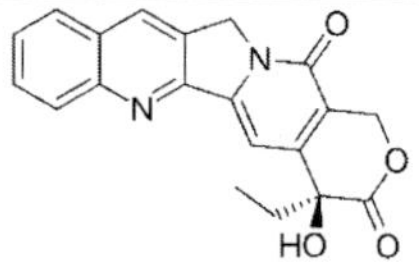	27% Full sunlight	Increase	*C. acuminate*
Phenols	Asiatic acid	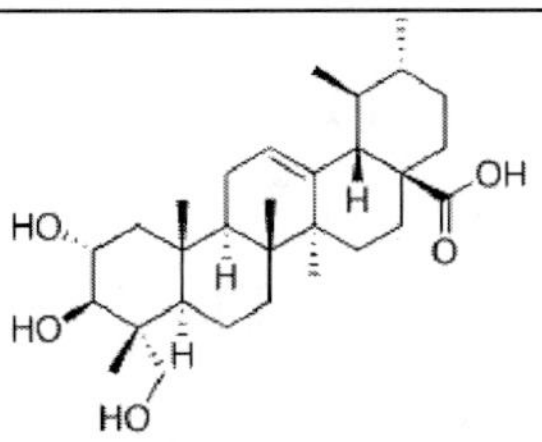	70% Shade	Increase	*C. asiatica*
Phenols	Asiaticoside	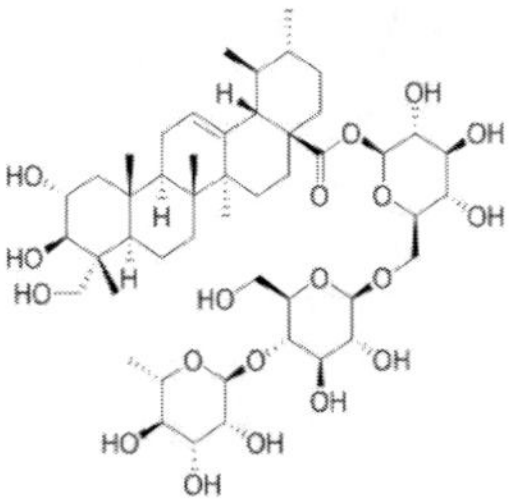	Full sunlight	Increase	*C. asiatica*
Phenols	Chlorogenic acid	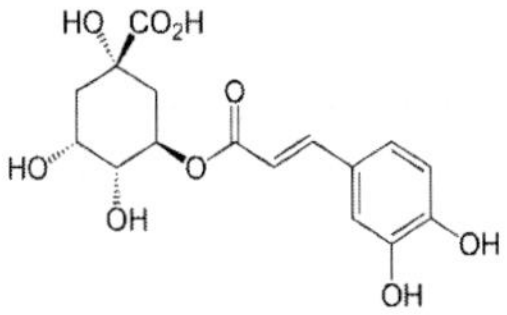	Full sunlight	Increase	*V. myrtillus*

There has been considerable public and scientific interest in the use of phytochemicals derived from dietary components to combat human diseases. They are naturally occurring substances found in plants. Ferulic acid (FA) is a phytochemical commonly found in fruits and vegetables such as tomatoes, sweet corn and rice bran. It arises from metabolism of phenylalanine and tyrosine by Shikimate pathway in plants. It exhibits a wide range of therapeutic effects against various diseases like cancer, diabetes, cardiovascular and neurodegenerative. Kaempferol (3,5,7-trihydroxy-2-(4-hydroxyphenyl)-4H-1-benzopyran -4-one) is a flavonoid found in many edible plants (e.g., tea, broccoli, cabbage, kale, beans,

Table 3. Light quality change on the content of various plant SMs [46-51]

Metabolite Class	Metabolite Name	Structural Image	Environment Factor	Concentration Change	Plant Species
Phenols	Ferulic acid	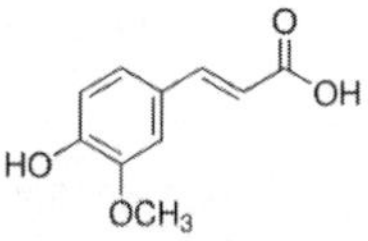	Increase red light	Decrease	*L. sativa*
Phenols	Kaempferol	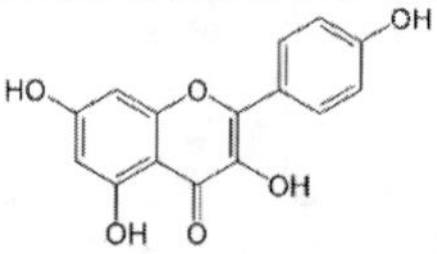	Increase red light	Decrease	*L. sativa*
Alkaloids	Catharanthine	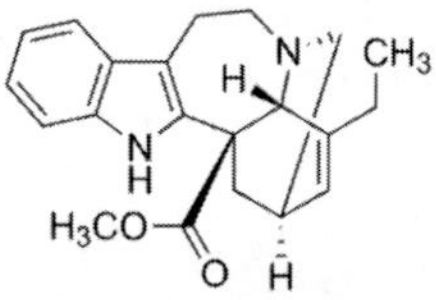	UV-B	Increase	*C. roseus*
Alkaloids	Vindoline	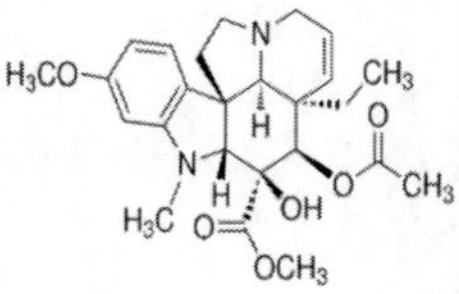	UV-B	Increase	*C. roseus*
Phenols	Rutin	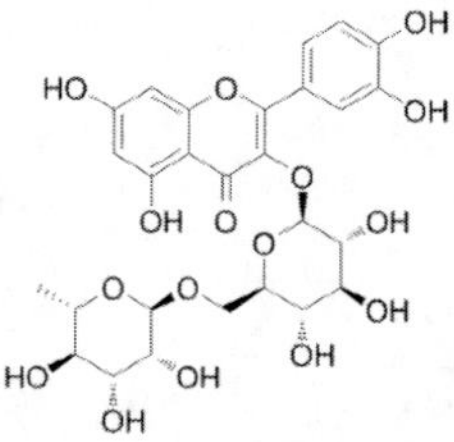	UV	Increase	*F. esculentum*
Phenols	Quercetin	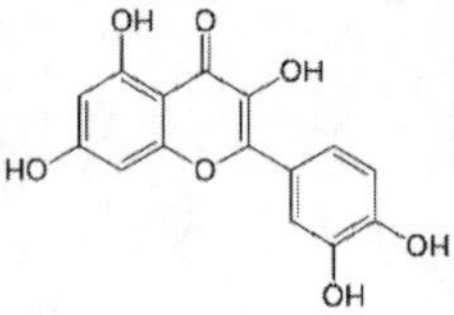	UV	Increase	*F. esculentum*
Phenols	Catechins	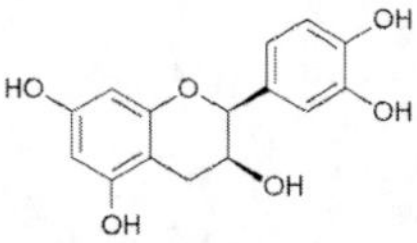	UV	Increase	*F. esculentum*

endive, leek, tomato, strawberries, and grapes) and in plants or botanical products commonly used in traditional medicine (e.g., Ginkgo biloba, Tilia spp, Equisetum spp, Moringa oleifera, Sophora japonica and propolis). Its anti-oxidant/anti-inflammatory effects have been demonstrated in various disease models, including those for encephalomyelitis, diabetes, asthma, and carcinogenesis. Moreover, kaempferol act as a scavenger of free radicals and superoxide radicals as well as preserve the activity of various anti-oxidant enzymes such as catalase, glutathione peroxidase, and glutathione-S-transferase. The anticancer effect of this flavonoid is mediated through different modes of action, including anti-proliferation, apoptosis induction, cell-cycle arrest, generation of reactive oxygen species (ROS), and anti-metastasis/anti-angiogenesis activities. Context Catharanthus roseus (L.) G. Don (Apocynaceae) is still one of the most important sources of terpene indole alkaloids including anticancer and hypertensive drugs as vincristine and vinblastine. These final compounds have complex pathway and many enzymes are involved in their biosynthesis. Indeed, ajmalicine and catharanthine are important precursors their increase can lead to enhance levels of molecules of interest. A direct coupling of cantharanthine with vindoline to provide vinblastine is detailed along with key mechanistic and labeling studies. With the completion of a first-generation total synthesis of vindoline that was extended to a series of related analogues. The antioxidant effects of the flavonoids rutin and quercetin inhibit oxaliplatin-induced chronic painful peripheral neuropathy.

10. Response of Plant SMs to Temperature

The modulation of temperature to alkaloids accumulation was reported, and high temperature preferable to induce the biosynthesis of alkaloids. The total accumulation of alkaloids (morphinane, phthalisoquinoline and benzylisoquinoline) in dry Papaver somniferum was restricted at low temperature [65]. In contrast, the total level of phenolic acids and isoflavonoid (genistein, daidzein and genistin) in soybean (Glycine max) roots increased after the treatment at low temperature for 24 h, and among which the highest increase of about 310% was observed in genistin after the treatment at 10°C for 24 h, in comparison to the control [52, 53].

In women, aging and declining estrogen levels are associated with several cutaneous changes, many of which can be reversed or improved by estrogen supplementation. Experimental and clinical studies in postmenopausal conditions indicate that estrogen deprivation is associated with dryness, atrophy, fine wrinkling, and poor wound healing.

Table 4. Temperature change on the content of various plant SMs [50, 54-58]

Metabolite Class	Metabolite Name	Structural Image	Environment Factor	Concentration Change	Plant Species
Alkaloids	Morphine	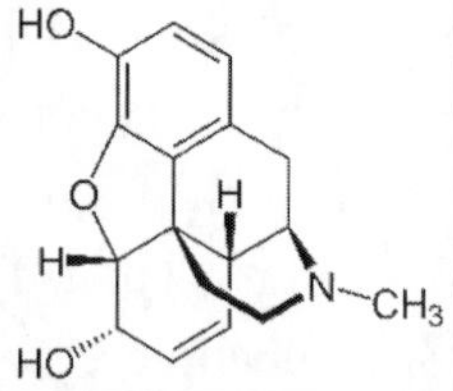	Low temperature	Decrease	*P. somniferum*
Phenols	Genistein	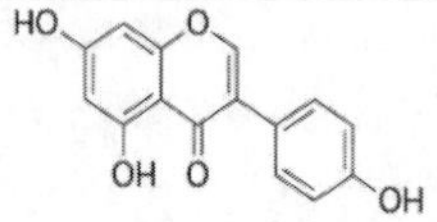	10°C for 24 h	Increase	*G. max*
Phenols	Daidzein	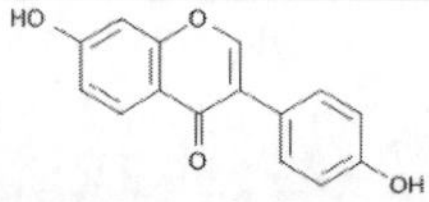	10°C for 24 h	Increase	*G. max*
Alkaloids	10-hydroxycamp-tothecin	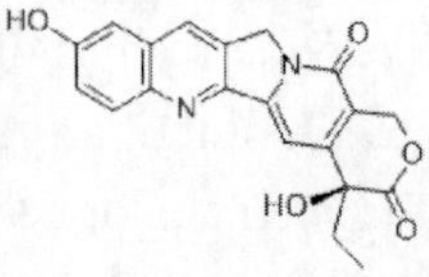	40°C for 2 h	Increase	*C. acuminata*
Alkaloids	Vindoline	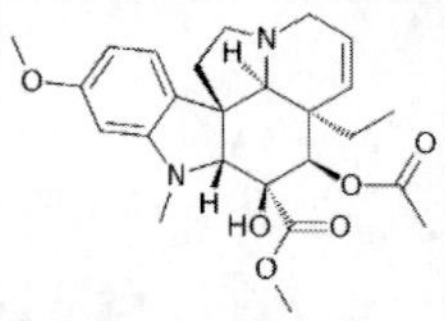	Short-term heat	Increase	*C. roseus*
Alkaloids	Catharanthine	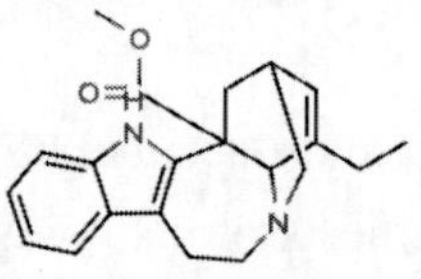	Long-term heat	Increase	*C. roseus*
Terpenes	Isoprene	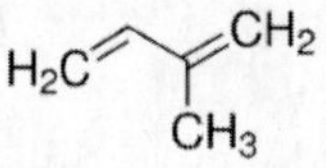	High temperature	Increase	*Q. rubra*
Terpenes	α-farnesene	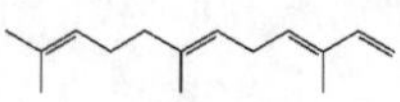	High temperature	Increase	*D. carota*
Phenols	Pelargonidin	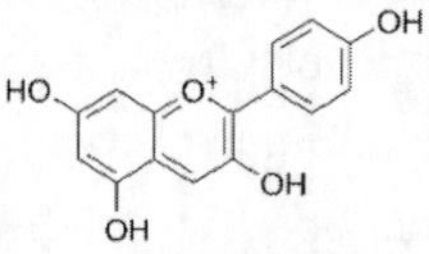	Low temperature	Increase	*Z. mays*

The isoflavone genistein binds to estrogen receptor β and has been reported to improve skin changes. In vitro data has shown that the soy isoflavones genistein and daidzein may even stimulate the proliferation of estrogen-receptor alpha positive (ERα+) breast cancer cells at low concentrations. 10-Hydroxycamptothecin (10-HCPT), an indole alkaloid isolated from a Chinese tree, Camptotheca acuminate, inhibits the activity of topoisomerase I and has a broad spectrum of anticancer activity in vitro and in vivo. However, its use has been limited due to its water-insolubility and toxicity with i.v. administration. Isoprene is synthesized through the 2-C-methylerythritol-5-phosphate (MEP) pathway that also produces abscisic acid (ABA). Increases in foliar free ABA concentration during drought induce stomatal closure and may also alter ethylene biosynthesis. This first report on α-farnesene synthesis in Y. lipolytica lays a foundation for future research on production of sesquitepenes in Y. lipolytica and other closest yeast species and will potentially contribute in its industrial production. Pelargonidin chloride is an anthocyanidin chloride that has pelargonidin as the cationic counterpart. It has a role as a phytoestrogen and a plant metabolite. It contains a pelargonidin.

11. Response of Plant SMs to Soil and Water

Water stress is one of the most important environmental stresses that can regulate the morphological growth and development of plants, and alter their biochemical properties. Severe water deficit has been considered to reduce the plants growth, but several studies have demonstrated that water stress may be possible to increase the amount of SMs in a wide variety of plant species [59, 60].

Salidroside is isolated from *Rhodiola rosea* and is one of the main active components in Rhodiola species. *Rhodiola rosea* has long been used as a medicinal plant and has been reported to have various pharmacological properties, including antifatigue and anti-stress activity, anticancer, antioxidant and immune enhancing and stimulating sexual activity, anti-inflammation, improvement of glucose and lipid metabolism, antiarrhythmic effect, and enhancement of angiogenesis. Tanshinone IIA (Tan-IIA) is derived from the dried roots of *Salvia miltiorrhiza* Bunge, a traditional Chinese medicine. Although *Salvia miltiorrhiza* has been applied for many years, the toxicity of the mono-constituent of *Salvia miltiorrhiza*, tanshinone IIA, is still understudied. Molecular evidence found with cryptotanshinone for treatment and prevention of human cancer. Synthesis of the compatible solute glycine betaine confers a considerable degree of osmotic stress tolerance to Bacillus subtilis. Recent study reveals that abietic acid can be developed as a wound-healing agent.

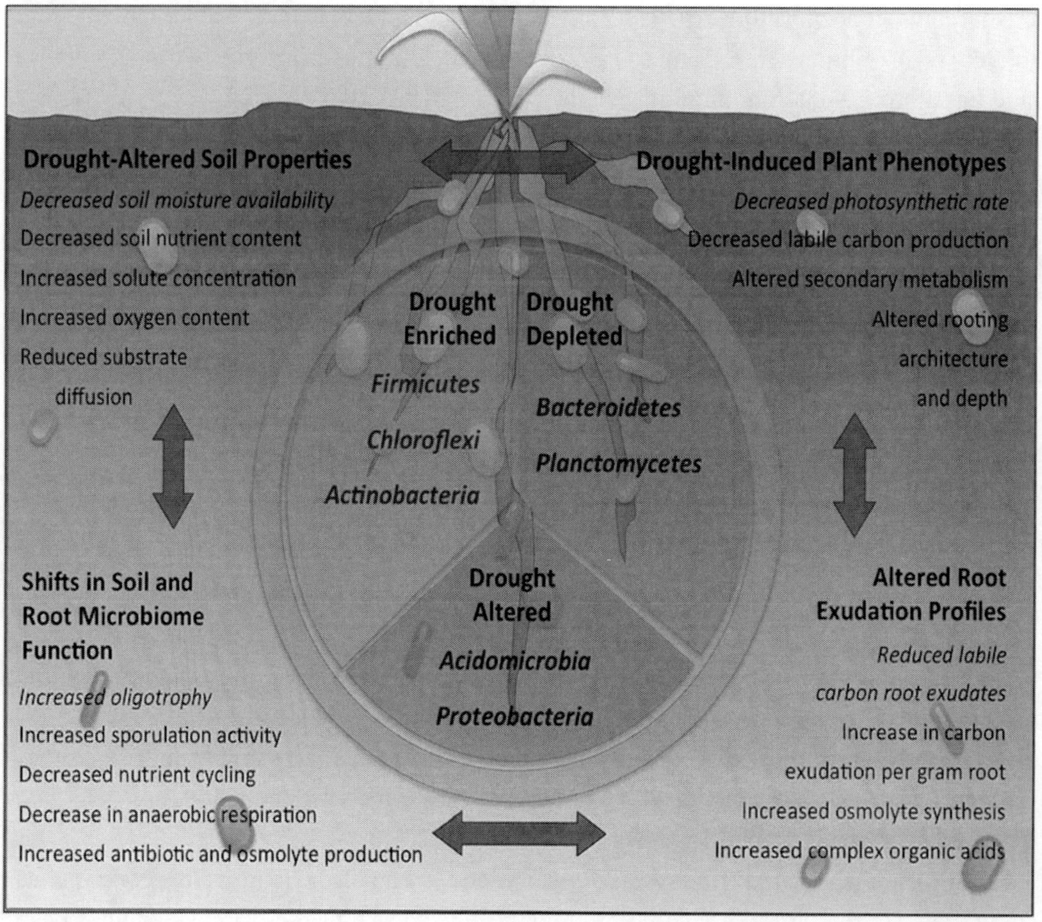

Figure 8. The effects of drought on soils, plants and their associated bacterial communities. Drought induces shifts in soil physicochemistry (upper left), plant phenotype (upper right), root exudation (lower right) and soil and rhizosphere microbiome function (lower left). These shifts are capable of influencing one other; for instance decreases in soil moisture availability (upper left) leads to a decrease in the rate of plant photosynthesis (upper right), which in turn leads to a reduction in the rate of labile carbon exudation to the rhizosphere (lower right) and a greater prevalence in bacteria with oligotrophic life-strategies (lower left), who are less reliant on such simple carbon sources. These shifts lead to a selection for specific phyla (center panel) within the soil, rhizosphere and root microbiome, including enrichment for many Gram-positive, oligotrophic (middle left) phyla, and concurrent depletion of many Gram-negative, copiotrophic (middle right) phyla. Members of other phyla exhibit a more balanced mixture of enrichment and depletion (middle bottom). (Source: Naylor D, Coleman-Derr D. Drought Stress and Root-Associated Bacterial Communities. Front. Plant Sci., 09 January 2018 | https://doi.org/10.3389/fpls.2017.02223.)

Table 5. Soil water change on the content of various plant SMs [61-64]

Metabolite Class	Metabolite Name	Structural Image	Environment Factor	Concentration Change	Plant Species
Phenols	Salidroside	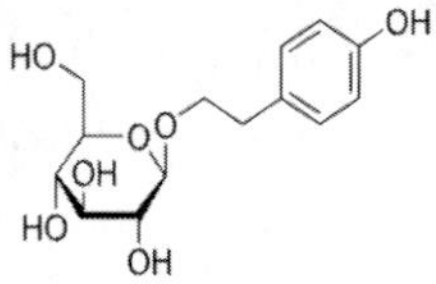	Soil moisture of 55–75%	Increase	*R. sachalinensis*
Phenols	Tanshinone	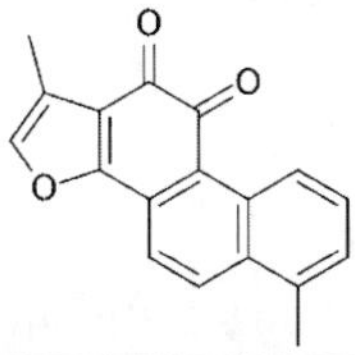	Severe drought	Increase	*S. miltiorrhiza*
Phenols	Cryptota-nshinone	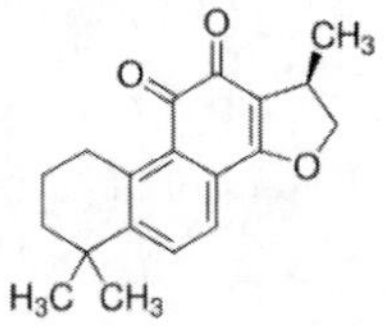	Severe drought	Increase	*S. miltiorrhiza*
Alkaloids	Codeine	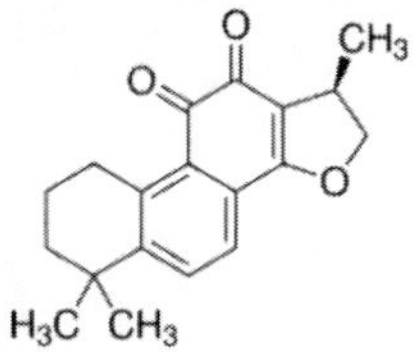	Drought	Increase	*P. somniferum*
Alkaloids	Glycine betaine	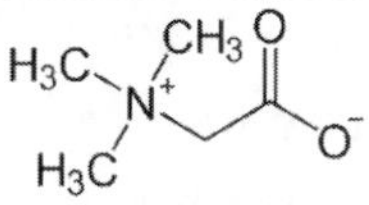	Drought	Increase	*C. roseus*
Phenols	Abietic acid	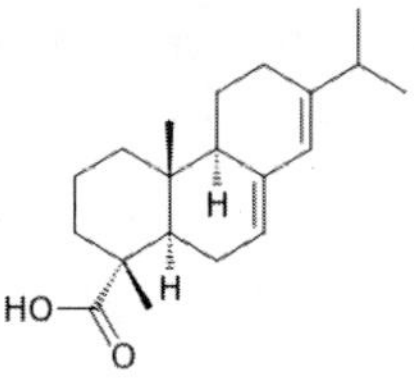	Severe drought	Increase	*P. sylvestris*

CONCLUSION

SMs are the useful natural products that are synthesized through secondary metabolism in the plants. The production of some secondary metabolites is linked to the induction of morphological differentiation and it appears that as the cells undergo morphological differentiation and maturation during plant growth. It is observed that in-Vitro production of secondary metabolites is much higher from differentiated tissues when compared to non-differentiated or less–differentiated tissues. There are lots of advantages of these metabolites like there is recovery of the products will be easy and plant cultures are particularly useful in case of plants which are difficult or expensive and selection of cell lines for high yield of secondary metabolites will be easy. Many other examples could be presented with plant metabolic engineering as this research area is developing actively. Metabolic engineering is probably a large step forward but playing on the genes will not solve all the problems that have prevented the development of commercial success in the field of plant secondary metabolites. And Advances in plant cell cultures could provide new means for the cost-effective, commercial production of even rare or exotic plants, their cells, and the chemicals that they will produce. Knowledge of the biosynthetic pathways of desired compounds in plants as well as of cultures is often still rudimentary, and strategies are consequently needed to develop information based on a cellular and molecular level. Because of the complex and incompletely understood nature of plant cells in-vitro cultures, case-by-case studies have been used to explain the problems occurring in the production of secondary metabolites from cultured plant cells. Advance research has succeeded in producing a wide range of valuable secondary phytochemical in unorganized callus or suspension cultures till to date; in other cases, production requires more differentiated micro plant or organ cultures.

SUMMARY

Medicinal plants constitute main resource base of almost all the traditional healthcare systems. Most of the herbal drugs produced currently in majority of the developing countries lack proper quality specification and standards. Herbal drugs used in traditional medicine may contain a single herb or combinations of several different herbs believed to have complementary and/or synergistic effects. Both the raw drugs and the finished herbal products manufactured contain complex mixtures of organic compounds, such as fatty acids, sterols, alkaloids, flavonoids, polyphenols, glycosides, saponins, tannins, terpenes etc. The quality of the finished product is based on the quality of the raw materials, which is again depends on mineral composition of soil, geographical area etc. As many as 35% of the medicinal plants used in Indian systems of medicine are highly cross pollinated which indicate the existence of a wide range of genetic variability in the populations of these medicinal plant species which in turn reflected in the variations in the composition of secondary metabolites. Ecological and edaphic as well as seasonal variations also cause changes in the chemical composition of medicinal plants. These facts have to be considered while developing quality parameters standards of medicinal plants and their finished products.

REFERENCES

[1] *Lehninger Principles of Biochemistry.* 6th Edition David L. Nelson & Michael M. Cox Publisher: W.H. Freeman, 2013.

[2] *Fundamentals of Biochemistry: Life at the Molecular Level,* Donald Voet, Judith G. Voet, Charlotte W. Pratt Publisher: Hoboken, NJ: John Wiley & Sons, 2016.

[3] *Trease and Evans Pharmacognosy.* William Charles Evans, Daphne Evans, George Edward Trease Publisher: St. Louis: Elsevier Health Sciences UK, 2014.

[4] *Pharmacognosy and Pharmacobiotechnology.* Author: James E Robbers; Marilyn K Speedie; Varro E Tyler. Publisher: Baltimore: Williams & Wilkins, ©1996.

[5] *Fundamentals of Pharmacognosy and Phytotherapy.* Author: Michael Heinrich; Joanne Barnes; Simon Gibbons; Elizabeth M Williamson Publisher: Churchill Livingstone, 2012.

[6] *Medicinal Plants: Ethno-Uses to Biotechnology Era.* Author: Aly Farag El Sheikha Affiliation: Department of Biology, McMaster University, 1280 Main St. West, Hamilton, ON, L8S 4K1, Canada.

[7] *Medicinal Plants: Chemistry and Properties.* M Daniel Publisher: CRC Press, Apr 19, 2016.

[8] Giweli AA, Džamić AM, Soković,M, Ristić M, Janaćković P, and Marin P. 2013. "The Chemical Composition, Antimicrobial and Antioxidant Activities of the Essential Oil of Salvia fruticosa Growing Wild in Libya." *Archives of Biological Sciences* 1 (65): 321-9.

[9] Bruno Leite Sampaio, RuAngelie Edrada-Ebel and Fernando Batista Da Costa. Effect of the environment on the secondary metabolic profile of Tithonia diversifolia: A model for environmental metabolomics of plants. *Sci Rep.* 2016; 6: 29265. doi: [10.1038/srep29265] PMCID: PMC4935878 PMID: 27383265.

[10] Claire Brittain, Claire Kremen, Andrea Garber, Alexandra-Maria Klein. Pollination and Plant Resources Change the Nutritional Quality of Almonds for Human Health. *PLoS One.* 2014; 9(2): e90082. doi: [10.1371/journal.pone.0090082] PMCID: PMC3937406 PMID: 24587215.

[11] Koppert Biological System. *Why do pollinators visit flowers?* URL: https://www.koppert.com/pollination/natural-pollination-bumble-bees/why-do-pollinators-visit-flowers/

[12] Ferris Jabr. Farming a Toxin to Keep Crops Healthy. *Scientific American.* The Sciences. September 3, 2013 Available From: https://www.scientificamerican.com/article/farming-a-toxin/

[13] *Forest Health Handbook.* North Carolina Forest Service 3rd Edition Publisher: Ryan A. Blaedow September 2011.

[14] *Crop Scouting Manual 2010 Field Crop Integrated Pest Management Program* - University of Wisconsin-Extension - Cooperative Extension Service.

[15] Douglas J. Futuymaa, and Anurag A. Agrawalb. Macroevolution and the biological diversity of plants and herbivores. *Proc Natl Acad Sci U S A.* 2009 Oct 27; 106(43): 18054–18061. doi: [10.1073/pnas.0904106106] PMCID: PMC2775342 PMID: 19815508.

[16] Marcia O. Mello and Marcio C. Silva-Filho Plant-insect interactions: an evolutionary arms race between two distinct defense mechanisms Braz. *J. Plant Physiol.* vol.14 no.2 Londrina May/Aug. 2002 http://dx.doi.org/10.1590/S1677-04202002000200001.

[17] *Plant Evolutionary Biology* Copyright Publisher Name Springer, Dordrecht Information Springer Science+ Business Media B.V. 1988 DOI https://doi.org/10.1007/978-94-009-1207-6.

[18] Neeraj Jain, Rajani S. Nadgauda Commiphora wightii (Arnott) Bhandari—A Natural Source of Guggulsterone: Facing a High Risk of Extinction in Its Natural Habitat. *American Journal of Plant Sciences,* Vol. 4 No. 6A, 2013, pp. 57-68. doi: 10.4236/ajps.2013.46A009.

[19] Nakuleshwar Dut Jasuja, Jyoti Choudhary, Preeti Sharama, Nidhi Sharma and Suresh C. Joshi A Review on Bioactive Compounds and Medicinal Uses of Commiphora mukul A Review on Bioactive Compounds and Medicinal Uses of Commiphora mukul. *Journal of Plant Sciences,* 7: 113-137. DOI: 10.3923/jps.2012.113.137.

[20] *Medicinal Plants Utilisation and Conservation.* 2nd Revised and Enlarged Edition Editor Prof. Pravin Chandra Trivedi, Publisher: Aavishkar Publishers, Distributors Jaipur 302 003 (Raj) India.

[21] Schäfer H, Wink M. Medicinally important secondary metabolites in recombinant microorganisms or plants: progress in alkaloid biosynthesis. *Biotechnol J.* 2009 Dec;4(12):1684-703. PMID:19946877 DOI: 10.1002/biot.200900229.

[22] Michael Wink Chapter 11 Importance of plant secondary metabolites for protection against insects and microbial infections. *Advances in Phytomedicine* Volume 3, 2006, Pages 251-268 https://doi.org/10.1016/S1572-557X(06)03011-X.

[23] Wink Michael. Plant breeding: importance of plant secondary metabolites for protection against pathogens and herbivores *Theoretical and Applied Genetics* January 1988, Volume 75, Issue 2, pp 225–233.

[24] Fumihiko Sato. *Plant Secondary Metabolism* DOI: 10.1002/9780470015902.a0001812.pub2.

[25] Zhang B. MicroRNA: a new target for improving plant tolerance to abiotic stress. *J Exp Bot.* 2015;66(7):1749-61.

[26] Singh R, Kumar M, Mittal A, Mehta PK. Microbial metabolites in nutrition, healthcare and agriculture. *3 Biotech.* 2017;7(1):15.

[27] Ashraf MA, Iqbal M and others: Chapter 8 - Environmental Stress and Secondary Metabolites in Plants: An Overview. *Plant Metabolites and Regulation Under*

Environmental Stress 2018, Pages 153-167. https://doi.org/10.1016/B978-0-12-812689-9.00008-X.

[28] Sulmon C, van Baaren J, Cabello-Hurtado F, Gouesbet G, Hennion F, Mony C, Renault D, Bormans M, El Amrani A, Wiegand C, Gérard C. Abiotic stressors and stress responses: What commonalities appear between species across biological organization levels? *Environ Pollut.* 2015 Jul;202:66-77. doi: 10.1016/j.envpol. 2015.03.013. Epub 2015 Mar 24. Review. PubMed PMID: 25813422.

[29] Rejeb IB, Pastor V, Mauch-Mani B. Plant Responses to Simultaneous Biotic and Abiotic Stress: Molecular Mechanisms. *Plants (Basel).* 2014;3(4):458-75. Published 2014 Oct 15. doi:10.3390/plants3040458.

[30] Saddique M, Kamran M, Shahbaz M. (2018) Differential Responses of Plants to Biotic Stress and the Role of Metabolites. *Plant Metabolites and Regulation under Environmental Stress,* pp. 69-87.

[31] Cragg GM, Newman DJ. Natural products: a continuing source of novel drug leads. *Biochim Biophys Acta.* 2013;1830(6):3670-95.

[32] Hussain MS, Fareed S, Ansari S, Rahman MA, Ahmad IZ, Saeed M. Current approaches toward production of secondary plant metabolites. *J Pharm Bioallied Sci.* 2012;4(1):10-20.

[33] Breitling R, Ceniceros A, Jankevics A, Takano E. Metabolomics for secondary metabolite research. *Metabolites.* 2013;3(4):1076-83. Published 2013 Nov 11. doi:10.3390/metabo3041076.

[34] Eibl R, Meier P, Stutz I, Schildberger D, Hühn T, Eibl D. Plant cell culture technology in the cosmetics and food industries: current state and future trends. *Appl Microbiol Biotechnol.* 2018;102(20):8661-8675.

[35] Wilson SA, Roberts SC. Recent advances towards development and commercialization of plant cell culture processes for the synthesis of biomolecules. *Plant Biotechnol J.* 2011;10(3):249-68.

[36] Yang L, Wen KS, Ruan X, Zhao YX, Wei F, Wang Q. Response of Plant Secondary Metabolites to Environmental Factors. *Molecules.* 2018;23(4):762. Published 2018 Mar 27. doi:10.3390/molecules23040762.

[37] dos Santos MD, Chen G, Almeida MC, et al. Effects of caffeoylquinic acid derivatives and C-flavonoid from Lychnophora ericoides on in vitro inflammatory mediator production. *Nat Prod Commun.* 2010;5(5):733-40.

[38] Skrovankova S, Sumczynski D, Mlcek J, Jurikova T, Sochor J. Bioactive Compounds and Antioxidant Activity in Different Types of Berries. *Int J Mol Sci.* 2015;16(10):24673-706. Published 2015 Oct 16. doi:10.3390/ijms161024673.

[39] Del Rio D, Stalmach A, Calani L, Crozier A. Bioavailability of coffee chlorogenic acids and green tea flavan-3-ols. *Nutrients.* 2010;2(8):820-33.

[40] Monteiro M, Farah A, Perrone D, Trugo LC, Donangelo C. Chlorogenic acid compounds from coffee are differentially absorbed and metabolized in humans. *J Nutr.* 2007 Oct;137(10):2196-201. PubMed PMID: 17884997.

[41] National Center for Biotechnology Information. *PubChem Compound Database;* CID=135, https://pubchem.ncbi.nlm.nih.gov/compound/135 (accessed Jan. 16, 2019).

[42] Hashimoto T, Yamada Y. Alkaloid biogenesis: Molecular aspects. *Annu. Rev. Plant Biol.* 1994;45:257–285. doi: 10.1146/annurev.pp.45.060194.001353.

[43] Vincent RM, Lopez-Meyer M, McKnight TD, Nessler CL. Sustained harvest of camptothecin from the leaves of Camptotheca acuminata. *J. Nat. Prod.* 1997;60:618–619. doi: 10.1021/np9700228.

[44] Gottschalk KW. Shade, leaf growth and crown development of quercus rubra, quercus velutina, prunus serotina and acer rubrum seedlings. *Tree Physiol.* 1994;14:735–749. doi: 10.1093/treephys/14.7-8-9.735.

[45] Liu Z, Carpenter SB, Constantin RJ. Camptothecin production in Camptotheca acuminata seedlings in response to shading and flooding. *Can. J. Bot.* 1997;75:368–373. doi: 10.1139/b97-039.

[46] Kim OT, Jin ML, Lee DY, Jetter R. Characterization of the Asiatic Acid Glucosyltransferase, UGT73AH1, Involved in Asiaticoside Biosynthesis in Centella asiatica (L.) *Urban. Int J Mol Sci.* 2017;18(12):2630. Published 2017 Dec 6. doi:10.3390/ijms18122630.

[47] Liu LF, Desai SD, Li TK, Mao Y, Sun M, Sim SP. Mechanism of action of camptothecin. *Ann N Y Acad Sci.* 2000;922:1-10. Review. PubMed PMID: 11193884.

[48] Srinivasan M, Sudheer AR, Menon VP. Ferulic Acid: therapeutic potential through its antioxidant property. *J Clin Biochem Nutr.* 2007 Mar;40(2):92-100. doi: 10.3164/jcbn.40.92. PubMed PMID: 18188410; PubMed Central PMCID: PMC2127228.

[49] Benyammi R, Paris C, Khelifi-Slaoui M, Zaoui D, Belabbassi O, Bakiri N, Meriem Aci M, Harfi B, Malik S, Makhzoum A, Desobry S, Khelifi L. Screening and kinetic studies of catharanthine and ajmalicine accumulation and their correlation with growth biomass in Catharanthus roseus hairy roots. *Pharm Biol.* 2016 Oct;54(10):2033-43. doi: 10.3109/13880209.2016.1140213. Epub 2016 Mar 17. PubMed PMID: 26983347.

[50] Ishikawa H, Colby DA, Boger DL. Direct coupling of catharanthine and vindoline to provide vinblastine: total synthesis of (+)- and ent-(-)-vinblastine. *J Am Chem Soc.* 2008;130(2):420-1.

[51] Azevedo MI, Pereira AF, Nogueira RB, et al. The antioxidant effects of the flavonoids rutin and quercetin inhibit oxaliplatin-induced chronic painful peripheral

neuropathy. *Mol Pain.* 2013;9:53. Published 2013 Oct 23. doi:10.1186/1744-8069-9-53.

[52] Bernáth J, Tétényi P. The Effect of environmental factors on growth. Development and alkaloid production of Poppy (Papaver somniferum L.): I. Responses to day-length and light intensity. *Biochem. Physiol. Pflanzen.* 1979;174:468–478. doi: 10.1016/S0015-3796(17)31342-2.

[53] Janas KM, Cvikrová M, Pałagiewicz A, Szafranska K, Posmyk MM. Constitutive elevated accumulation of phenylpropanoids in soybean roots at low temperature. *Plant Sci.* 2002;163:369–373. doi: 10.1016/S0168-9452(02)00136-X.

[54] Irrera N, Pizzino G, D'Anna R, et al. Dietary Management of Skin Health: The Role of Genistein. *Nutrients.* 2017;9(6):622. Published 2017 Jun 17. doi:10.3390/nu9060622.

[55] Poschner S, Maier-Salamon A, Zehl M, et al. The Impacts of Genistein and Daidzein on Estrogen Conjugations in Human Breast Cancer Cells: A Targeted Metabolomics Approach. *Front Pharmacol.* 2017;8:699. Published 2017 Oct 5. doi:10.3389/fphar.2017.00699.

[56] Ping YH, Lee HC, Lee JY, Wu PH, Ho LK, Chi CW, Lu MF, Wang JJ. Anticancer effects of low-dose 10-hydroxycamptothecin in human colon cancer. *Oncol Rep.* 2006 May;15(5):1273-9. PubMed PMID: 16596197.

[57] Yang X, Nambou K, Wei L, Hua Q. Heterologous production of α-farnesene in metabolically engineered strains of Yarrowia lipolytica. *Bioresour Technol.* 2016 Sep;216:1040-8. doi: 10.1016/j.biortech.2016.06.028. Epub 2016 Jun 11. PubMed PMID: 27347651.

[58] National Center for Biotechnology Information. *PubChem Compound Database;* CID=67249, https://pubchem.ncbi.nlm.nih.gov/compound/67249 (accessed Jan. 16, 2019).

[59] Zobayed SMA, Afreen F, Kozai T. Phytochemical and physiological changes in the leaves of St. John's wort plants under a water stress condition. *Environ. Exp. Bot.* 2007;59:109–116. doi: 10.1016/j.envexpbot.2005.10.002.

[60] Zhu Z, Liang Z, Han R, Wang X. Impact of fertilization on drought response in the medicinal herb Bupleurum chinense DC: Growth and saikosaponin production. *Ind. Crops Prod.* 2009;29:629–633. doi: 10.1016/j.indcrop.2008.08.002.

[61] Zhang BC, Li WM, Guo R, Xu YW. Salidroside decreases atherosclerotic plaque formation in low-density lipoprotein receptor-deficient mice. *Evid Based Complement Alternat Med.* 2012;2012:607508.

[62] Wang T, Wang C, Wu Q, Zheng K, Chen J, Lan Y, Qin Y, Mei W, Wang B. Evaluation of Tanshinone IIA Developmental Toxicity in Zebrafish Embryos. *Molecules.* 2017 Apr 21;22(4). pii: E660. doi: 10.3390/molecules22040660. PubMed PMID: 28430131; PubMed Central PMCID: PMC6154573.

[63] Chen W, Lu Y, Chen G, Huang S. Molecular evidence of cryptotanshinone for treatment and prevention of human cancer. *Anticancer Agents Med Chem.* 2013;13(7):979-87.

[64] Park JY, Lee YK, Lee DS, Yoo JE, Shin MS, Yamabe N, Kim SN, Lee S, Kim KH, Lee HJ, Roh SS, Kang KS. Abietic acid isolated from pine resin (Resina Pini) enhances angiogenesis in HUVECs and accelerates cutaneous wound healing in mice. *J Ethnopharmacol.* 2017 May 5;203:279-287. doi: 10.1016/j.jep.2017.03.055. Epub 2017 Apr 4. PubMed PMID: 28389357.

Chapter 3

INDIAN HERBS OF PHARMACOLOGICAL INTEREST

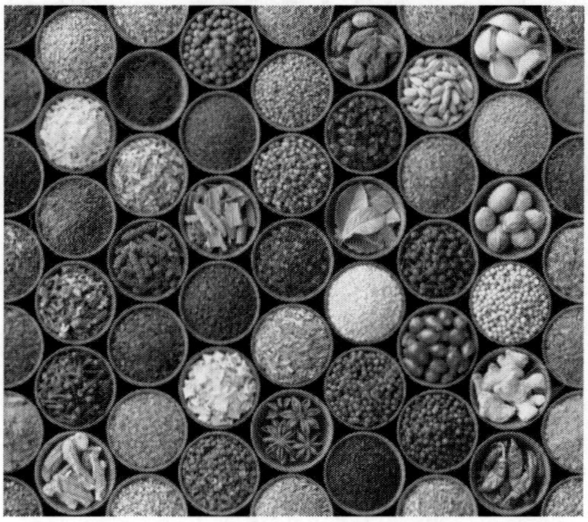

1. BACKGROUND

Plants produce a wide variety and high diversity of secondary metabolites, which are not required for the immediate survival of the plant but which are synthesized in response to stress as a means to protect themselves from organisms, diseases or the environment. Medicinal uses of plants have been documented in approximately 10,000 to 15,000 of world's plants and roughly 150-200 have been incorporated in western medicine. And, it is currently estimated that approximately 420,000 plant species exist in nature. A good number of secondary metabolites from plants possess interesting biological activities with various applications, such as pharmaceutical ingredients, insecticides, dyes, flavors, and fragrances. Despite decades of research, active compounds of plant remain poorly characterized. Usage of natural substances as therapeutic agents in modern medicine has sharply declined from the predominant position held in the early decades of last century, but search for bioactive molecules from plants continues to play an important role in fashioning new medicinal agents. With the advent of modern techniques, instrumentation and automation in isolation and structural characterization, we have on hand an enormous repository of natural compounds. In parallel to this, biology has also made tremendous progress in expanding its frontiers of knowledge. The interplay of these two disciplines constitutes the modern thrust in research in the realm of compounds elaborated by nature.

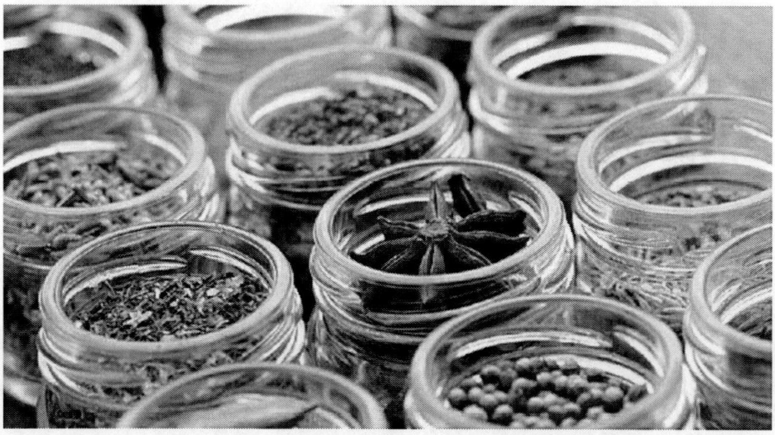

Figure 1. Spices and herbs that can help you stay healthy. (Source: Pagán CN. Spices and herbs that can help you stay healthy. WebMD LLC January 03, 2019.)

Exhibit 1. Scientific and local names of selected Indian spices

S. No	Name of Spice	Scientific Name	Local Name
1	Red chillies	*Capsicum annuum* L. & *Capsicum frutescens* L.	*Lal mirch*
2	Turmeric	*Curcuma longa* L.	*Haldi*
3	Cumin seeds	*Cuminum cyminum* L.	*Zeera*
4	Coriander seeds	*Coriandrum sativum* L.	*Dhania*
5	Mustard seeds	*Brassica juncea* L.Czern	*Rai*
6	Fenugreek seeds	*Trigonella foenum-graecum* L.	*Mehthi*
7	Black pepper	*Piper nigrum* L.	*Kali mirch*
8	Cloves	*Syzygium aromaticum*	*Lavang*
9	Cardamom	*Elettaria cardamomum* Maton	*Ilaichi*
10	Cinnamon	*Cinnamomum zeylanicum* Breyn	*Dalchini*
11	Caraway seeds	*Carum carvi* L.	*Shahzeera*
12	Carom seeds	*Trachyspermum ammi* L.	*Ajwain*
13	Nutmeg	*Myristica fragrans*	*Jaiphal*
14	Mace	*Myristica fragrans*	*Japatri*
15	Fennel	*Foeniculum vulgare* Mill.	*Saunf*
16	Asafoetida	*Ferula asafoetida*	*Hing*
17	Star Anise	*Illicium verum*	*Anasphal*

Source: Siruguri V, Bhat RV. Assessing intake of spices by pattern of spice use, frequency of consumption and portion size of spices consumed from routinely prepared dishes in southern India. Nutr J. 2015;14:7. Published 2015 Jan 11. doi:10.1186/1475-2891-14-7.

2. Abstract

The term of medicinal plants includes a various type of plants used in herbalism with medicinal activities. These plants are considered as rich resources of ingredients which can be used as complementary and alternative medicines and, also in drug developments and synthesis. In addition, some plants regarded as valuable origin of nutrition. Thus, all these plants are recommended as therapeutic agents. Information related to medicinal plants and herbal drugs accumulated over the ages are scattered and unstructured which make it prudent to develop a curated database for medicinal plants. The knowledge base of pharmacy medicine is changing. Even five decades ago rural people used to visit folk healers for traditional medication mostly obtained from the roots and leaves of the remote plants (As seen in old dramas and movies). During 70's to 8o', a modern allopathy system taken over most of it and plant medicines were completely became obsolete. The Indian traditional medicine is a unique conglomerate of different ethnomedical influences. Due to the geographic location and sociocultural characteristics of the country, it involves traditionally rooted elements influenced by local indigenous people and close-by Indian Ayurveda and Unani medicine. Given its inexpensive, easily accessible and well-established health services, the use of traditional medicine is an integral part of public health services in India with its providers being deeply embedded within the local community. Recent data suggest that the utilization of traditional medicine health services in India is widespread and plays a crucial role in providing health care for poor people, people in rural areas and for tribal people.

Keywords: medicinal plants, medical pluralism, folk healers, spiritual healing, herbal drugs

Abbreviations

TMs	Traditional medicines;
TCM	Traditional Chinese Medicine;
TKM	Traditional Korean Medicine;
CDs	Communicable Diseases;
WAPIC	West African Power Industry Convention.

3. Introduction

The concept of ethnopharmacology was first defined in 60's which describes an approach to the discovery of single biologically active molecules that has been used ever since the first compounds were isolated from plant material. It should also be noted that the discovery of new drugs might derive from a wider use of plants than for strictly medical purposes alone. Thus, materials used as poisons, in pest control, in agriculture, as cosmetics, in fermentation processes and for religious purposes might also yield active substances that can be exploited as leads for drug development. However, traditional plants of India and their use because of the greater interest of general people, surprisingly, around 80% of the population of developing countries (according to WHO) now partially or fully dependent upon herbal drugs for primary healthcare. It should be remembered that Since the ingredients used are herbal, not only the ingredients often have added benefits that overall improve your health but there are chances of side effects.

4. Traditional Medicines (TMs): Contribution to Modern Medicine

Since prehistoric times, humans have used natural products, such as plants, animals, microorganisms, and marine organisms, in medicines to alleviate and treat diseases. According to fossil records, the human use of plants as medicines may be traced back at least 60,000 years. The use of natural products as medicines must, of course, have presented a tremendous challenge to early humans. It is highly probable that when seeking food, early humans often consumed poisonous plants, which led to vomiting, diarrhea, coma, or other toxic reactions—perhaps even death. However, in this way, early humans were able to develop knowledge about edible materials and natural medicines. Subsequently, humans invented fire, learned how to make alcohol, developed religions, and made technological breakthroughs, and they learned how to develop new drugs. TMs make use of natural products and are of great importance. Such forms of medicine as TCM, Ayurveda, Kampo, TKM, and Unani employ natural products and have been practiced all over the world for hundreds or even thousands of years, and they have blossomed into orderly-regulated systems of medicine. In their various forms, they may have certain defects, but they are still a valuable repository of human knowledge.

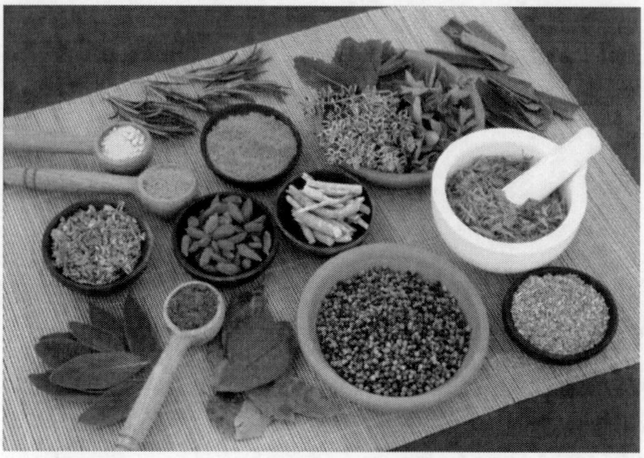

Figure 2. Ayurveda medicines. (Source: Chitnis R. Best Ayurvedic Treatment to Cure Infertility. Web Parenting.FirstCry.com.)

4.1. Ayurveda

With the term "Ayurveda" (AYUR means life, VEDA means Knowledge) translating to the 'science of life', this traditional medical system is based on the belief that the human mind and body are deeply interconnected [1, 2]. It reveals disease has been considered for fold (Body, mind, external factors and natural intrinsic causes). Being one of the oldest medical systems in the world, Ayurveda has its roots from the Vedic culture of India. The motto is simple- if you want to be healthy, your mind and bodily systems must be in balance and at harmony with each other [3, 4]. Ayurvedic doctors prescribe a combination of medicines that often include essential oils, diet supplements and breathing exercises based on your DOSHA's. They are ultimate irreducible basic metabolic elements of living beings, determines the process of growth and decay. The TRIDOSHIC system was the fundamental concept of Ayurveda. They are classified into VATA (Air, causes emaciation, tremors, distention, constipation etc.), PITTA (Bile, which governs digestion, hunger, courage etc.) and Kapha (Phlegm, that holds together, gives lubrication, stability, causes nausea, cough and lethargy when becomes excess) [5]. The '*Samhitas*', or encyclopedia of medicine, were written during the post Vedic era, and include '*Charka Samhita*' (900 BC), '*Sushruta Samhita*' (600 BC) and *Ashtanga Hridaya*' (1000 CE). Utilization of plants was mentioned in Rigveda and Ayurveda (Veda, 3 types, there was also a Juju Veda). *Charka Samhita* was the first recorded treatise on Ayurveda (8 sections divided into 150 chapters, describing 341 medicinal plants. Another treatise of Ayurveda was Shushruta Samhita with special emphasis on surgery, although describing 395 medicinal plants, 57 drugs from animal origin and 64 minerals and metals as drugs [6, 7].

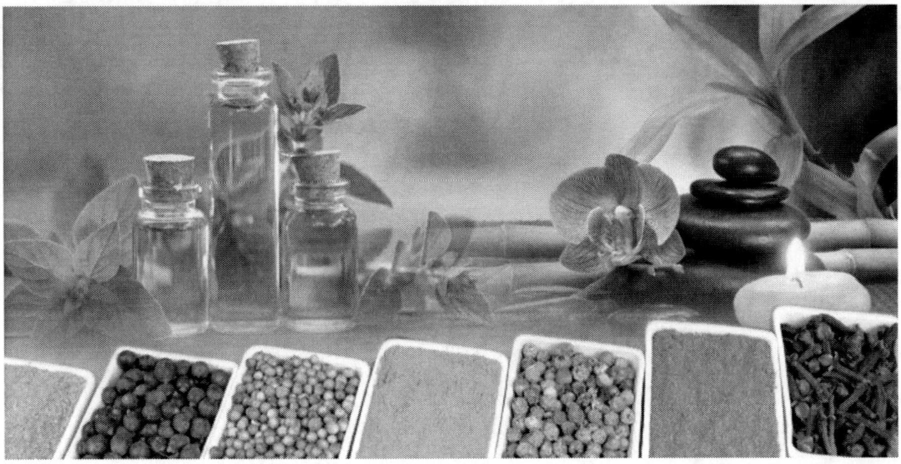

Figure 3. Unani medicine system. (Source: Mittal A. Unani Medicine Gaining Acceptance as an Substitute System of Medicine. Web pitnit.com.)

4.2. Unani

Contribution of Unani medical system to modern pharmacy is beyond description. In between 7th to 8th centuries, Arabs conquered a greater part of ancient civilized world, extending empire from Spain to India. During the reign of Caliph Harun-Al-Rashid (786-814 A.D), some Indian physicians were invited to Baghdad. Manaka, one of those physicians translated some book of Sanskrit to Arabic. Juhanna Ibn Masawaih translated Greek manuscripts to Arabic and wrote a medical book, 1st London Pharmacopoeia was largely based on his formulae. The Arabs greatly improved pharmaceutical products and made them more elegant and palatable. Their pharmacy and Materia Medica were followed for a long time. Arab pharmacists mixed rose water and perfumes with medicines. They invented tinctures, confections, syrups, pomade, plasters and ointments [7, 8].

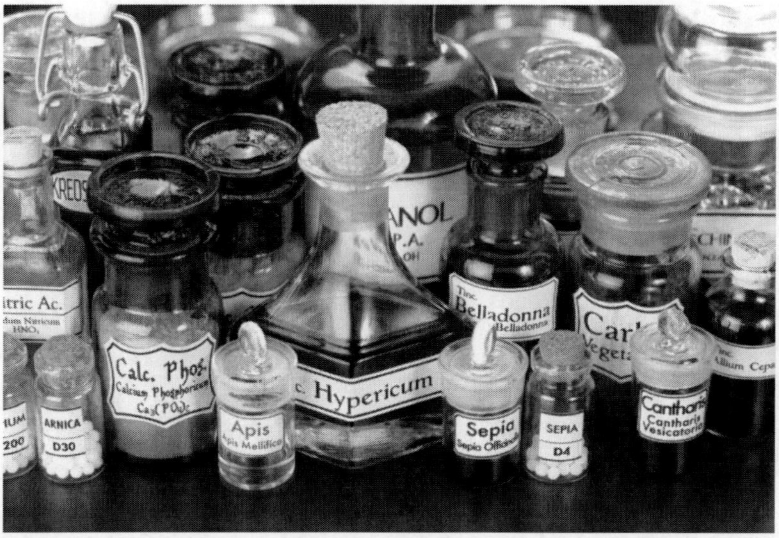

Figure 4. Homeopathy medicines. (Source: Wanjek C. What is Homeopathy? Szasz-Fabian Ilka Erika Shutterstock.)

4.3. Homeopathy

According to Homeopathy system until the potency governing the on the body of a human being is powerful and controls the functions of all organs. A disease produced in the body and brain will affect the other body organs, truly reveals modern day doctors saying, if your heart is weak, it will affect your kidneys someday. Or the ultimate untreated rheumatoid arthritis affects heart in a long run. However, there are three essential processes involved in preparation of remedies; serial dilution, succession and trituration (methods by which mechanical energy is delivered to our preparations in order to imprint the pharmacological message of the original drug upon the molecules of the diluent).

Homeopathy's roots emerge from the findings, teachings and writings of Dr. Samuel Hahnemann (1755-1843). It was when Hahnemann began working on a project to translate William Cullen's Materia Medica into German that he began his quest for a better way of providing healthcare using the principles of "Similars". While working on this project, he became fascinated with a species of South American tree-bark (cinchona) which was being used to treat malaria-induced fever. Hahnemann ingested the bark and discovered that it caused symptoms similar to malaria. He continued his research into "cures" and the idea of "similar suffering," and began compiling his findings. Similia similibus curentur, the Latin phrase meaning "let likes be cured by likes," is the primary principle of homeopathy [9]. Today, nearly all French pharmacies sell homeopathic remedies and medicines; and homeopathy has a particularly strong following in Russia, India, Switzerland, Mexico, Germany, Netherlands, Italy, England, and South America. Homeopathy is also rising again in the United States. This resurgence has been documented by the National Center for Homeopathy in Virginia, which stated that Americans spent 230 million dollars on homeopathic remedies in 1996. It has also been said that sales are rising rapidly at about 12 – 15% each year.

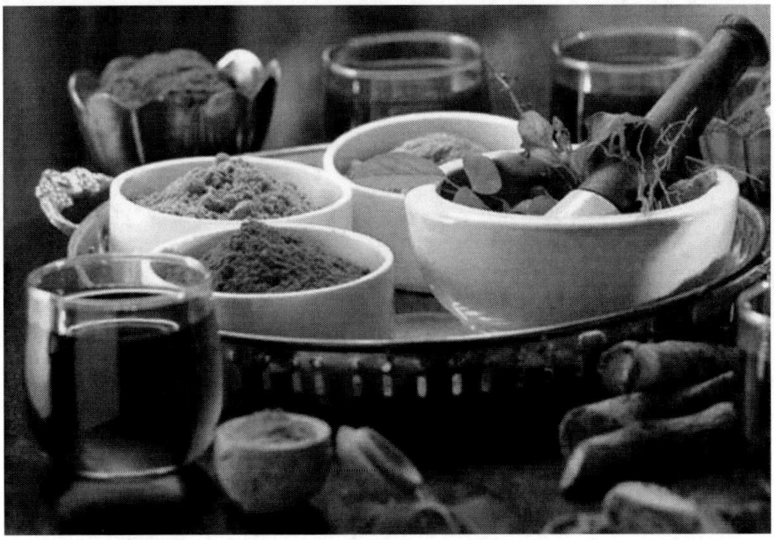

Figure 5. Sidhdha medicine preparation. (Source: Ayurveda Vs Siddha system. Web The Hans India.)

4.4. Siddha System of Medicine

An ancient system of medicine, uses minerals and metals, mainly but some products of vegetable and/or animal origin also used. The Siddha system is based on a combination of ancient medicinal practices and spiritual disciplines as well as alchemy and mysticism. Hence medicine of the human is produced from PONCHOBUTA (PONCHOBOTI DAWAKHANA concept, mostly called in India) theory (Gold, Lead, Copper, Iron and

Zinc), where Gold and lead imparts maintenance of the body; Iron and Zinc generates electricity, employed in medicines that are administered for life extension. Copper used for heat preservation and other metals for body detoxification. Traditionally, it is taught that the siddhas laid the foundation for this system of medication. Siddhas were spiritual adepts who possessed the ASHTA siddhis, or the eight supernatural powers. Siddha medicine has been used for the management of chronic diseases and degenerative conditions, such as rheumatoid arthritis, autoimmune conditions, collagen disorders, and conditions of the central nervous system. Its effectiveness in those situations has varied [7, 10].

It is important to know that drugs are collected from various parts (Table 5 and Table 6) of these plants for example: Barks (Cinnamon, Cinchona, Asoka); Roots (Podophyllum, Rauwolfia); Rhizomes (Ginger, Turmeric, Dioscorea); Leaves (Senna, Tulsi, Vasaka, Digitalis); Flowers (Saffron, Datura, Rose, Arnica); Fruits (Amla, Bael, Bahera, Almond, Cardamom); Seeds (Ispaghula, Linseed, Nux-vomica); Herbs (Chirata, Kalmegh, Pudina) [12].

Table 1. Classification of plant drugs [11]

Base of Classification	Brief Detail
Alphabetical	Although suitable for quick reference it gives no indication of interrelationships between drugs.
Taxonomic	It allows for a precise and ordered arrangement and accommodates any drug without ambiguity.
Morphological	These groupings have some advantages for the practical study of crude drugs; the identification of powdered drugs is often based on micro-morphological characters.
Therapeutic	This classification involves the grouping of drugs according to the pharmacological action of their most important constituent or their therapeutic use.
Biogenetic	The important constituents, e.g., alkaloids, glycosides, volatile oils, etc., or their biosynthetic pathways, form the basis of classification of the drugs

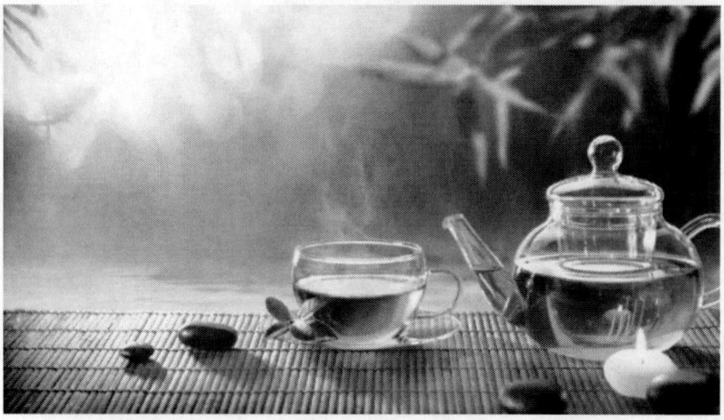

Figure 6. Herbal tea. Fights the cold; improves digestion; boosts immune system; reduces inflammation; anti-aging; relieve stress and anxiety; lower blood pressure; great for skin health. (Source: Ferguson T. 8 Health Benefits of Herbal Tea. Web GROSCHE International Inc. May 22, 2018.)

5. Traditional Plants in Treating Major/Minor Ailments

Through the centuries, sick people have been helped over and over again by remedies that did not arise out of the formal doctrines and procedures of the medical profession. The use of plants (Tables 2-5) to treat sickness is probably as old as mankind; formal medicine and medical degrees are, of course, much more recent. Yet if medicine is broadly defined as the attempt to treat and cure human illness, then the human beings who first grew and collected plants they thought useful, herbalists, and the first people to try to heal by the use of herbs, also called herbalists or herb doctors, must surely rank as pioneers of modern medicine [13].

Many Western medicines are based on traditional knowledge from Europe and the Mediterranean region. This is why interest is rapidly increasing in Indian and Chinese medicine, both of which represent a very long tradition of apparently safe use. However, these healthcare systems are different from Western medicine, so novel methods are required to verify the efficacy and safety of the therapies [15].

Table 2. Frequently used traditional drugs in different ailments [7, 14]

Disorders	Plants Used
Cough & Cold	Leaves of Angelica, Garlic, Tulsi, *Eucalyptus* sp. dried stigma of Saffron, Ginger
GI Disorders	Ispaghula husk, Senna leaves, honey (constipation), bark of Cascara, Cardamom, Cinnamon, Chirata (stomachic)
Urinary disorders	Kalmegh, Picrorhiza, Jar-amla (Cholagogue disorders); Arjuna, Punarnava (Diuretic ailments)
Anti-arthritic agents	Rasna (Rheumatism), Gugul resin (anti-arthritic)
Sedative & Tranquilizers	Ashwagandha, Belladonna, Datura, Cannabis, Hyoscyamus, Wild Cherry bark (Mild sedative)
Cardiac	Sarpagandha (hypotensive), Strophanthus (Cardiotonic)
Others	Chenopodium oil (Anthelmintic) Vasaka (Anti-asthmatic), Turmeric, Punarnava, Ashwagandha (Anti-inflammatory)

Table 3. Frequently used traditional drugs based on pharmacological action [11]

Pharmacological Action	Plant/Plant Part Used
Anti-amoebic	Ipecuc root, Kurchi bark
Anti-Asthmatic	Ephedra, Vasaka, Tylophora
Anti-spasmodic	Belladonna, Datura, Hyoscyamus
Analgesic	Opium, Cannabis
Carminative	Cinnamon bark, Cardamom seed, Nutmeg fruit, Clove, Saffron
Purgative	Cascara bark, Senna leaf, Rhubarb
Bitter Tonic	Nux-vomica, Gentian, Picorhiza, Chirata, Kalmegh
Cardiotonic	Digitalis, Squill, Strophanthus
Tranquilizers	Rauwolfia Roots
Expectorant	Benzoin, Tolu Balsam, Vasaka
CNS action	Ergot, Belladonna, Stramonium, Ephedra, Physostigma

Table 4. Individual plants/plant parts with active contents for intended medicinal use [7, 16]

Plant	Biological Source	Plant Part in Use	Important Content	Use
Punarnava	*Boerhaavia diffusa*	Root	Alkaloids, Xanthenes, Ursolic acid	Diuretic, useful in nephritic syndrome, chronic edema & liver diseases
Vasaka	*Adhatoda vaska*	Dried/fresh leaves	Vasicine, Vasicinone (alkaloid)	Cough & cold, chronic bronchitis & asthma, expectorant
Anantamul	*Hemidesmus indicus*	Root	Essential Oil, Saponin, Resin, Tannins, Sterols and glucosides.	Tonic, diuretic, demulcent, diaphoretic, carminative
Arjun	*Tarminalia arjuna*	Leaves & bark	Tannins, β-sitosterols, saponin	As cardio tonic in angina pain, diuretic in palpitations
Chirata	*Gentiana chirayita*	Entire dried plant	Gentiopicrin (bitter glycoside)	Bitter tonic, febrifuge, stomachic & laxative
Picrorhiga	*Picrirhiga kurroa*	Dried rizomes	Picrorhigin (Glycoside)	Bitter tonic, cathartic, stomachic used in dyspepsia, anti-periodic & colagogue
Kalomegh	*Andrographis paniculata*	Leaves or entire aerial part	Kalmeghin (bitter crystalline diterpin lactone)	Febrifuge, astringent, anthelmintic. Useful in cholera, piles, gonorrhea, dyspepsia and general weakness
Amla (Triphala)	*Phylanthus emblica*	Dried fruit	Vit C (20 times more than in orange)	Cooling, refrigerant, diuretic & laxative, promotes hair growth
Asoka	*Saraca indica*	Dried bark	Tannins, catechol, sterols	Astringent used in uterine affections, dyspepsia, dysentery, colic, piles, ulcer.
Bahera	*Terminalia belerica*	Dried ripe fruit	20% tannins, phyllembin, mannitol	Bitter tonic, astringent, laxative, antipyretic used in dysentery, piles, leprosy
Haritaki	*Terminalia Chebula.*	Fruit	Triterpenes & conjugated coumarins	Carminative, appetite stimulant used in leprosy, anemia, piles, intermittent fever, heart disease, diarrhea
Tulsi	*Ocimum sanctum*	Leaves	Eugenol (essential oil), carvacrol	Expectorant, diaphoretic, antiperiodic, antiseptic & spasmolytic
Neem	*Azadiachta indica*	Leaves & seed oil	Nimbin, nimbinene, nimbandiol (indole alkaloids)	Stimulant, antiseptic used in rheumatism & skin diseases
Betel nut	*Areka catechu*	Seed	acrecoline and other alkaloids	emmenagogue, digestive aid, mitotic, nervine, cardiotonic, and astringent.
Garlic	*Alium stivum*	Bulb	Designated allicin	Used in hypertension, stimulating bile production, common cold, acceleration in wound healing
Spirulina	*Spirulina maxima*	Blue-green algae	Protein & Vit B_{12}	Weight loss
Ginseng	*Panax quinquefolius*	Root	Complex mixture of triterpenoid saponins	Aphrodisiac
Aloe	*Aloe barbadensis*	Dried latex juice of leaves	Barbaloin (anthraquinine glycosides	Benzoin tincture, cathartic

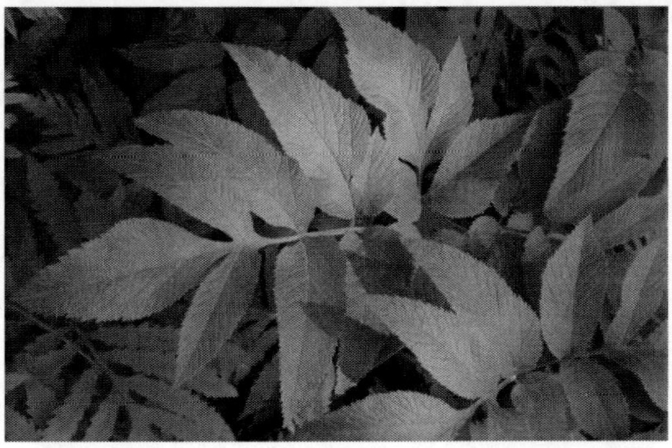

Figure 7. Angelica leaves. Widely used as a traditional Indian and Chinese herbal medicine, functional food and cosmetic product ingredient, mostly because of the high furanocoumarin compounds in roots. The root of Angelica is a traditional medicine known for its antipyretic and analgesic properties since thousands of years ago. The multiple pharmacological effects of Angelica root extracts include antioxidation, anti-inflammatory, antiproliferative, skin whitening, anti-tumor, antimicrobial and anti-Alzheimer effects. (Source: Liang WH, Chang TW, Charng YC. Influence of harvest stage on the pharmacological effect of *Angelica dahurica*. Bot Stud. 2018;59(1):14. Published 2018 May 15. doi:10.1186/s40529-018-0230-1.)

Table 5. Plants/plant parts with active contents' chemical class [7, 18]

Plants/Plant Parts as Source	Chemical Class	Active Contents	Major Uses
Agar, Acacia, Tragacanth	Carbohydrates	Gums and Mucilages	Suspending Agents
Aloe (Ghritokumari)	Anthaquinone Glycosides	Aloin, Resin, Emodin, Volatile Oils	Laxative
Digitalis (Fox/Fairy Gloves)	Cardio-active Glycosides	Digitoxin, Gitoxin, Gitaloxin	Cardiac Stimulant and Tonic
Hazel Leaves	Tannin	Hemamelitannin, Ca-Oxalate	Astringent in hemorrhoidal products and treating insect bites and tings
Olive Oil	Lipid	Oleic acid, Palmitic acid, Linoleic acid	Pharmaceutic aid, demulcent, emollient, laxative
Coconut Oil	Lipid	Caprylic acid and Capric acid	Weight loss aid, skin moisturizer
Dried bark of Cinnamon	Volatile Oil	Cinnamic Aldehydes, Lemonene, p-cymen	Carminative, Pungent Aromatic
Capsicum Fruit	Resin	Capsaicin, Volatile and Fixed Oil	Irritant, Carminative, Rubefacient
Ginger	Volatile Oil	Bisabolene, Zingiberene, Zingiberol	Condaminant, Stimulant, Carminative
Belladonna Leaves	Alkaloids	Hyoscyamine, Atropine	Parasympathetic depressants, Adjunct in PUD
Ipecac Roots	Alkaloids	Emetin, Cephaeline, Psychotrine	Emetic
Arnika Dried Flowering Heads	Alkaloids	Sesquiterpinoid lactones	Treating abrasion, bruises and sprains
Angelica	Volatile Oils	Furocoumarins	Aromatic Stimulant, Bronchial Tonic, Diaphoretic
Ginseng Roots	Glycosides	Triterpenoid Saponins	Tonic, Stimulant, Diuretic

In the case of China, Western medicine was introduced in the sixteenth century, but it did not undergo any development until the nineteenth century. Before that, traditional medicine was the dominant form of medical care and still now plays an important role in China, and it is constantly being developed.

In the early development of modern medicine, biologically active compounds from higher plants have played a vital role in providing medicines to combat pain and diseases. For example, in the British Pharmacopoeia of 1932, over 70% of organic monographs were on plant-derived products. However, with the advent of synthetic medicinal and subsequently of antibiotics, the role of plant derived therapeutic agents significantly declined in the economically developed nations [17]. Even in developed countries a variety of natural products enjoy their well-deserved recognition in the therapeutic arsenal. However, their actual and precise method of production is more or less an extremely individualized aspect.

6. Commonly Practiced Home Remedies with Traditional Medicines

India and a significant part of South Asia possess a vibrant and thriving medical pluralism. Traditional medicine continues to be a valuable source of remedies (Table 6) that have been used by millions of people around the world to secure their health. The various diseases treated included gastrointestinal disorders, jaundice, leucorrhea, tooth and gum disorders, helminthiasis, allergy, respiratory tract disorders, skin diseases, anemia, pain, and diabetes [19].

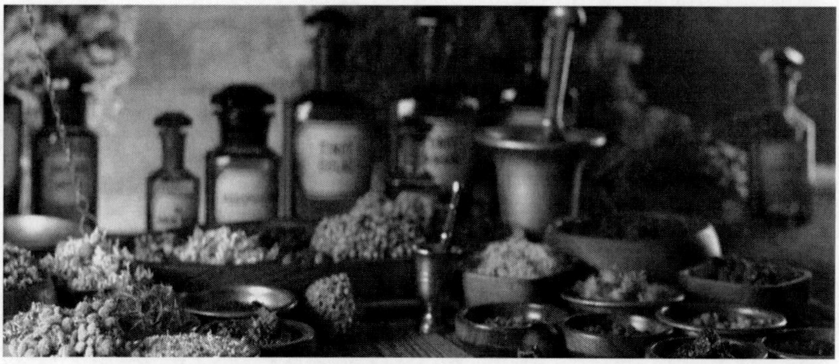

Figure 8. Home remedies with traditional medicines. Generally, the first line of defense for hypertension is drug therapy. But before starting drug therapy, try lifestyle changes and some home remedies for high blood pressure. Medications can be harsh, and while best avoided if possible, if you are on them, know that natural remedies can interfere with their functioning. Learn how to lower high blood pressure with home remedies. (Source: Eli Ben-Yehuda. Natural ways to lower blood pressure. Web RESPeRATE, August 18, 2018.)

Table 6. Popular home remedies with traditional medicines [20]

Plant Local Name	Scientific Name	Commonly Used Plant Part	Remedial Option (s)
Mango	*Mangifera indica*	Bark	Mango Juice with ginger for aid in Jaundice
Turmaric (Holud)	*Curcuma longa*	Rhizome	Gastric Disorder
Bael	*Aegle marmelos*	Fruit	Leucorrhea and Stomachache
Arjun	*Terminalia arjuna*	Bark	Cardiotonic and anemia Treatment
Pineapple	*Ananas comosus*	Fruit	Helminthiasis, should be taken in empty stomach
Helencha	*Enhydra fluctuans*	Leaves	Along with ginger for Jaundice
Thankuni	*Centella asiatica*	Leaves	Gum Infection
Supari	*Areca catechu*	Root	Root Juice for Helminthiasis
Boitha shak	*Chenopodium album*	Leaves	Cold with coughs
Bashok	*Adhatoda vasaka*	Leaves	Cough and Cold
Telakuchi	*Coccinia grandis*	Roots/leaves	Roots for arthritic joint pain and leaves for lowering blood sugar level
Neem	*Antelaea azadirachta*	Leaves and bark	Gingivitis, Stomach upset
Shankhapushpi	*Convolvulus pluricaulis*	Whole aerial part	Brain tonic
Ginger	*Zingiber officinale*	Rhizome	Cough and cold
Anantamul	*Tylophora indica*	Leaves	Emetic, diaphoretic and expectorant
Chirata	*Swertia chirata*	Bitter stick	Bitter tonic, febrifuge, laxative
Asoka	*Saraca indica*	Dried bark	Uterine affections, biliary colic, pimples and menorrhagia
Amla	*Embelic myrobalan*	Dried fruit	Promote hair Growth
Tulsi	*Ocimum sanctum*	Leaves	Expectorant, diaphoretic. Antiperiodic
Ispaghula	*Plantago ovata*	Seeds	Managing Constipation

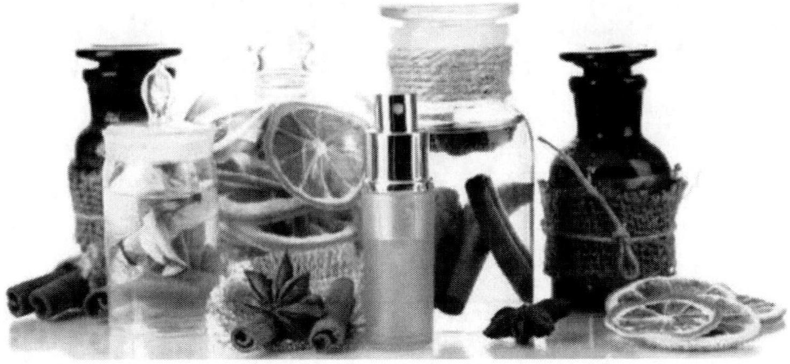

Figure 9. Herbal hair care and skin care products. Effective botanical antioxidant compounds are widely used in traditional medicine and include tocopherols, flavonoids, phenolic acids, nitrogen containing compounds (indoles, alkaloids, amines, and amino acids), and monoterpenes. As the topical supplementation of antioxidants has been shown to affect the antioxidant network in the skin, applying aromatherapy formulations that are rich in antioxidants offers interesting avenues for future research. The next step has been to look at other cultural remedies and to dissect the ethnopharmacy of countries around the world and to use our knowledge to assign chemicals that might be responsible for the skin benefits. Many new active molecules have been discovered and there are many more to be discovered. (Source: Korać RR, Khambholja KM. Potential of herbs in skin protection from ultraviolet radiation. Pharmacogn Rev. 2011;5(10):164-73.)

7. Cosmetic Uses of Traditional Medicine

It is claimed that herbal cosmetics are natural and free from all the harmful synthetic chemicals which otherwise may prove to be toxic to the skin. Instead of traditional synthetic products different plant parts and plant extracts are used (Table 7) in these products, e.g., aloe vera gel and coconut oil. There are a rising number of consumers who demand more natural products with traceable and more natural ingredients, free from harmful chemicals and with an emphasis on the properties of botanicals.

Table 7. Popular cosmetic uses of traditional medicines [21, 22]

Plant/Plant Part	Scientific Name	Active Component	Intended Use
Coconut oil	*Cocos nucifera*	Glycerides of lower chain fatty acids	Skincare, Promotes Hair growth
Sunflower oil	*Helianthus annuus*	lecithin, tocopherols, carotenoids and waxes.	Skincare
Aloe vera (Ghrtokumari)	*Aloe indica*	leucine, isoleucine, saponin glycosides, vitamins	Skincare, hair growth
Jojoba oil	*Simmondsia chinenesis*	Palmitic acid, stearic acid, oleic acid	Replenishes skin and hair lose
Carrot	*Daucus carota*	β-carotene	Anti-ageing
Gingko	*Ginkgo biloba*	flavone glycoside quercetin and kaempferol	Anti-ageing
Green tea	*Camellia sinensis*	(2)-epicatechin (EC), EGC, (2)-EC-3-gallate, EGCG	Skin protection and Anti-ageing
Calendula	*Calendula officinalis*	α-thujene, α-pinene, 1,8-Cineole, dihydrotagetone and T-muurolol	Anti-oxidant, skin repair
Turmeric	*Curcuma longa*	zingiberene, curcumol, curcumenol, eugenol, tetrahydrocurcumin	UVB induced sunburn
Henna Leaves (Mehendi)	*Lawsonia inermis*	Lawsone, gallic acid, glucose, mannitol, fats, resin	Staining hair, nails and beard
Rose oil	*Rosa damascena*	citronellol, phenyl ethanol, geraniol, nerol, farnesol	clearing, cleansing, and purifying effect on the female sex organs
Ginseng	*Panax ginseng*	Triterpenoid Saponins	skin's metabolism, reduce keratinization, alleviate wrinkling and enhance skin whiteness
Onion	*Allium cepa*	flavonoids (quercetin and kampferol)	externally as a poultice for acne, boils, abscesses and blackheads, speed healing.
Rosemary	*Rosmarinus officinalis*	caffeic acid and rosmarinic acid	to stimulate growth of hair as a rinse
Cucumber	*Cucumis sativa*	vitamin C, vitamin K, and potassium	soothing to irritated skin and treatment of hyperpigmentation
Eucalyptus oil	*Eucalyptus cinerea*	Eucalyptol, limonene, α-pinene, α-phellandrene, β-pinene	Tingling Hair Conditioner, promoted hair growth
Pumpkin	*Cucurbita pepo*	linoleic, oleic, palmitic and stearic acid	Syphilitic sores, herpes lesions, pimples and blackheads

8. Traditional Medicines as Potential Antidotes

Thousand claims of traditional medicines for anti-venom or antidotes (Table 8). Both spiritual healing (rituals) and plant medicines are practiced to detoxify and manage poisons of plant and animal origin. Folk medicines must be documented, validated and their practice be encouraged for the benefit of rural mass. Food-medicines overlap exhibited in many cultures can be an interesting area of investigation.

Table 8. Common traditional plants as anti-venoms [23, 24]

Plant Name	Plant Part in Use	General Practice
Allium sativum	Leaves	First aid for snake bite
Achyranthes aspera	Roots, Leaves and Stem	Snake bite
Abelmoschus moschatus	Roots	Snake bite
Averrhoa Carambola	Fruits	Datura poisoning
Capsicum frutescens	Leaves	Applied locally in bee sting
Citrus limon	Stem and Fruit	Snake bite
Curcuma longa	Rhizome	Applied in leech bites to heal the wound
Datura metel	Fruit	Given once daily to patient for dog bite
Oryza sativa	Grain	Rubbed on the body in caterpillar allergy
Nicotiana tabacum	Leaves	Crushed leaves for removing leeches
Xanthium strumarium	Leaves	Food poisoning
Saccharum bengalense	Root	Taken orally or applied locally thrice daily till recovery in snake bite.

9. Alternative Medicine Dispensing by the Folk Medicine Practitioners

Medical pluralism has led to an intrinsic feature of its medical system in historical and contemporary contexts. Folk medicines are widely practiced for primary healthcare, underlying factors such as economy, education, religion, culture, and environment. The KAVIRAJI treatment is also known as BONOJO CHIKTSYA (treatment by wild forest herbs) or VESHOJO CHIKITSYA (herbal treatment). They primarily use different Barks, Roots, Rhizomes, Leaves, Flowers, Fruits, Seeds, Herbs or other common items available in and around their homestead, collected from remote hills/forests or grown through cultivation. In some cases, they also perform rituals based on faiths, and recite holy verses (mantras). Three factors which legitimize the role of the folk healers include: their own beliefs, the beliefs of the community and the success of their actions. Nearly 40% of rural community members have superstitions/misbeliefs or strong beliefs on herb and approximately 15% treats simple ailments with herbs. They mostly use different plant extracts for different diseases. Some of the kavirajes also use snakes' blood, birds or other animal parts, fish or fish oil and others chemicals as ingredients of their medicines. Dilution, dose, administration time and mixture played a significant role in need of combinations of useful extracts by the traditional practitioners [25].

10. Global Disease Burden

Diseases have been grouped as communicable or non-communicable based on the involvement or otherwise of a transmissible biologic disease-causing agent. Until recently, communicable diseases (CDs) were the major causes of ill-health and deaths in the developing (low and middle resource) countries while non-communicable diseases were prevalent in the developed (high resource) countries, where improvement in living conditions and widespread deployment of technology had brought the CDs under control. However, the optimism that communicable diseases would be less of a health problem in the developed countries appears to have been misplaced with the appearance of new infectious diseases and re-emergence of older disease agents. Similarly, non-communicable diseases are already a major cause of morbidity and mortality as a consequence of globalization and changing lifestyle in developing countries. Globally therefore, NCDs and CDs account for about equal quantities of morbidity and mortality, thus making all countries to currently face the double disease burden. The overall picture is, however, graver for low- and middle-income countries in terms of the health and socio-economic impacts. The growing importance of medicinal plants can be appreciated from the economic stand point when the following facts are considered:

- Global trade in herbs is over USD 100 Billion per annum
- India and China's medicinal plant trade is about two to five billion US dollars annually
- In Germany, it is over one billion US dollars annually
- Rose Periwinkle which is endemic to Madagascar fetches US$100 million per annum
- China trades in 7,000 species and 700,000 tons of medicinal plants per annum
- India trades in 7,000 species of medicinal plants
- Morocco exports 58.7 tons of medicinal plants annually
- In the last 5 years, sales of medicinal plants doubled in China, tripled in India and grew by 25% in Europe.

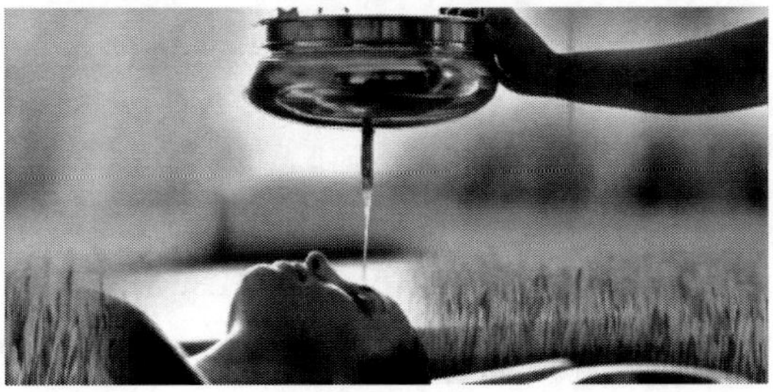

Figure 10. Ayurveda massage. CAM centers of the Faculty of Public Health of different Hungarian universities at Szeged, Pecs, Miskolc, Nyiregyhaza started offering short courses on Ayurveda. Private organizations like Maharishi College from the Netherlands also started few courses and training programs. Indian government facilitated training courses on Ayurveda massage and beauty treatments for experts from Hungarian thermal spas. The Indian Embassy organized series of lectures under the theme 'Ayurveda for All' to promote interest amongst doctors, medical workers, vets, students and common people. (Source: Healing with Ayurvedic Herbs | Panchakarma Treatment Centre in Croydon London/Wele A. The Hungarian initiative for Ayurveda: European Institute of Ayurvedic Sciences. J Ayurveda Integr Med. 2018;9(2):155-158.)

11. Misuse and Abuses of Traditional Medicine

Traditional medicine has its own limitations. It takes time to cure the patient and restore health. Or there should be enough study using these drugs in specific indication or any sorts of well-being like anti-ageing or antioxidant properties. Different tea combinations of Tulsi, Ginger, pepper and neem suggested by fitness trainers as slimming aids and people are spending a lot as well [28]. Another worsening feature is heavy metal toxicity by the marketed products having poor prior quality control. Herb extracts are best while taken fresh, dried and long-term preservation gives rise poisoning from the preservatives in use [29]. Some concerned people noticed that ginseng preparations are endowed with Sildenafil (VIAGRA) and claiming sexual enhancement, whereas ginseng is best known for anti-ageing activities. Substance use among women and children is increasingly becoming the focus of attention and merits further research. Abrupt use of herbal cosmetics and frequent use of herbal cough syrups thinking that natural means safe also reported. After caffeine, alcohol, and nicotine, betel nut (PAAN) is the fourth most abused substance in the world, chewed alone or in a mixture of other spices for its stimulant effect [30]. And Aloe Vera is blindly taken by so called health conscious people. The poisonous effects of these abuses and misuses will be discussed later part of this article.

12. Industrial Production of Herbal Drugs

Despite the advantages and the past successes, many large pharmaceutical companies decreased the use of natural products in drug discovery screening in last few decades. This has been because of the perceived disadvantages of natural products (difficulties in access and supply, complexities of natural product chemistry and inherent slowness of working with natural products, and concerns about intellectual property rights), and the hopes associated with the use of collections of compounds prepared by combinatorial chemistry methods. The process in natural product drug discovery usually required several separation circles and structure elucidation and was thus time consuming. However, Drug discovery from natural products has reclaimed the attention of the Pharma industry and is on the verge of a comeback due to new technological inputs that promise better returns on investment. In addition to their chemical structure diversity and their biodiversity, the development of new technologies has revolutionized the screening of natural products in discovering new drugs. Applying these technologies compensates for the inherent limitations of natural products and offers a unique opportunity to re-establish natural products as a major source for drug discovery. An integrative approach by combining the various discovery tools and the new discipline of integrative biology will surely provide the key for success in natural product drug discovery and development. Natural products can be predicted to remain an essential component in the search and development for new, safe and economical medicaments [42].

Table 9. Important bioactive molecules from medicinal plants and their biological activity [42]

Drug	Plant	Biological Activity
Achyranthine	*Achyranthes aspera*	Diuretic
Aegelin, Marmelosin	*Aegle marmalos*	Bowel diseases
Ajmalicine	*Rauwolfia canesocence*	Hypotensive
Allicin	*Allium sativum*	Hypolipidemic
Aloin	*Aloe vera*	Demulcent, Skin diseases
Andrographolide	*Andrographis paniculata*	Hepatoprotective
Arboreol	*Gmelina arborea*	Tonic, Stomachic
Artemisinin	*Artemisia annua*	Antimalarial
Asiaticoside	*Centella asiatica*	Memory enhancer
Asparanin A, Asparanin B, Sarasapogenin	*Asparagus adscendens*	Fertility enhancer
Atropine	*Solanaceae spp.*	Anticholinergic
Bacoside	*Bacopa monneri*	Memory enhancer
Berberine	*Berberis lycium*	Antiemetic
Boeravinones	*Boerrhavia diffusa*	Hepatoprotective
Boswellic acid	*Boswellia seratta*	Antiinflammatory
Caffeine	*Camellia sinensis*	CNS stimulant
Camphor	*Cinnamomum camphora*	Aromatic
Camptothecin	*Camptotheca acuminata*	Anticancer
Capsiacin	*Capsicum annum*	Counter irritant
Cocaine	*Erythroxylum coca*	Analgesic
Codeine	*Papaver somniferum*	Anaesthetic
Colchicine	*Colchicum luteum*	Antiinflammatory
Conessine	*Holarrhena antidysentrica*	Antiamoebic
Curcumin	*Curcuma longa*	Antioxidant

Drug	Plant	Biological Activity
Diosogenin	*Dioscorea deltoidea*	Base for steroids
Embelin	*Embelia ribes*	Anthelmintic
Emetine	*Cephaelis ipecacuanha*	Antiamoebic
Ephedrine	*Ephedrae herba*	Hypertensive
Ergotamine	*Claviceps purpurea*	Hemorrhage
Etoposide/Tenopside	*Podophyllum hexandrum*	Anticancer
Forskolin	*Coleus forskolin*	Cardiotonic
Galanthamine	*Leucojum aestivum*	Anticholinesterase
Glycyrrhizin	*Glycyrrhiza glabra*	Antiviral
Gossypol	*Gossypium herbaceum*	Contraceptive
Guggulsterones/Gugallipid	*Commiphora wightti*	Hypocholeromic
Hydroxy citric acid	*Garcinia cambogia*	Antiobesity agent
Hyoscine/Hyoscyamine	*Hyoscyamus niger/H. muticus*	Parasympatholetic
Hypericin	*Hypericum perforatum*	Anti-HIV
Ipecac	*Cephaelis angustifolia*	Emetic
Liquiritigenin, Isoliquiritigenin	*Pterocarpus marsupium*	Anti-diabetic
Lycopene	*Lycopersicon esculentum*	Antioxidant
Methoxsalen	*Ammi majus/Heracleum candicans*	Leucoderma
Monoterpenes, Sesquiterpenes	*Ocimum sanctum*	Respiratory diseases, Immunomodulatory
Morphine/Papaverine	*Papaver somniferum*	Sedative
Polyphenolics, Tannins	*Phyllanthus emblica*	Antioxidant
Protodioscin	*Tribulus terrestris*	Diuretic, Anabolic, Aphrodisiac
Psoralen	*Psoralea corylifolia*	Antileucoderma
Quinine/Quinidine	*Cinchona officinalis*	Antimalarial
Reserpine	*Rauwolfia serpentina*	Hypotensive
Sennoside	*Cassia angustifolia*	Laxative
Shatavarin	*Asparagus racemosus*	Galactogogue, Tonic
Silymarin	*Silybium marianum*	Hepatoprotective
Strychnine	*Strychnose nux-vomica*	Central stimulant
Taxol	*Taxus wallichiana*	Anticancer
Tinosporic acid, Cordifolioside	*Tinospora cordifolia*	Immunomodulatory
Trigonellin	*Trigonella foenum-graecum*	Anti-diabetic
Tubocurarine	*Chondodendron tomentosum*	Muscle relaxant
Tylophorine	*Tylophora indica*	Bronchodilator
Vasacine	*Adhatoda vasica*	Vasodilatory
Vinblastine/ Vincristine	*Cathranthus roseus*	Anticancer
Valepotriates	*Valeraina wallachi*	Sedative
Withanolides	*Withania somnifera*	Immunomodulatory

13. Poisonous and Serious Side Effects Found with Traditional Plant Medicines

WAPIC reported undiluted essential oils on sensitive skin or in the nostrils can irritate or burn in children. Certain marketed products reported kidney or liver damage (Table 9), and are sometimes adulterated with steroids, pesticides, antibiotics or harmful metals.

Chronic use of betel nut can cause addiction, as well as red staining of the teeth and gums and the potential for oral cancers. Mushroom poisoning is said to be most severe though no fatal incidents have been reported despite the lack of modern medical facilities.

Table 10. Poisoning reported with commonly used herbs

Local Name	Scientific Name	Poisonous Effects
Kuchila	*Strychnos nux-vomica*	Respiratory failure, nausea, muscle twitching [31]
Antamul	*Tylophora indica*	Plant juice causes vomiting, unconsciousness, and death [31]
Aloe Vera	*Aloe indica*	Nephrotoxicity and group 2B carcinogenic [32]
Eucalyptus oil	*Eucalyptus globulus*	Irritation of skin and nostril of children [33]
Betel Nut	*Areca catechu*	Nausea, vomiting, dizziness, chest discomfort [34]
Coconut oil	*Cocos nucifera*	Oxidative stress, hyperlipidemia [35]
Ginseng	*Panax ginseng*	cardiovascular and renal toxicity, hepatotoxicity, reproductive toxicity [36]
Henna	*Lawsonia inermis*	Hemolytic crisis in individuals deficient in glucose-6-phosphate dehydrogenase (G6PD) [37]
Green Tea	*Camellia sinensis*	restlessness, confusion, psychomotor agitation, EGCG (component of green tea) has anti-folate activity [38]
Cucumber	*Cucumis sativus*	Hair loss [39]
Rosemary	*Rosmarinus officinalis*	Not safe in pregnancy [40]
Turmeric	*Curcuma longa*	Not safe in pregnancy [41]

Again, herbal medicines contain a combination of pharmacologically active plant constituents that are claimed to work synergistically to produce an effect greater than the sum of the effects of the single constituents. Even it is a single drug, it is pharmacologically active, might interact with other drugs (Table 10) by compete any receptor or enzymatic system.

Table 11. Drug interaction reported with common HDS [42]

HDS	Interaction Possibility	Potential Impact
Acacia	Amoxicillin	Reduce absorption due to presence of oleoresin.
Aloe Vera	Digoxin	Increased Digoxin Toxicity
American ginseng	Warfarin, Enalapril, Nitroglycerin, Spironolactone	Lowers effects of warfarin and increased others hypotensive effects due to glycoside contents similar to digoxin
Ginkgo	Aspirin, cilostazol, clopidogrel, dipyridamole, heparin, ibuprofen, naproxen, ticlopidine, warfarin	Increases risk of bleeding
Green tea	Ephedrine	Risk of stimulatory adverse effects
Evening primrose	Warfarin	Risk of bleeding
Garlic	Ritonavir, Saquinavir, Warfarin	Reduce antiviral effects and risk of bleeding

14. Safety Issues and Recommendations

Lack of side effects do not mean taking a medicine without any expert's recommendations. One should always take medicine consulting an expert of allied field. Moreover, opt for well-known trusted sources when it comes to buying medicines. With traditional medicine, there is always risk of counterfeits. And while their effectiveness varies from person to person, such traditional medicinal systems are often the last resort for people, especially when the western ones fail them. Definitely we get energized with a number of active herbal ingredients posing on the package but a little but relevant question rise how all these ingredients are altogether found at a time as plant constituents varies in different seasons. Moreover, some plants should not be found anytime and every time.

Table 12. Medicinal plants used by Indian tribes [43]

State Name/ Tribal Communities	Botanical Name/Local Trial Name	Disease	Part Used	Mode of Administration
Chhatisgarh/ Gond, Bhunjia, Baiga, Bisonhom, Maria Parghi	*Aloe barbadensis* Linn.(Gaur patha)	Annonaceae	Leaves	One teaspoonful of leaf juice with sugar
	Vitex negundo Linn.(Sambhalu)	Abortion	Leaves	Leaves powder with cow milk
	Haldinia cordifolia (Haldu)	Body pain	Stem bark	Paste is applied on body for 3 days.
	Moringa pterygosperma Gaern (Munga)	Cold and cough	Leaves	Leaf powder with mustard oil is given orally for 3 days.
Meghalaya/Bala magre, Modupara and Dumnigaon	*Aegle marmelos* Correa. (Selpri)	Burning sensation	Pulp of fruit	The pulp of unripe fruit is dipped in ginger oil for a week, and this mixture is applied over body.
	Artocarpus lakoocha Roxb (Arimu)	Anaemia	Fruit	Fresh fruit are use.
	Averrhoa carambola L. (Amillenga)	Jaundice	Fruit and Leaves	Juice of fruit and leaf are used for treatment.
	Dillenia pentagyna Roxb (Agatchi)	Diabetics and stomachache	bark	Powder of Bark is used.
Uttarakhand/Tharu, Bhotia, Jaunsari, Raji	*Allium sativum* L. (Lehsun)	Diarrhoea, earache	Plant part	Bulbs of garlic are boiled in Till oil; after cooling it is pour into ear.
	Aconitum heterophyllum Wall.(Atees)	Abdominal pain and vomiting	Dry Root	½ tablespoon dry root powder is boiling in water during fever. Root is also chewed twice a day.
	Bergenia ligulata (Wall) Engl. (Pashanbhed)	Kidney stone	Root	Dry form of rhizome is chewed
Kerala/ Paniya, Kurich, Adiyan, Kattunaika	*Acorus calamus* L. (Vayambus)	Abdominal pain and diarrohea	Whole Plant	Juice of plant and tuber paste is taken orally to control abdominal pain blood circulation respectively.

Table 12. (Continued)

State Name/ Tribal Communities	Botanical Name/Local Trial Name	Disease	Part Used	Mode of Administration
	Baliosperm montanum (Nagadenth)	Piles	Root	Root paste is applied over piles.
	Chonemorpha fragrans (Perumkurumba)	Skin diseases, blood purification	Root	Paste is applied over skin.
Rajasthan/ Bhils, Lohars, Sanshi, Meena, Raibari,Gadarias	*Capparis sepiaria* (Kather)	Itching	Leaves	Bath with leaf decoction.
	Cucumis colossus Rotl. (Cogn)	Finger infection	Fruit	An infected finger is placed into the hole made in fruit, into some time intervals.
	Solanum nigrum Linn	kama	Leaves	Crushed leaves and fruits are used to treat infection.
W.Bengal/ Santhali and Pahari	*Dendropthae falcate* Linn (Shibphul)	Antibacterial	leaves	Decoction of the plant use
	Tectona grandis (Sagoan)	Skin infection	Wood	Wood oil used for treatment.
	Cassia sophera (kalkasunda)	Skin disease	leaves	Leaf juice is applied inn ringworm
Tripura/Auchai, Kabiraj, Ozai	*Crotalaria albida* Heyne ex Roth (Banatasi)	Body swelling	Root	One cup root decoction mixed with 2-3 spoon ginger extract is taken regularly in empty stomach
	Cuscuta reflexa Roxb. (Bannalata)	Jaundice, cough and diabetes	Whole plant	Plant juice mixed with coconut water is taken early morning for 2 weeks.
	Euphorbia hirta L. (Shyamkhai)	Skin disease	Leaves	Leaf paste of plant and *Achyranthus aspera (Apang)* along with sulfur (gandhi), copper sulphate and mustard oil in 6:2:1:1:2 is applied on the skin for one hour before bath.

And if we are convinced with the fact that they collected and stored for selling year-round, where's the guaranty that they were stored in a prescribed manner, in India where BSTI seal creates doubts sometimes. A mushrooming of folk healer's shops clearly visible with their unusual claim of complete recovery from ulcer, cancer, asthma, erectile dysfunctions, alopecia, AIDS and by born complications. A common scenario of roadside hawkers surrounded by a lot of many unprivileged people claiming leeches' oils for stronger penile erection, whereas leeches do not possess oil at all. Plants have provided us with some of our most effective drugs, including aspirin, made from willow bark. Moreover, at least 7,000 medical compounds in the modern pharmacopoeia are derived from plants. Nearly two thirds of traditional medicinal plants are as effective as medical drugs but it is still difficult to get a sound advice. A growing number of people are looking for guidance on the Internet while others believe dishonest ads. It is strictly recommended that plant drugs are miraculous, better avoid plant drugs as food supplements, they can't be always safe as they are natural and taking expert's advice before use.

Conclusion

Safety is when any drug is ingested following an expert. Indiscriminate use of plant medicine may rise to severe long-term poisoning and short-term adverse events. A doctor or a pharmacist is the legally qualified and professionally competent person to handle drugs and allied supplies required for the patients. It is a matter of regret that the government of our country is taking very little effort to employ highly skilled pharmacy personnel in different sectors of the health services. But in the developed countries, Pharmacists are in unique position in this regard. So, the governmental health policy should be modified by incorporation Pharmacist in different areas. So that a rational use of traditional, as well as allopathic medicines are promoted, distributed and used. Lastly, traditional plants have vast opportunities to explore, conducting extensive research necessary for their rational use in India and abroad. Companies with big reserve can invest further to bring qualified researchers from abroad to see their further scope of extension for both business purpose and mankind.

References

[1] Warrier M. Seekership, Spirituality and Self-Discovery: Ayurveda Trainees in Britain. *Asian Med* (Leiden). 2009;4(2):423-451.

[2] Markbunn. *Ayurveda & Vedic Science: The Science of Life.* Friday, 29 May 2015.

[3] Proma AM. The magic of Ayurvedic medicines. *The Daily Star* July 10, 2018.

[4] Agrawal DP, Tiwari L. Ayurveda: *The Traditional Indian Medicine System and its Global Dissemination.* Available From: https://www.infinityfoundation.com/mandala/t_es/t_es_agraw_ayurveda_frameset.htm.

[5] Banyan Botanicals. Vata, Pitta, and Kapha. *An Introduction to Three Energetic Forces of Nature.* Learning Ayurveda Updated 2018. Available From: https://www.banyanbotanicals.com/info/ayurvedic-living/learning-ayurveda/vata-pitta-and-kapha.

[6] Copper H2O. *Ayurvedic Medicine Origin, History and Principles.* Available From: https://www.copperh2o.com/blogs/blog/ayurvedic-medicine-origin-history-and-principles.

[7] Mohammed A. *Textbook of Pharmacognosy (Second Edition).* Publisher: CBS Publishers & Distributors Pvt. Ltd. Publication Date: 2012.

[8] Masic I, Skrbo A, Naser N, et al. Contribution of Arabic Medicine and Pharmacy to the Development of Health Care Protection in Bosnia and Herzegovina - the First Part. *Med Arch.* 2017;71(5):364-372.

[9] WholeHealthNow. *History of Homeopathy. The Founder of Homeopathy.* © WholeHealthNow 2018.

[10] The Editors of Encyclopaedia Britannica. *Siddha Medicine*. Available From: https://www.britannica.com/science/Siddha-medicine.

[11] Tyler VE, Brady L, Robbers JE. *Pharmacognosy.* 8th edition. Philadelphia, PA 19106. https://doi.org/10.1002/jps.2600710445.

[12] Alamgir ANM. *Therapeutic Use of Medicinal Plants and Their Extracts:* Volume 1 Pharmacognosy.

[13] Ashraf MA, Khatun A, Sharmin T, et al. MPDB 1.0: a medicinal plant database of India. *Bioinformation.* 2014;10(6):384-6. Published 2014 Jun 30. doi:10.6026/97320630010384.

[14] Rakotoarivelo NH, Rakotoarivony F, Ramarosandratana AV, et al. Medicinal plants used to treat the most frequent diseases encountered in Ambalabe rural community, Eastern Madagascar. *J Ethnobiol Ethnomed.* 2015;11:68. Published 2015 Sep 15. doi:10.1186/s13002-015-0050-2.

[15] Yuan H, Qianqian M, Ye L and Piao G. The Traditional Medicine and Modern Medicine from Natural Products. *Molecules* 2016, 21, 559; doi:10.3390/molecules21050559.

[16] Web WHO (2007). WHO guidelines on good manufacturing practices (GMP) for herbal medicines.

[17] Tripathi IP. Chemistry, Biochemistry and Ayurveda of Indian Medicinal Plants. Publisher: International E Publication, 2010.

[18] USA Forest Service. *Active Plant Ingredients Used for Medicinal Purposes.* Available From: https://www.fs.fed.us/wildflowers/ethnobotany/medicinal/ingredients.shtml.

[19] Sheikh H. Alternative medicine in India. Stethoscope. *The Independent* 24 September, 2018.

[20] *WHO Traditional Herbal Remedies for Primary Health Care.* Available From: apps.who.int/medicinedocs/documents/s22298en/s22298en.pdf.

[21] Joshi LS and Pawar HA. Herbal Cosmetics and Cosmeceuticals: An Overview. *Nat Prod Chem Res* 3: 170. doi:10.4172/23296836.1000170.

[22] Aburjai T and Natsheh FM. Plants Used in Cosmetics. *Phytother. Res.* 17, 987–1000 (2003) DOI: 10.1002/ptr.1363.

[23] Teron R, Borthaku SK. *Folklore claims of some medicinal plants as antidote against poisons among the Karbis of Assam*, India.

[24] Jahan R, Jannat K, Islam MMM and others. A Review of Two Plants Used Traditionally in India for Treatment of Snake Bites. *J Pharmacol Clin Toxicol* 6(3):1113.

[25] Rashid S. Chapter 5. Heritage, Folk Medicine and Kaviraji Treatment in India. *Traditional Medicine Sharing Experiences from the Field.* Eivind Falk. Available From: http://www.ichngoforum.org/wp-content/uploads/2018/01/Traditional-Medicine-Final-Web-3.pdf.

[26] Lang JJ, Alam S, Cahill LE, et al. Global Burden of Disease Study Trends for Canada from 1990 to 2016. *CMAJ.* 2018;190(44):E1296-E1304.

[27] Yoon SJ, Kim YE, Kim EJ. Why They Are Different: Based on the Burden of Disease Research of WHO and Institute for Health Metrics and Evaluation. Biomed Res Int. 2018; 2018:7236194. Published 2018 Apr 23. doi:10.1155/2018/7236194Ekor M. The growing use of herbal medicines: issues relating to adverse reactions and challenges in monitoring safety. *Front Pharmacol.* 2014;4:177. Published 2014 Jan 10. doi:10.3389/fphar.2013.00177.

[28] Tchounwou PB, Yedjou CG, Patlolla AK, Sutton DJ. Heavy metal toxicity and the environment. *Exp Suppl.* 2012;101:133-64.

[29] Bhat SJ, Blank MD, Balster RL, Nichter M, Nichter M. Areca nut dependence among chewers in a South Indian community who do not also use tobacco. *Addiction.* 2010;105(7):1303-10.

[30] Basher A, Islam QT. Plants and Herbal Poisoning in India. *Clinical Toxinology* 2014, pp 1-19 DOI 10.1007/978-94-007-6288-6_28-1.

[31] Guo X, Mei N. Aloe vera: A review of toxicity and adverse clinical effects. *J Environ Sci Health C Environ Carcinog Ecotoxicol Rev.* 2016 Apr 2;34(2):77-96. doi: 10.1080/10590501.2016.1166826. PMID: 26986231.

[32] Kumar KJ, Sonnathi S, Anitha C, Santhoshkumar M. Eucalyptus oil poisoning. *Toxicol Int* 2015; 22:170-1.

[33] Jou-Fang D, Ger J, Wei-Jen T, Wei-Fong K, and Chen-Chang Y. Acute Toxicities of Betel Nut: Rare but Probably Overlooked Events. *Clinical Toxicology,* 39(4), 355–360 (2001).

[34] BoemekeL, Marcadenti A, Busnello FM, Bertaso C, Gottschall A. Effects of Coconut Oil on Human Health *Open Journal of Endocrine and Metabolic Diseases,* 5, 2015, 84-87. Available From: http://dx.doi.org/10.4236/ojemd.2015.57011.

[35] Paik DJ and Lee CH. Review of cases of patient risk associated with ginseng abuse and misuse. *J Ginseng Res.* 2015 Apr; 39(2): 89–93. doi: 10.1016/j.jgr.2014.11.005 PMID: 26045681.

[36] Hazra A. Adverse reactions to henna. *Indian Journal of Pharmacology* 2002; 34: 436-437.

[37] Nawab A, Farooq N. Review on green tea constituents and its negative effects. *The Pharma Innovation Journal* 2015; 4(1): 21-24.

[38] Assouly P. *Hair Loss Associated With Cucurbit Poisoning JAMA Dermatol.* 2018; 154(5):617-618. doi:10.1001/jamadermatol.2017.6128.

[39] *WebMD Vitamins and Supplements.* Available From: https://www.webmd.com/vitamins/ai/ingredientmono-154/rosemary.

[40] *WebMD Vitamins and Supplements.* Available From: https://www.webmd.com/vitamins/ai/ingredientmono-662/turmeric.

[41] Tsai HH, Lin HW, Simon PA, Tsai H. Y., Mahady GB. Evaluation of documented drug interactions and contraindications associated with herbs and dietary supplements: a systematic literature review *Ernst. Int J Clin Pract* 2012; 66: 1019-20. doi.org/10.1111/j.1742-1241.2012.03008.

[42] Kumar S, Paul S, Walia YM and others. Therapeutic Potential of Medicinal Plants: A Review. *J. Biol. Chem. Chron.* 2015, 1(1), 46-54.

[43] Rautela I. Traditional medicine used by Tribal Communities of India. Health in: *Web Scientific India Magazine* 30 Apr – 2018.

Chapter 4

ALTERNATIVE TREATMENTS FOR MINOR GI AILMENTS

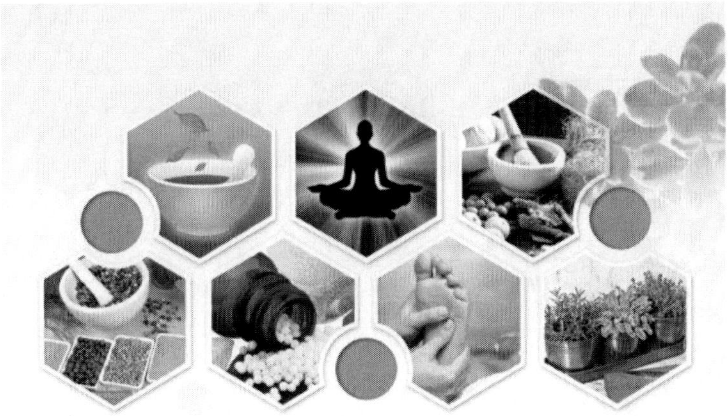

1. ABSTRACT

About 80% of the population worldwide use a variety of traditional medicine, including herbal medicines, for the diagnosis, prevention and treatment of illnesses, and for the improvement of general well-being. Total consumer spending on herbal dietary supplements in the United States reached an estimated $8.085 billion in 2017. In addition, the 8.5% increase in total sales from 2016 is the strongest growth for these products in more than 15 years. The main reason to use herbal products in these countries is the assumption of a better tolerability compared to synthetic drugs. Whereas in developing countries herbal medicines are mostly the only available and affordable treatment option. Surveys from industrialized countries reveal as main health areas in which herbal products are used upper airway diseases including cough and common cold; other leading causes are gastrointestinal, nervous and urinary complaints up to painful conditions such as rheumatic diseases, joint pain and stiffness. Gastrointestinal disorders are the most widespread problems in health care. Many factors may upset the GI tract and its motility (or ability to keep moving), including: eating a diet low in fiber; lack of motion or sedentary lifestyle; frequent traveling or changes in daily routine; having excessive dairy products; anxiety and depression; resisting the urge to have a bowel movement habitually or due to pain of hemorrhoids; misuse of laxatives (stool softeners) that, over time, weaken the bowel muscles; calcium or aluminum antacids, antidepressants, iron pills, narcotics; pregnancy. About 30% to 40% of adults claim to have frequent indigestion, and over 50 million visits are made annually to ambulatory care facilities for symptoms related to the digestive system. Over 10 million endoscopies and surgical procedures involving the GI tract are performed each year. Community-based studies from around the world demonstrate that 10% to 46% of all children meet the criteria for RAP. Gastrointestinal disorders such as chronic or acute diarrhea, malabsorption, abdominal pain, and inflammatory bowel diseases can indicate immune deficiency, present in 5% to 50% of patients with primary immunodeficiencies. The gastrointestinal tract is the largest lymphoid organ in the body, so it is not surprising that intestinal diseases are common among immunodeficient patients. Gastroenterologists therefore must be able to diagnose and treat patients with primary immunodeficiency. Further, pathogens do influence the gut function. On the other hand, dietary habits and specific food types can play a significant role in the onset, treatment, and prevention of many GI disorders. Many of these can be prevented or minimized by maintaining a healthy lifestyle, and practicing good bowel habits.

Keywords: herbs, bowel, gastric mucosa, probiotics, economic burden, HRQoL

Abbreviations

ACG	The American College of Gastroenterology
GERD	Gastroesophageal Reflux Disease
PPIs	Proton Pump Inhibitors
RAP	Recurrent Abdominal Pain
FGIDs	Functional gastrointestinal disorders
PDS	Postprandial Distress Syndrome
CAM	Complementary and Alternative Medicine
FD	Functional Dyspepsia
CC	Chronic Constipation
QoL	Quality Of Life
ESPGHAN	European Society for Paediatric Gastroenterology Hepatology and Nutrition
NASPGHAN	North American Society for Pediatric Gastroenterology, Hepatology and Nutrition
CSID	Congenital Sucrase-Isomaltase Deficiency
FODMAPs	Fermentable Oligosaccharides, Disaccharides, Monosaccharides and Polyols
SIBO	Small Intestinal Bacterial Overgrowth
NCGS	(Nonceliac Gluten Sensitivity
ATIs	α-Amylase/Trypsin Inhibitors
Ni ACM	Nickel Allergic Contact Mucositis
HRQoL	Health-Related quality of life

HRU	Healthcare Resource Utilization
5-HT3	5-Hydroxytryptamine-3 Receptor
FAO	Food and Agriculture Organization of the United Nations
DOH	Department of Health
ALE	Artichoke Leaf Extract
IBD	Inflammatory Bowel Disease
PD	Parkinson's Disease
CD	Crohn's Disease
UC	Ulcerative Colitis
DS	Dietary Supplement
EIMs	Extraintestinal Manifestations
CDAI	Crohn's Disease Activity Index
SES-CD	Simple Endoscopic Score for Crohn's Disease
PUD	Peptic Ulcer Disease
EGD	Esophagogastroduodenoscopy
BPAE	Bauhinia Purpurea Aqueous Extract
HDS	Herbal Dietary Supplements
GRAS	Generally Regarded As Safe
QPS	Qualified Presumption of Safety
EFSA	European Food Safety Authority
MAP	Mitogen-Activated Protein
ERK	Extracellular Signal-Regulated Kinase
SCFAs	Short-Chain Fatty Acids
CagA	Cytotoxin-associated gene A
SIBO	Small Intestinal Bacterial Overgrowth

1.1. Article Highlights

1. About 80% of the population worldwide use a variety of traditional medicine.
2. Sales of HDS in US passed $8 billion in 2017, with 8.5% increase in total sales from 2016.
3. In community settings, almost 50% of patients with FGIDs used CAM therapies.
4. GERD affects up to 40% of the population, 40%-50% of patients with GERD have abnormal peristalsis.
5. 20–30% continue to experience reflux symptoms despite PPI treatment.
6. Dyspepsia affects 20% of the global population, 30–70% of the patients with functional dyspepsia experience delayed gastric emptying.
7. Dyspepsia prevalence was 30.4% in India, 24% in Spain and 45% in Nigeria.
8. The prevalence of functional dyspepsia is 12-15% in patients with IBS.

9. 30% of the general population experiences constipation during life time but incidence sometimes rises up to 80% in critically ill patients.
10. The economic burden of IBS in the U.S. is estimated at $28 billion annually, 32% of IBS-C patients suffer depression as their condition almost every day in the previous month.
11. Sexual dysfunction is positively associated with perceived GI symptom severity and HRQoL.

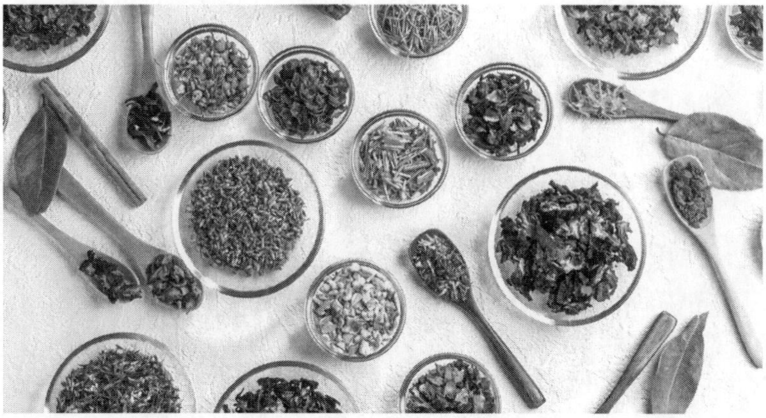

Figure 1. Herbs for GI disorders.

2. INTRODUCTION

The digestive system is dedicated to breaking down food and allowing its nutrients to be absorbed into the bloodstream, from where they are then carried to every part of the body. Spices and herbal remedies have been used since ancient times to treat a variety of disorders. It has been experimentally demonstrated that spices, herbs, and their extracts possess antimicrobial, anti-inflammatory, antirheumatic, lipid-lowering, hepatoprotective, nephroprotective, antimutagenic and anticancer activities, besides their gastroprotective and anti-ulcer activities. Nowadays, several experimental studies and, to a lesser extent, clinical trials have also emphasized the role of herbs in the treatment of a variety of disorders. Several herbs and herbal extracts have been shown to possess antibacterial properties. For instance, onion, garlic, ginger, pepper and mustard have demonstrated antimicrobial activity against several types of bacteria. Tayel and El-Tras have recently reported a potent antibacterial activity of cinnamon and clove against several bacterial strains. Some spices possess antifungal activity. Beside their antifungal activity, herbs have also shown vermicidal, nematocidal and molluscicidal potential. In addition, gingerol, the active ingredient of ginger, and eugenol have shown anti-inflammatory and antirheumatic activity. More recent studies have also demonstrated anti-inflammatory and antirheumatic properties of herbs. Furthermore, gingerol and curcumin have also shown lipid-lowering potential in experimental animals as well as in clinical trials. The mechanism of epigastric pain and dyspepsia induced by red and black pepper is not well-defined. However, it is believed to be a consequence of inhibition of gastric surface hydrophobicity, enhancement of surface wettability and activation of intramucosal pain receptors. Some spices may stimulate acid secretion and have deleterious effects on the gastric mucosal lining. Intragastric perfusion of albino rats with aqueous extracts of red pepper, fennel, omum/ajwain, cardamom, black pepper, cumin and coriander have stimulated a cholinergic response, and/or via other mechanism(s) have induced acid secretion with a respectively.

3. GERD

The AGC guidelines define GERD as "symptoms or complications resulting from the reflux of gastric contents into the esophagus or beyond, into the oral cavity (including larynx) or lung. GERD is one of the most common diseases in society, affecting up to 40% of the population [22]. A systematic review demonstrated that the prevalence of GERD ranged from 18.1% to 27.8% in North America, 8.8% to 25.9% in Europe, 2.5% to 7.8% in East Asia, 8.7% to 33.1% in the Middle East, 11.6% in Australia, and 23.0% in South America [1]. The cardinal symptoms of GERD are heartburn and regurgitation. However, GERD may present with a variety of other symptoms, including water brash, chest pain or discomfort, dysphagia, belching, epigastric pain, nausea, and bloating. In addition, patients may experience extraesophageal symptoms like cough, hoarseness, throat clearing, throat pain or burning, wheezing, and sleep disturbances [2]. Approximately 50% of the patients presenting with heartburn have erosive esophagitis on upper endoscopy, up to 70% of these patients have normal endoscopy findings. Furthermore, 40% of those with normal endoscopy findings and normal pH test results have reflux hypersensitivity (a positive correlation between symptoms and reflux events), and 60% have functional heartburn [8]. Impaired aspects of quality of life are disturbed sleep, reduced vitality, generalized body pain, unsatisfactory sex life, and anxiety. Nocturnal symptoms caused by reflux appear to have a particularly marked influence on quality of life and the burden of illness imposed by GERD also has an impact on work productivity [23]. Studies have demonstrated that symptom frequency, severity, or combination of both are not predictive of any specific phenotypic presentation of GERD [3]. However, elderly patients with GERD appear to experience a more severe mucosal disease that is associated with overall milder and more atypical symptoms [4]. 40%-50% of patients with GERD have abnormal peristalsis. This dysmotility is particularly severe in about 20% of patients because of very low amplitude of peristalsis and/or abnormal propagation of the peristaltic waves (ineffective esophageal motility) 17]. Other symptoms of GERD include: sore throat; sour taste in the back of the mouth; asthma symptoms (prevalence of GERD found in 30% to 65% patients with asthma), dry cough; trouble swallowing [18, 19]. Psychological comorbidity (anxiety, hypervigilance, depression, and somatization) does play an important role in patients with refractory heartburn [7]. GERD has emerged as a comorbidity of asthma and COPD. The prevalence of GERD in asthma patients has ranged from 25% to 80%, 38% of asthma patients had GERD in another study [1, 44]. The prevalence of GERD in COPD ranges from 17% to 78%. Although GERD is usually confined to the lower esophagus in some individuals, it may be associated with pulmonary micro-aspiration of gastric contents [45]. The overall prevalence of IBS symptoms in the GERD population ranges from 10-74% [64].

Exhibit 1. Non-drug treatment options of GERD [10, 20, 30]

1.	Elevation of the bed head (15 cm)
2.	Moderation in the ingestion of the following foods (based on symptom correlation): fatty foods, citrus, coffee, alcoholic and/or carbonated beverages, mint, peppermint, tomato, chocolate
3.	Refraining from wearing tight-fitting clothes: Clothes that are tight around the waist can put extra pressure on your stomach. This added pressure can then affect the LES, increasing reflux.
4.	Avoidance of lying down in the 2 h following meals. Lying down too soon after meals can induce heartburn.
5.	Eliminate distractions at mealtime. Avoid reading, checking phone, or watching television while eating. Chew each bite thoroughly. Eat smaller meals rather than big meals. Overeating puts more pressure on lower esophageal sphincter.
6.	Quitting of smoking
7.	Reduction of body weight, if overweight

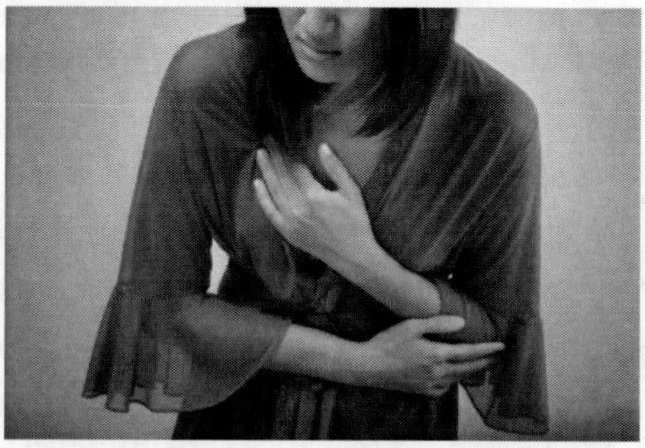

Figure 2. Gastroesophageal reflux disease. This disorder mainly affects the lower esophageal sphincter, a muscle section between the stomach and the esophagus. Stomach contents are refluxed or sent back upwards into the esophagus resulting in acid indigestion, heartburn and other maladies. Many Doctors believe that a weak lower esophageal sphincter causes GERD. It opens back up after food enters the stomach and allows the stomach's contents to move up back into the esophagus. Doctors also believe that hiatal hernias cause the reflux disease as well and are caused by pregnancy, obesity, severe straining of the body, extreme and rapid physical exertion, coughing and vomiting. It is also important to note that smoking contributes to the relaxation of the lower esophageal sphincter which leads to GERD. (Source: Causes and Treatment of Gerd: Gastroesophageal Reflux Disease. Web ercare24.com April 9th, 2017.)

3.1. GERD Expenditure

GERD is a common, chronic, relapsing symptom. Often people self-diagnose and self-treat it even though health-related quality of life is significantly impaired. In the lack of a valid alternative approach, current treatments focus on suppression of gastric acid secretion by the use of PPIs, but people with GERD have a significantly lower response rate to therapy [9], approximately 20–30% continue to experience reflux symptoms despite PPI treatment [11]. 30–40% of patients receiving medical therapy with PPIs experience troublesome breakthrough symptoms, and recent evidence suggests that this therapy is related to increased risk of complications [12]. In the US alone, overall spending on all GI diseases is estimated to be $142 billion (in 2009 US dollars) per year in direct and indirect costs. GERD accounts for approximately $15–20 billion of these direct and indirect costs. It has been estimated that prescribed medications for GERD, primarily PPIs, account for over 50% of prescriptions for all digestive diseases, resulting in around $10 billion in annual direct health care costs [25, 26]. Extraesophageal manifestations of reflux, including LPR, asthma, and chronic cough, have been estimated to cost $5438 per patient in direct medical expenses in the first year after presentation and $13,700 for 5 years [28].

3.2. Herbs for GERD Management

Some research has also shown improved symptoms in people with GERD who take peppermint oil. Historically, ginger has been used to treat other gastrointestinal ailments, including heartburn. This may reduce overall swelling and irritation in the esophagus. Caraway, garden angelica, German chamomile flower, greater celandine, licorice root, lemon balm, milk thistle and turmeric have little clinical evidence to support their effectiveness [29]. Fermented foods, like kimchi (alkaline), can be incredibly helpful for digestive system. Consuming a spoonful of mustard during the onset of acid reflux symptoms of heartburn by balancing pH levels. Many patients have seen significant benefits from snacking tasty nuts (especially almond), to be consumed raw, organic and salt-free. Both bananas and apples contain natural antacids that can help relieve or prevent an onset of acid reflux [26]. Marshmallow (*Althea officinalis* L.) contains a mucilage quality (may interfere with the absorption of other medications) which helps to coat the esophagus and stomach lining, creating a protective barrier against stomach acid. It's an effective stimulator of cell physiology of epithelial cells which can prove the traditional use of Marshmallow preparations for treatment of irritated mucous membranes within tissue regeneration [31, 32]. Chewing DGL (deglycyrrhizinated licorice) also helps boost enzyme production, allowing for easier and quicker digestion as well as better absorption of nutrients [32]. Use of low doses of pure glycyrrhetinic acid and bilberry anthocyanosides, together with alginic acid as addon therapy, substantially improves symptoms in patients with nonerosive reflux disease without increasing side effects or worsening tolerability or compliance [33]. To add to all that nutrition, papaya is an excellent treatment for acid reflux. It contains a proteolytic enzyme that breaks down proteins in the digestive system into amino acids. The active ingredient, papaine, is helpful to the digestion of fats and carbs. It aids in digestion and allows body to make acid. The potassium in papaya (*Carica papaya* L.) also introduces healthy bacteria into intestines. This can prevent stomach from working as hard and helps to stop indigestion and reflux. Papaya is used as a natural remedy in abnormal digestion in tropical and industrialized countries [34-36]. The fenugreek fiber effects were generally similar to the results produced by an OTC antacid medication (ranitidine at 75 mg, twice a day). 2 weeks intake of a fenugreek fiber product, taken 30 min before two meals/day, diminished heartburn severity [37]. The cytoprotective effect of the seeds seemed to be not only due to the anti-secretory action but also to the effects on mucosal glycoproteins. The fenugreek seeds also prevented the rise in lipid peroxidation induced by ethanol presumably by enhancing antioxidant potential of the gastric mucosa thereby lowering mucosal injury. Histological studies revealed that the soluble gel fraction derived from the seeds was more effective than omeprazole in preventing lesion formation [38]. An involvement of *Opuntia ficus-indica* mucilages (mainly cultivated in the Mediterranean region and in Central America) has been hypothesized, mainly formed by arabinogalactan and galacturonic acid, forming a defense layer in these gastroprotective effects. The mucilage is strongly viscous which because of the negative charges causes strong intermolecular repulsion, resulting in expansion of the molecules. It is believed that this changing in molecular shape could be responsible for the protection of the gastric mucosa [13-15]. Olive leaf extract possesses antioxidant properties, which can positively influence gastroprotection. The main iridoide monoterpene oleuropein contained in olive leaf was usually thought to be responsible for pharmacological effects but it was recently observed that olive leaf is as a stable source of bioactive flavonoids. In fact, the contribution of flavonoids to the overall radical scavenging activity of olive leaf extracts has been investigated and luteolin 7-O-glucoside was found to be one of the dominant scavengers (8–25%) [16]. Turmeric (*Curcuma longa*) and its compounds (especially Curcumin) should be considered as a promising alternative for patients who suffer from digestive disorders because it is safe, inexpensive, and ubiquitously available. Curcumin has been defined as the most active component in C. longa and has considerable gastroprotective and antiulcerogenic effect. Improvement in clinical scores of GERD and GERD Activity Index is proven with turmeric [39, 40]. German chamomile (*Matricaria recutita*) (contains flavonoids, in particular apigeningastric shown protective effect in clinical trial) and bismuth have known gastric protective properties, and *Atropa belladonna* contains anticholinergic agents that have bronchodilatory effect. Complementary treatments containing these ingredients could be used to treat patient with asthma patients having GERD, and if effective, could be an additional treatment tool that could also reduce the use of long-term inhaled corticosteroids and proton pump inhibitor treatment and thus their side effects [41]. Although a number of toxic effects have been attributed to bismuth compounds in humans: nephropathy, encephalopathy, osteoarthropathy, gingivitis, stomatitis and colitis. Whether hepatitis is a side effect, however, is open to dispute [42]. Aloe Vera was safe and well tolerated and reduced the frequencies of all the assessed GERD symptoms, but nephrotoxicity and hepatotoxicity (also human carcinogen, Group 2B) is keeping its use in a controversial position [46-49].

4. Dyspepsia

Dyspepsia is common, affecting approximately 20% of the global population, and is frequently encountered in primary care. Functional dyspepsia (FD) is one of the most prevalent gastrointestinal disorders, and is defined as a chronic disease with persistent upper gastrointestinal symptoms without any explanatory organic or metabolic causes [50]. Dyspepsia is a very common GI complaint, with up to one in five individuals affected worldwide. Of those with dyspepsia, around 40% will seek the advice of their primary care physician. Almost 15% of patients with dyspepsia are referred to secondary care for further investigation and management [58]. When broadly defined, dyspepsia occurs in 40%, leads to GP consultation in 5% and referral for endoscopy in 1% of the population annually. In patients with signs or symptoms severe enough to merit endoscopy, 40% have functional or non-ulcer dyspepsia, 40% have GERD and 13% have some form of ulcer [62]. Heartburn and acid regurgitation are no longer considered to be symptoms of dyspepsia, but of GER. Both the underlying causes and progress of functional dyspepsia are still unknown. That is largely true of GERD as well [65]. One-third of patients who visit general physician practices are patients with dyspepsia syndrome; and half of patients who visit gastroenterologists are also patients with dyspepsia syndrome [66]. The prevalence of functional dyspepsia was UK (21%), US (26%), Jordan (60%), western Iran (18%), China (18.4%) found in a 2014 study [51]. In a German study, around one third of the normal persons interviewed reported dyspeptic symptoms, including acute dyspepsia in 6.5% and chronic dyspepsia in 22.5% of cases [52]. 8%-30% and 8%-23% of Asian people suffer from of uninvestigated dyspepsia and FD, respectively [53]. Dyspepsia prevalence was 30.4% in India, 5% in Scandinavian countries, 24% in Spain and 45% in Nigeria estimated [68]. Smoking might affect all gastrointestinal functions including those of the esophagus, stomach, and colon, resulting in susceptibility to several kinds of FGIDs including GERD, FD, and IBS [54]. Potential lifestyle factors associated with dyspepsia include tobacco, alcohol, and analgesic consumption. Furthermore, dietary habits that include consumption of smoked food, fast food, salty food, coffee/tea, and spicy food were associated with aggravating the symptoms of dyspepsia; while fruits, vegetables, and water were noted to improve the symptoms [68]. FD is more prevalent in women (24.4%) than men (16.6%)

and its occurrence was found to increase significantly with age [69, 70]. Typical dyspeptic symptoms include postprandial fullness, early satiety, epigastric pain, and epigastric burning [55]. Visceral hypersensitivity, impaired gastric accommodation and impaired gastric emptying are commonly reported by patients with functional dyspepsia. Involvement of duodenal hypersensitivity to the luminal contents, small bowel dysmotility, psychological disturbances, central nervous system disorders and Helicobacter pylori infection also been reported [56]. Delayed gastric emptying has been reported by gastric scintigraphy in a large proportion (up to 45%) of dyspeptic patients, especially those with PDS [57]. About 30–70% of the patients with functional dyspepsia experience delayed gastric emptying [86]. The overall costs to the health service associated with managing dyspepsia are considerable, estimated to be over $18 billion per annum in the United States. Moreover, when one considers that dyspepsia impacts on physical, mental, and social aspects of health-related quality of life, the true overall costs to society are likely to be far higher, and also encompass loss of economic productivity due to sickness-related absence from work [58-60]. The risk of malignancy predominantly relates to increasing age, and so guidelines have previously recommended upper GI endoscopy to routinely investigate dyspepsia only when patients are aged 55 years and older [61]. The prevalence of functional dyspepsia (after normal upper endoscopy) is 12-15% in patients with IBS [64].

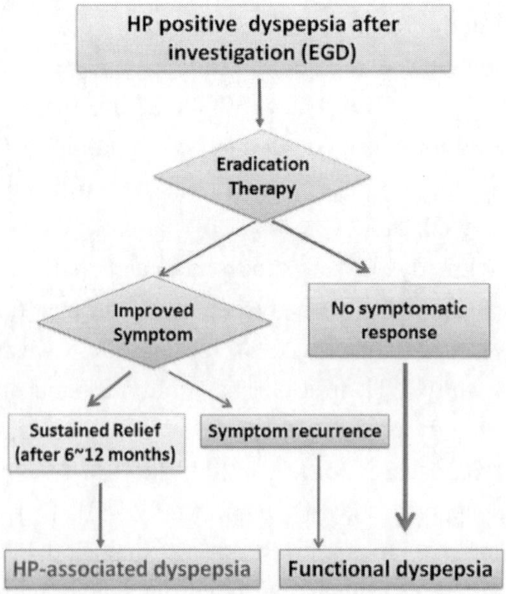

Figure 3. Diagnostic algorithm of Helicobacter pylori-associated dyspepsia. Patients with dyspeptic symptoms after negative routine laboratory and upper gastrointestinal endoscopy except for positive H. pylori tests, should undergo eradication therapy. If sustained symptomatic relief is obtained, their dyspeptic symptoms are considered as H. pylori-associated dyspepsia. On the other hand, if dyspeptic symptoms do not resolve or recur after eradication therapy, they are judged to have functional dyspepsia. EGD, oesophagastroduodenoscopy. (Source: Sugano K, Tack J, Kuipers EJ on behalf of faculty members of Kyoto Global Consensus Conference, et al. Kyoto global consensus report on Helicobacter pylori gastritis Gut 2015;64:1353-1367.)

Exhibit 2. Alarm features in patients with dyspepsia [61]

1.	Age > 55 years with new onset dyspepsia*
2.	Evidence of overt gastrointestinal bleeding including melaena or haematemesis
3.	Dysphagia, particularly if progressive, and odynophagia
4.	Persistent vomiting
5.	Unintentional weight loss
6.	Palpable abdominal or epigastric mass or abnormal adenopathy
7.	Family history of upper gastrointestinal cancer
8.	Evidence of iron deficiency anemia after blood testing

* ACG/CAG guidelines now recommend an age threshold of 60 years or older.

4.1. Rationale of Alternative Treatments with Dyspepsia

Prokinetics are recommended for the treatment of functional dyspepsia (FD) but systematic reviews give conflicting results on the efficacy of these agents [62]. Although several PPI-related adverse effects have been reported, their clinical relevance is not yet clear. Again, their beneficial effects for functional dyspepsia have not been fully confirmed [63]. The popularity of CAM in treating FGIDs has steadily increased in Western countries. In community settings, almost 50% of patients with FGIDs used CAM therapies. Herbal remedies consist of multi-component preparations, whose mechanisms of action have not been systematically clarified. Few studies analyzed the effectiveness of acupuncture in Western countries, yielding conflicting results and possibly reflecting a population bias of this treatment. Hypnosis has been extensively used in irritable bowel syndrome, but few data support its role in treating FD [67].

Exhibit 3. Adverse events reported in patients treated with proton pump inhibitors [63, 84]

Adverse Events Unrelated to Acid Inhibition	Adverse Events Related to Acid Inhibition
Allergic reaction to drug chemicals	Pneumonia
Collagenous colitis	Gastrointestinal infection
Acute interstitial nephritis	Gastric carcinoid tumor
Chronic kidney disease	Gastric fundic mucosal hypertrophy
Drug interaction	Changes in gut microbiome
Dementia	Small intestinal bacterial overgrowth
Cerebral ischemic diseases	Iron deficiency
Ischemic cardiac diseases	Bone fracture; decrease calcium absorption; Vitamin B12 deficiency; Hypomagnesemia; Gastric fundic gland polyps; Gastric & Colon cancer; Spontaneous bacterial peritonitis; Hepatic encephalopathy; Drug interaction

4.1. Herbs and Probiotics for Dyspepsia

Flavonoid rich phytochemical composition of the root extract of *Glycyrrhiza glabra*, revealed significant decrease in symptoms scores of dyspepsia [71]. Adjuvant supplementation of honey-based formulation of Black Seed/ black caraway (*Nigella sativa*) can cause significant symptomatic improvement of patients with functional dyspepsia whom received the standard anti-secretory therapy [72]. Basil Leaf (*Ocimum basilicum* L) strengthens stomach, nervous system and is also carminative, also has been demonstrated to decrease acid and pepsin outputs, widely used as a spice and a typical ingredient of the healthy Mediterranean diet [73, 74]. The fruit of Amla (Phyllanthus emblica L.) has cytoprotective acid-reducing features, prevents indigestion, and controls acidity and well tolerated [75-77]. *Pistacia lenticus* Desf. (Mastaki) act against different microorganisms (Mustic gum) specially Helicobacter pylori, positively affect liver function, could be effective as an alternative regime in patients unwilling to undergo eradication with the triple therapy regime [78, 79]. Rhizome of Ginger (*Zingiber officinale* Roscoe) is stomach tonic, protective, antiulcer and is effective for digestion problems, bloating, and nausea, stimulated gastric emptying and antral contractions in patients with functional dyspepsia [80-83]. Iberogast (commercial preparation of 9 herbal extracts including bitter candy tuft, lemon balm leaf, chamomile flower, caraway fruit, licorice root, angelica root, milk thistle fruit, peppermint leaf, and greater celandine herb) has been shown to protect against the development of ulcers with decreased acid production, increased mucin production, an increase in prostaglandin E2 release, both safe and effective for treatment of functional dyspepsia and IBS in Children [21]. Licorice root, the dried rhizome or extracts of *glycyrrhiza glabra*, has long been used in botanical medicine for treatment of gastric inflammation, showed a significant decrease in total symptom scores ($p < 0.05$) and improvement in quality of life with functional dyspepsia [77]. Red pepper as a drug is given in atonic dyspepsia and flatulence due to increasing the motility in the gastric antrum, duodenum, proximal jejunum and colon. It can also increase parietal, pepsin, and bile acid secretions. Chilies are known to protect against gastrointestinal ailments including dyspepsia, loss of appetite, gastroesophageal reflux disease and gastric ulcer due to the several mechanisms such as reducing the food transition time through the gastrointestinal tract and anti-*Helico pylori* effects [85]. Celery (Apiumgraveolens), radish (Raphinussativus L.), rocket (*Eruka sativa*), and marjoram (Origanummajorana L.) demonstrated anti-ulcer effect in experimental investigations [86]. Probiotics appear effective in the treatment of FD through the normalization of gastric microbiota. The finding of an FD-type phylum profile can be used to characterize patients with FD and may serve as an objective biomarker for both the diagnosis and treatment of FD. Probiotics could be effective treatment for the indigestion via the reduction of Escherichia/Shigella, major source of toxic lipopolysaccharides in the upper GIT [98].

5. CONSTIPATION

Constipation is a common gastrointestinal problem, which causes many expenses for the community with an estimated prevalence of 1% to 80%, worldwide. Various factors are involved in the pathogenesis of the disease, including type of diet, genetic predisposition, colonic motility, absorption, social economic status, daily behaviors, and biological and pharmaceutical factors. Acute constipation may cause closure of the intestine, which may even require surgery. Chronic constipation is a complicated condition among older individuals, which is characterized by difficult stool passage [87]. To better characterize the condition, physicians conceive constipation objectively using defecation frequency, with a normal range of between three and 21 bowel movements per week [94]. Factors that may contribute to functional constipation include pain, fever, dehydration, dietary and fluid intake, psychological issues, toilet training, medicines, and family history of constipation [88]. Pathogenesis is multifactorial with focusing on the type of diet, genetic predisposition, colonic motility, and absorption, as well as behavioral, biological, and pharmaceutical factors. Furthermore, low fiber dietary intake, inadequate water intake, sedentary lifestyle, IBS, failure to respond to urge to defecate, and slow transit have been revealed to be associated with predisposition [87, 90]. About 30% of the general population experiences problems with constipation during life time. with elderly people and women being mostly affected. Constipation is also reported to occur in 2% to 25% of healthy people, but the incidence sometimes rises to 80% in critically ill patients [101].

Exhibit 4. Common causes of secondary constipation [90]

Drugs	Anabolic steroids, analgesics, opioids (codeine), NSAIDs, anticholinergics, anticonvulsivants, antidepressants, antihistamines, antihypertensives (verapamil e clonidine), anti-Parkinsonian, diuretics, antiacids containing calcium or alluminium, cholestyramine.
Neuropathic and myopathic disorders	Amyloidosis, Chagas disease, connective tissue disorders, CNS lesions, autonomic diabetic neuropathy, Hirschprung's disease, multiple sclerosis.
Idiopathic	Paraneoplastic syndromes, Parkinson's disease, dementia, scleroderma, post-viral colon-paresis, intestinal pseudo-obstruction, spinal or ganglion tumor, ischemia.
Electrolytic balance alterations	Hypokalemia, hypercalcemia
Organic intestinal diseases	Obstruction/stenosis: adenoma, cancer, diverticolitis, rectocele, hernia, foreign bodies, faecal impaction, IBD and complications.
	Anorectal abnormalities: anal stenosis or fissures, proctitis, rectocele, haemorrhoids.
Endocrine-metabolic causes	Hypothyroidism, diabetes mellitus, pregnancy and childbirth, dehydration, low fibers intake diet, hyperglycemia

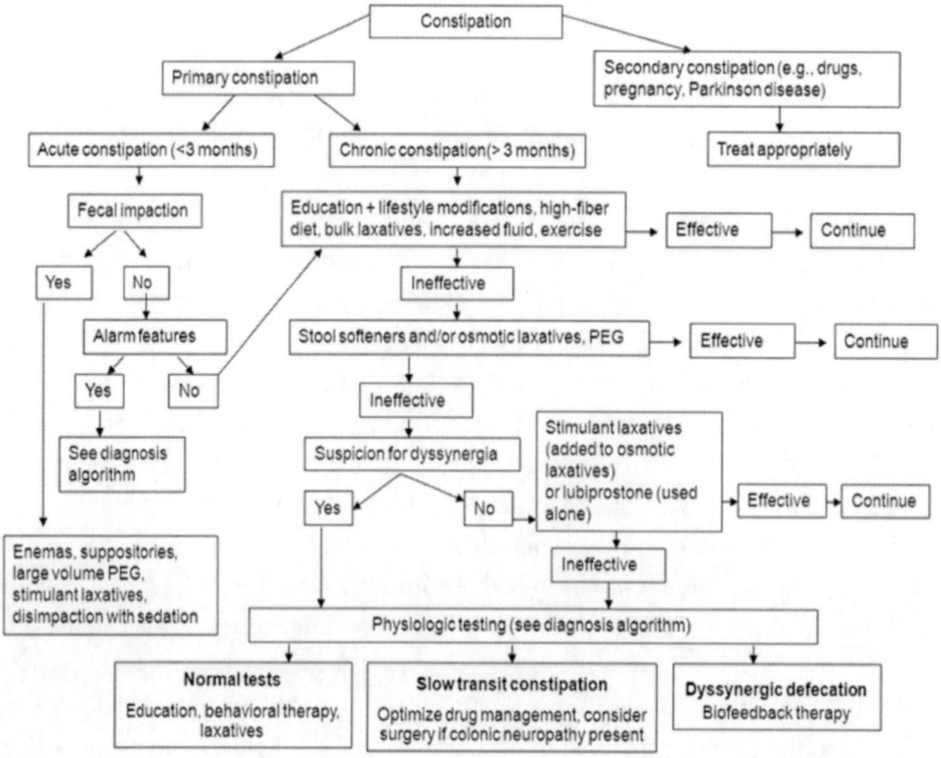

Figure 4. Initial management of acute primary constipation (symptoms <3 months). (Source: Constipation in adults: Treatment Practice. BMJ Best Practice). When constipation presents acutely, it is important to consider possible secondary causes, including colorectal cancer. Further investigations may be performed to exclude secondary causes. Enemas, suppositories, large volume polyethylene glycol solution (PEG), stimulant laxatives, or disimpaction with sedation may be required if there is fecal impaction. If fecal impaction is absent and secondary causes are excluded, the treatment is the same as for patients with chronic constipation. Initial steps in the management of chronic primary constipation are: Patient education; Lifestyle modifications; High-fiber diet; Increased fluid; Regular exercise; Bulk laxatives. Dietary and lifestyle changes may be helpful. Patients are advised to increase their daily dietary fiber and calorie intake (in patients with low caloric intake). Patients are advised on adequate fluid intake and encouraged to get regular nonstrenuous exercise. Modest exercise can help relieve constipation, especially if patients are sedentary or generally inactive. Patients are advised to dedicate time for bowel movements and to avoid postponing bowel movements when an urge for defecation is felt.

5.1. Prevalence and Economic Burden

Functional constipation is a prevalent condition in childhood, about 29.6% worldwide. Up to 84% of functionally constipated children suffer from fecal incontinence, while more than one-third of children present with behavioral problems primary or secondary due to constipation [88]. However, only a minority of patients (approximately 25%) uses medical treatments, whereas a considerable proportion relies on alternative solutions, following advices given in pharmacies or herbalist's shops [91, 92]. A population-based study of outpatient clinic and emergency department visits found outpatients taking five or more drugs had an 88% increased risk of experiencing an adverse drug effect compared to those who were taking fewer drugs [93]. According to reports from Western countries, the prevalence of CC in the general population ranges from 2% to 28%, with an increasing trend over years. Moreover, severe constipation is frequently observed in elderly women, with rates of 2 to 3 times higher than that of their male counterparts [95]. FGIDs, including chronic constipation (CC), are among the most frequent illnesses seen by gastroenterologists and account for up to one-half of patient care time (1). CC is a remarkably common and costly condition that can negatively impact the QoL, and result in a major social and economic burden [96]. 66,287 people in the UK were admitted to hospital with constipation as the main condition in 2014/15, equivalent to 182 people a day. 48,409 were unplanned e emergency admissions (this is equivalent to 13 3 per day). The total cost to hospitals for treating unplanned admissions due to constipation was £145 million in 2014/15. The figure is likely to be much higher for total NHS expenditure on constipation when including GP visits, home visits and prescriptions. The prescription cost of laxative costs is £101 million (Over the counter costs of laxatives will undoubtedly be higher). 1 in 7 adults are affected by constipation at any one time in UK [97]. Pregnancy predisposes women to developing constipation owing to physiologic and anatomic changes in the gastrointestinal tract. For instance, rising progesterone levels during pregnancy and reduced motilin hormone levels lead to increases in bowel transit time. Also, there is increased water absorption from the intestines, which causes stool to dry out. Decreased maternal activity and increased vitamin supplementation (eg, iron and calcium) can further contribute to constipation. Later in pregnancy, an enlarging uterus might slow onward movement of feces. Constipation can result in serious complications such as fecal impaction, but such complications are rare [107].

5.2. Herbs and Probiotics for Constipation

Cascara sagrada used (hydroxyanthraquinone glycosides found in the dried bark) to be approved by the U.S. FDA as an OTC drug for constipation. However, over the years, concerns were raised about its safety and effectiveness (causes nausea, vomiting and griping abdominal pain) [98-100]. Psyllium is the most commonly used bulking agent in Canada. In placebo-control trials, psyllium has been shown to decrease stool transit time, and improve stool frequency, consistency and weight; when psyllium was compared with lactulose, the magnitude of effects on stool frequency was similar, associated benefit of dietary fiber in reducing coronary heart disease and lowering low-density lipoprotein cholesterol, it is generally recommended as the initial conservative treatment for chronic constipation [100]. Recently, maintenance of intestinal motility has become an important issue in intensive-care medicine. Although drugs such as metoclopramide, erythromycin, neostigmine, and others are reported to resolve incompetent intestinal motility [101], there are problems with drug tolerance. Rhubarb has been widely used as a traditional Chinese herbal medicine since ancient times. Sennoside A and other dianthrone derivatives are reported to be the active ingredients causing rhubarb's laxative effect. To induce its laxative effect, rhubarb needs to be metabolized to rhein anthrone by β-glucosidase, which is produced by gut microbiota [102]. Improvement in intestinal motility can prevent sepsis of gut origin [103]. Rhubarb contains dianthrone glucosides (sennosides A to F) and anthraquinones (e.g., rhein, aloe-emodin, emodin, physcion, chrysophanol); Among these components, sennosides (i.e., stimulant laxatives), have been well documented for their pharmacological action on constipation [104]. Senna is used to treat constipation and clear the bowel before some medical procedures.it should only be used in the short term and at the recommended doses. Long-term and high-dose use has been reported to cause liver damage [105]. Senna induced dermatitis is rare, but may occur when patients need a higher dose. Pediatric caregivers should advise families of the rare side effect of skin blistering and educate them to change the diaper frequently in children who are not toilet- trained to reduce stool to skin exposure. Senna is a safe treatment option for constipation in children [106]. Until more data are available, the use of probiotics for the treatment of constipation should be considered investigational.

Exhibit 5. Summary of randomized controlled trials of probiotics for the management of chronic constipation [114]

Population	Intervention	Comparator	Author's Conclusion
n = 159 (control n = 80, intervention n = 79)	*B. lactis* DN-173 010	Acidified milk without probiotics	Increased stool frequency, but not statistically significant compared with control group
n = 44 (control n = 22, intervention n = 22)	*L. reuteri* DSM 17938	Identical placebo	Increased bowel frequency
n = 30 (control n = 15, intervention n = 15)	*B. lactis* Bi-07	Fresh cheese without probiotics	Beneficial effects
n = 126 (control n = 63, intervention n = 63)	*B. lactis* DN-173010	Acidified milk without probiotics	Beneficial effects on stool frequency, defecation condition and stool consistency
n = 17 (cross-over design)	*B. lactis* GCL2505	Milk-like drink	Beneficial effects
n = 100 (control n = 34, Intervention: high dose n = 33 low dose n = 33)	*B. lactis* HN019	Capsules with rice maltodextrin	Decreased whole gut transit time in a dose-dependent manner
n = 90 (control n = 43, intervention n = 47)	*L. casei* Shirota	Fermented milk without probiotics	Improvement in constipation severity
n = 20 (cross-over design)	*L. paracasei* IMPC 2.1	Artichokes without probiotics	Beneficial effects
n = 70 (control n = 35, intervention n = 35)	*L. casei* shirota	Beverage without probiotics	Beneficial effects on self-reported severity of constipation and stool consistency

Current ESPGHAN/NASPGHAN recommendations that probiotics should not be used in the treatment of functional constipation in children [113]. The bacterial endotoxin lipopolysaccharide may influence intestinal motility by delaying gastric emptying and inducing sphincteric dysfunction. Human colonic gases produced by microflora may also be associated with changes in gut motility. For example, breath methane excretion in patients with slow-transit constipation was greater than in healthy subjects or patients with normal-transit constipation, supporting the idea that methane can slow gut transit. Collectively, the altered intestinal microbiota may play an essential role in the pathogenesis of chronic constipation [114].

5.3. Herbs in Pregnancy Induced Constipation

It has been estimated that approximately 11% to 38% of pregnant women experience constipation, which is generally described as infrequent bowel movements or difficult evacuation [107]. The prevalence of herbal medicine utilization in pregnancy ranges between 7% and 55% in different geographical, social and cultural settings, and ethnic groups [108]. The majority of the studies reported the highest use of herbs during the first trimester with the frequency varying from 17.3% to 67.5% in Middle East [107]. It is a well-documented fact that the risk in pregnancy is unknown for 91.2% of the approved medications. The use of herbal products which are not usually tested in clinical trials during pregnancy could result in immense risk to the mother and fetus [109, 110]. Since herbal medicines are a part of traditional medicine, they are not included in the FDA pregnancy categories giving a false impression of safety. The whole extracts of these herbal drugs contain numerous active molecules that could elicit adverse effects including teratogenicity [111, 112].

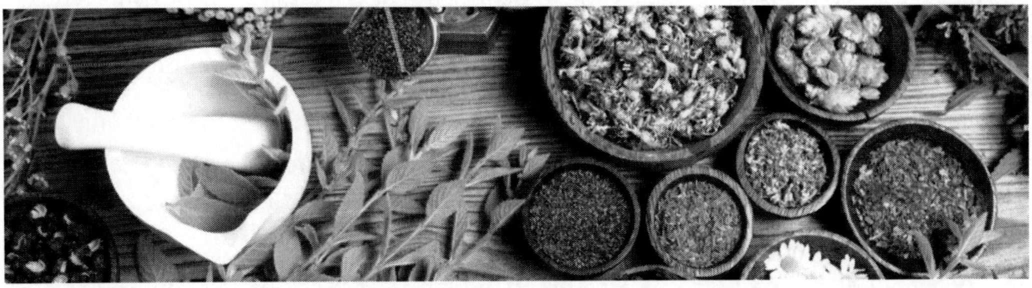

Figure 5. Herbs in pregnancy. Although medicine has replaced most natural supplements with a synthetic substitute, there are many who still look to natural herbs and vitamins to provide essential nutrition and relief of common discomforts for pregnant women. The FDA urges pregnant women not to take any herbal products without talking to their health-care provider first. Herbs may contain substances that can cause miscarriage, premature birth, uterine contractions, or injury to the fetus. (Source: Herbs and Pregnancy: Risks, Caution & Recommendations. Web American Pregnancy Association.)

6. Irritable Bowel Syndrome (IBS)

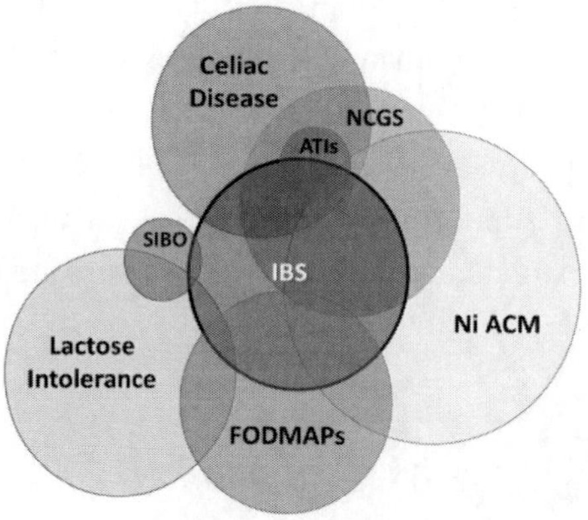

Figure 6. Clinical overlap between IBS and IBS-like disorders. IBS; FODMAPs; SIBO; NCGS; ATIs; Ni ACM. FODMAPs have been shown to share clinical characteristics and trigger foods with both lactose intolerance and Ni ACM. Specifically, many foods rich in FODMAPs are also high in lactose. Given the high prevalence of lactose intolerance, it is not surprising that a diet low in FODMAPs may reduce or even resolve gastrointestinal and extra-intestinal symptoms. The same thing can be true for foods rich in Ni, very numerous in the FODMAPs family, such as pears, cabbage, garlic, onion and legumes. Another important intersection exists between FODMAPs and NCGS, or even better between Ni ACM and NCGS: upon closer analysis, symptoms of suspected NCGS patients are actually triggered by associated Ni-rich ingredients or condiments (e.g., yeast or tomato), and not by gluten itself. As a consequence, foods such as bread, pasta with tomato sauce, pizza and bakery products turn into real traps for Ni-sensitive and/or lactose intolerant patients, in defiance of the Mediterranean diet, recently declared part of the UNESCO's Intangible Heritage List.

IBS is present in patients with symptoms of chronic abdominal pain and altered bowel habits but no identifiable organic etiology [113]. Patients with IBS often associate their symptoms to certain foods [115]. In CSID, recessive mutations in the SI gene (coding for the disaccharidase digesting sucrose and 60% of dietary starch) cause clinical features of IBS through colonic accumulation of undigested carbohydrates, triggering bowel symptoms [116]. Diagnosing IBS can be challenging due to the nonspecific nature of symptoms, overlapping upper and lower abdominal symptoms, and the frequent presence of somatic and psychological comorbidities. Despite these guidelines, there remains low awareness and little consensus on the use of diagnostic tests and surgical procedures in IBS. Furthermore, although surgery has no role in the recommended treatment approach for IBS, multiple studies have reported that this patient population is predisposed to unnecessary surgical procedures, suggesting a disconnect between the recommended best practices and real-world management of IBS [117]. Under certain ambiguous circumstances, an exclusive and pure diagnosis of IBS cannot be achieved because of food-dependent symptoms: in fact, up to 80% of IBS patients identify food as a possible trigger for their symptoms, so they increasingly ask for dietary and behavioral counseling [118]. Common practices for IBS management begin with diet and lifestyle modification, and in more severe cases, pharmacotherapy (e.g., antidepressants, smooth muscle antispasmodics, or secretagogues) [119].

6.1. Prevalence and Economic Burden

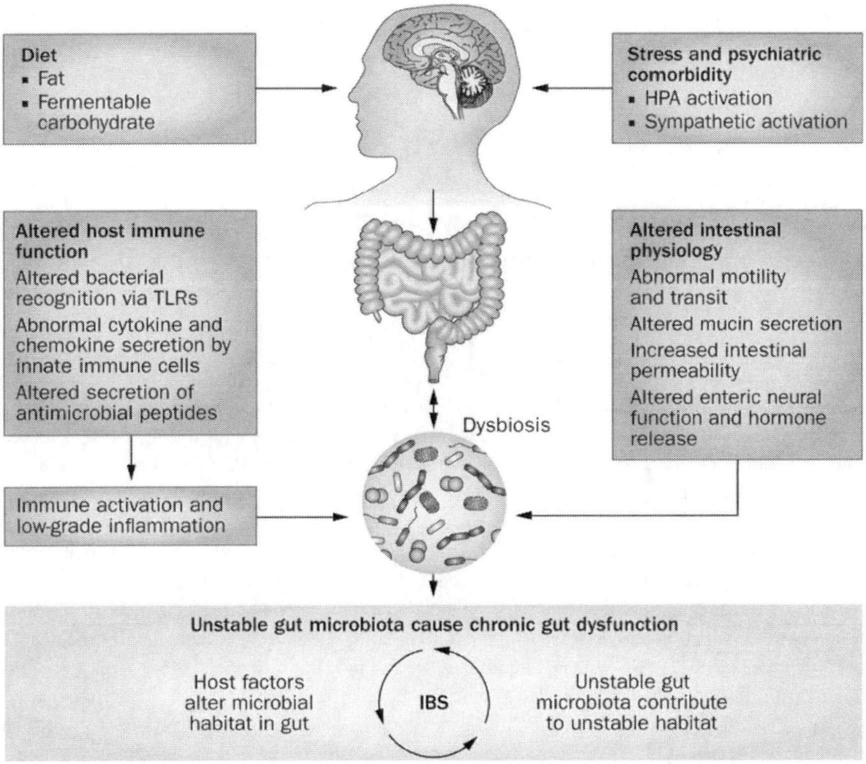

Figure 7. Unstable gut microbiota responsible for chronic gut malfunction. Studies reveal the gut microbiota in not only the expression of the intestinal manifestations of IBS, but also the psychiatric morbidity that coexists in up to 80% of patients with IBS. It is a condition for which investigators have long been in search of plausible underlying pathogeneses and it is inevitable that altered composition or function of the gut microbiota will be considered as a potential etiological factor in at least a subset of patients with IBS. (Source: Collins SM. A role for the gut microbiota in IBS. Nature Reviews Gastroenterology & Hepatology volume 11, pages 497–505 (2014).)

IBS affects both men and women of all ages. It is thought only a fraction of individuals with symptoms of IBS seek medical attention. The prevalence of IBS globally is 11%, however, it is thought that IBS often remains underdiagnosed. A survey of patients with IBS (both with and without a formal diagnosis) conducted by the Gastrointestinal Society in Canada showed that 46% had missed work or school due to IBS symptoms [120]. Its estimated prevalence is 10%–20%, although marked variation may exist based on geographical location; for example, its prevalence is 21% in South America versus 7% in Southeast Asia. It is nearly twice more common in women than men [118]. Various studies have reported prevalence to be approximately 8 to 12% in children, and 5 to 17% in adolescents [125]. IBS causes a significant burden on healthcare systems, due in part to the high level of HRU associated with IBS. Direct medical costs attributed to IBS in the US, excluding prescription and OTC medicines, were estimated at US $1.5–$10 billion per year in 2005. According to University at Buffalo, the economic burden of IBS in the U.S. is estimated at $28 billion annually [124]. A portion of these costs may be related to unnecessary and high-frequency tests, although few studies have assessed the factors underlying frequent tests and procedures among patients with IBS [117]. In IBS, it has been reported that 50% to 90% of patients have or had at some point one or more common psychiatric condition, including major depressive disorder, generalized anxiety disorder, social phobia, somatization disorder, or posttraumatic stress disorder [123].

Exhibit 6. Subtypes of IBS are recognized by the Rome IV criteria based on the person's reported predominant bowel habit, when not on medications [118, 120-122]

IBS-C	With predominant constipation. The symptoms most frequently reported for IBS-C are: abdominal pain, bloating and constipation. 32% of IBS-C respondents reported feeling depressed because of their condition almost every day in the previous month. HRQoL for those with IBS-C is low compared to those with chronic conditions such as diabetes, heart failure and heart defects, who have a high rate of mortality, and also those with asthma, migraine and rheumatoid arthritis, with well-known morbidity.
IBS-D	With predominant diarrhea. The symptoms most frequently reported for IBS-D are: abdominal pain and discomfort, abdominal bloating, distension, urgency and diarrhea. 47% of respondents with IBS-D stated that they had little or no ability to predict their symptoms on a daily basis. When asked how IBS-D affects them, 81% stated that they avoided situations where there was no nearby washroom.
IBS-M	With both constipation and diarrhea. In the United States, patients are equally distributed among IBS with diarrhea (IBS-D), IBS with constipation (IBS-C), and IBS with a mixed bowel pattern (IBS-M), whereas in Europe, studies have found either IBS-C (45.9%) or IBS-D (50%) as the main pattern group. IBS-M is a heterogeneous symptom group and thus requires that subclassification criteria be better defined. Use of laxative/antidiarrheal medications adds to the diagnostic complexity in a potentially more severe subset of IBS-M and should be assessed for accurate subclassification.
IBS-U	Un-subtyped IBS, has a lower prevalence (17.8%). Un-subtyped IBS subjects had the highest HR-QOL compared to other subtypes.

6.2. Lifestyle Modification

An important lifestyle adjustment that should be recommended to IBS patients is regular exercise. Mild exercise or physical activity has been shown to reduce IBS symptoms and alleviates bloating and gas production in several studies. Since regular exercise also helps to increase gastrointestinal motility it is beneficial in IBS-C patients with primary low GI movement and hard stools. As part of exercise, yoga has been investigated due to its low impact on joints and its relatively targeted postures that can help to reduce GI symptoms. Pranayama yoga administered twice daily has been shown to increase sympathetic tone and may benefit IBS-D patients that present with decreased sympathetic activity to the same degree than daily loperamide administration in the control group [127]. Fiber is defined as non-starch polysaccharides in agreement with FAO/WHO/DOH measurement methods. It includes β-glucans, pectins, gums, mucilages and some hemicelluloses. Dietary sources include oats, psyllium, ispaghula, nuts and seeds, some fruit and vegetables and pectins. An increase in fiber has often been suggested as an initial treatment for IBS [131].

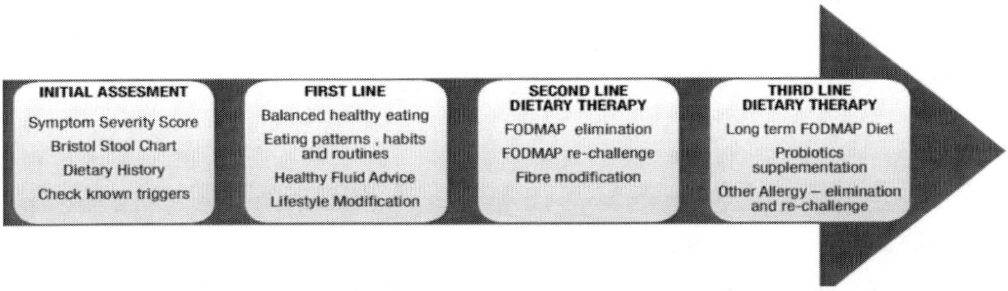

Figure 8. IBS Dietary Treatment Pathway. In the last 10 years, evidence has emerged for the restriction of a group of short chain fermentable carbohydrates which have collectively become known as FODMAPs. The common factor in these foods is the size and chain length of these carbohydrate molecules, as they all contain between 1 and 10 glucose molecules. This group of short-chain carbohydrates is susceptible to colonic fermentation by a number of possible mechanisms, which have been shown to exacerbate IBS symptoms. There is strong evidence to support three mechanisms of action: 1. Augmentation of small intestinal water 2. Increased colonic fermentation 3. Immune modulation. (Source: Jankovich E, Watkins A. Case Study: The low FODMAP diet reduced symptoms in a patient with endometriosis and IBS. S Afr J Clin Nutr 2017;30(4):32-36.)

6.3. Herbs and Probiotics for IBS

Pharmacological treatment of IBS varies from antidepressants including tricyclic antidepressants and selective serotonin reuptake inhibitors, to antispasmodics, 5-HT3 antagonists, 5-HT4 agonists, antibiotics, probiotics, and melatonin. But involvement of numerous factors in pathophysiology and a very significant placebo effect cause therapy of this disease to be more complex. Due to disappointing results with conventional IBS treatments, complementary and alternative medicines are becoming attractive options for many patients [126]. CAM alone and in conjunction with pharmacological treatments as an integrative approach to manage patients with IBS and improve their quality of life. Prokinetics are not specific to IBS and increase gastrointestinal motility in general by acting via dopamine and 5-HT3 receptors as antagonists or 5-HT4 receptors as agonists. Lubiprostone, a 5-HT4 agonist, has been recently approved to treat IBS-C in women through activation of chlorine channels leading to increased water secretion into the lumen which decreased transit time and associated visceral pain in patients. The common use of 5-HT3 receptor antagonists such as ondansetron and granisetron to reduce visceral pain perception in IBS-D patients has shown some benefits but is also limited by side effects [127]. Novartis has agreed to continue to supply Zelnorm® (Tegaserod maleate) for use in emergency situations, due to an increased cardiovascular risk [128, 129]. Glaxo Wellcome

(Now GSK) has informed the US FDA that it will voluntarily withdraw Lotronex® (alosetron) tablets (for IBS-D) from the market [130]. Clinical benefits of supposed spasmolytic (anti-spasmodic) agents may relate more to effects on visceral sensation than motility. A mixture of dried powdered slippery elm bark, lactulose, oat bran, and licorice root significantly improved both bowel habit and IBS symptoms in patients with constipation-predominant IBS [132]. There is a growing body of evidence which indicates therapeutic properties for ALE. Furthermore, 96% of patients rated ALE as better than or at least equal to previous therapies administered for their symptoms, and the tolerability of ALE was very good [133]. In IBS, the gastrointestinal flora may undergo both qualitative and quantitative changes and the most common finding is a decrease in the population of 'good bacteria' such as *Bifidobacteria* and *Lactobacilli* and the faecal microflora has increased numbers of facultative organisms. Probiotics may be useful in the management of IBS, however dose and specific bacterial strain are important. In vivo studies have identified some of the variables that determine the survival of probiotics through the GI tract, and some have attempted to quantify the degree of survival of the dose administered. This was found to vary from 10 to 50% depending on the probiotic species used and the dose administered [131].

Exhibit 7. Herbs used for treatment of irritable bowel syndrome [125, 127]

Herbal Medicine	Type of Study	Results
Artichoke (Whole plant)	Post-marketing surveillance study	Significant reductions in the severity of symptoms
	Open dose-ranging study	"Alternating constipation/diarrhea" toward "normal", significant improvement in total quality-of-life (QOL) score
Fumaria officinalis (Whole plant)	Double-blind, placebo-RCT	No difference between treatment and placebo groups
Curcuma longa (Rhizome)	Pilot study, partially blinded, RCT randomized,	No difference between treatment and placebo groups
Iberogast ®	Randomized, double-blind, placebo-controlled	Significantly improves quality of life and reduces abdominal pain in IBS patients
Hypericum perforatum (HP) (Aerial parts)	Open-label, uncontrolled trial	Autonomic nervous system to different stressor, improvement of Gastrointestinal symptoms of IBS
	Double-blind, placebo-RCT	No difference between treatment and placebo groups
Mentha piperita (MP) (Oil/Essence)	Double-blind, placebo-RCT	Peppermint-oil was effective and well tolerated
	Prospective double-blind, placebo-RCT	Improves abdominal symptoms
	Double-blind, placebo-RCT	Significantly improved the quality of life, improves abdominal symptoms
Plantago psyllium (Seed)	Placebo, RCT	Decrease Symptom severity significantly in the psyllium group, no differences in QOL
Carmint (Mentha spicata leaf, Melissa officinalis leaf, Coriandrum sativum fruit)	Double-blind, placebo-RCT	Severity and frequency of abdominal pain/discomfort were significantly lower in the Carmint group than the placebo group

7. Inflammatory Bowel Disease (IBD)

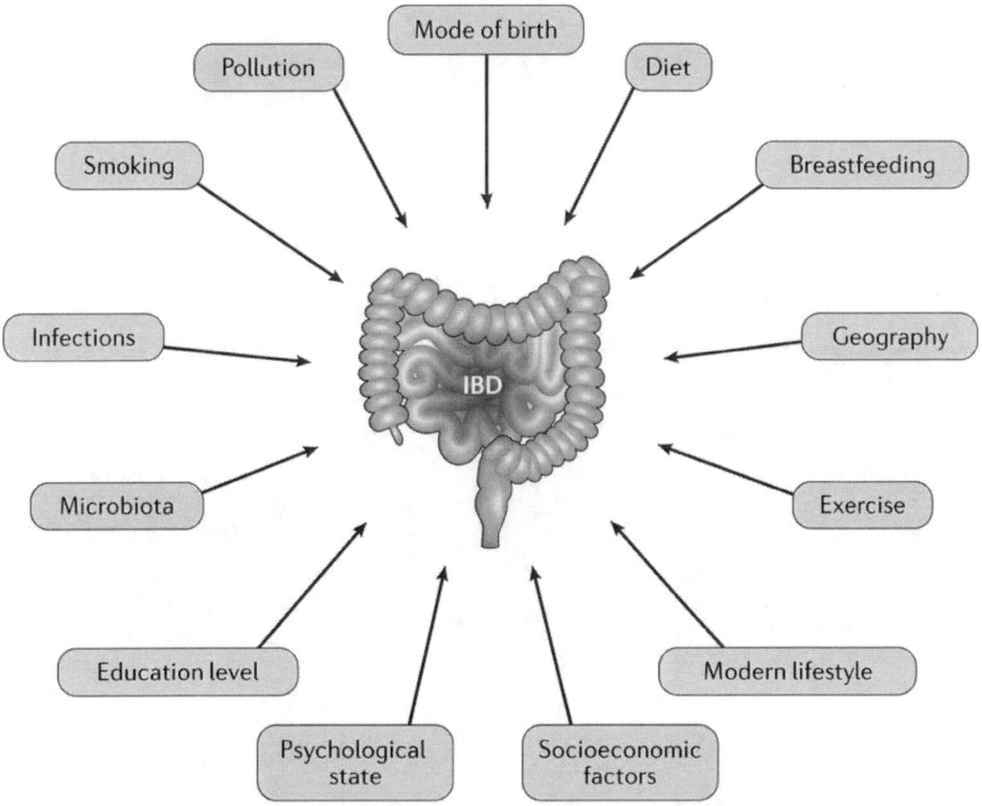

Figure 9. Environmental triggers in IBD. A wide variety of environmental triggers have been associated with IBD pathogenesis, including the gut microbiota, diet, pollution and early-life factors. Smoking remains the most widely studied and replicated risk factor, contributing to increased risk and severity of CD while conferring protection against UC. Lower plasma vitamin D is associated with an increased risk of Crohn's disease, and vitamin D supplementation may prevent relapse of disease. Several medications including oral contraceptives, post-menopausal hormone replacement, aspirin, NSAIDs, and antibiotics may increase risk of CD or UC with the mechanisms of effect remaining inadequately defined. There is continuing evidence that depression and psychosocial stress may play a role in the pathogenesis of both CD and UC, while at the same time also increasing risk for disease flares. There is also a growing understanding of the role of diet on IBD, in particular through its effect on the microbiome. Animal protein intake and n-6 fatty acids may increase risk of UC while n-3 fatty acids and dietary fiber may confer protection. The effect of diet on established disease remains poorly studied. There is need for routine measurement of a spectrum of environmental exposures in prospective studies to further our understanding. (Source: Ananthakrishnan AN. Environmental triggers for inflammatory bowel disease. Curr Gastroenterol Rep. 2013;15(1):302.)

IBS, a common gastrointestinal disorder involving the gut-brain axis; IBD, a chronic relapsing inflammatory disorder. Both have significant overlap in terms of symptoms, pathophysiology, and treatment, suggesting the possibility of IBS and IBD being a single disease entity albeit at opposite ends of the spectrum [133]. A significant association between IBD and later occurrence of PD, which is consistent with recent basic scientific findings of a potential role of GI inflammation in development of parkinsonian disorders

[134]. An area of recent research interest where the role of adiposity is avidly discussed is in IBD, which presents mainly as Crohn's disease (CD) and ulcerative colitis (UC) [135]. IBD is a chronic illness, and sexual dysfunction is a well-recognized complication of chronic illness [136]. A subgroup of IBD patients considered diet to be a more important and successful managing tool than medication to relieve their disease symptoms [137].

7.1. Prevalence and Economic Burden of IBD

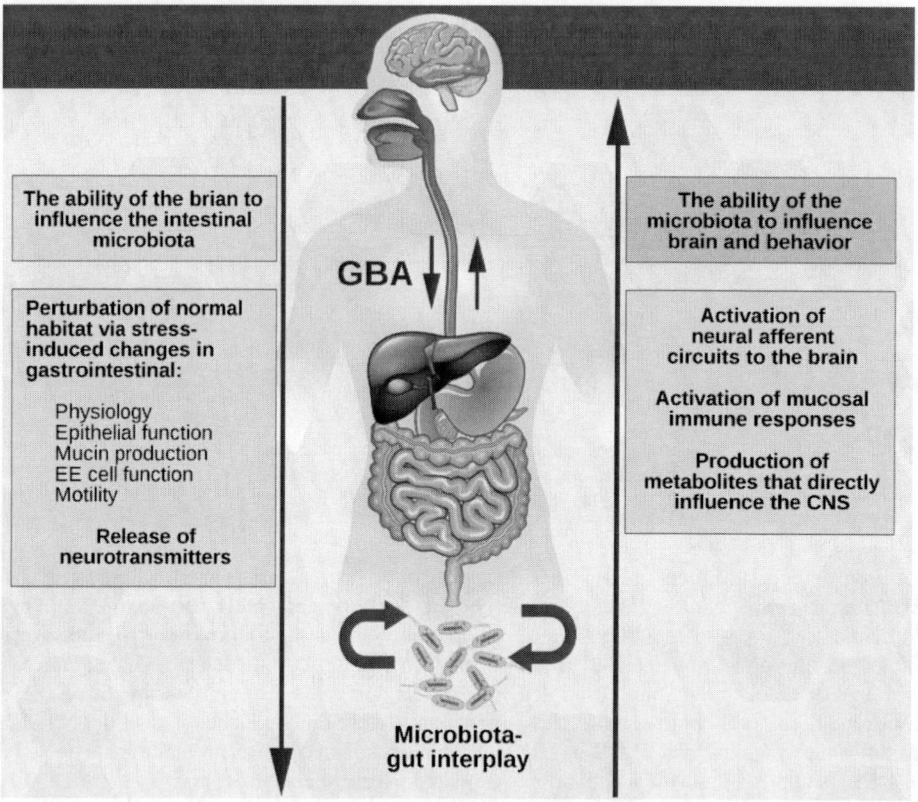

Figure 10. Integration of the microbiota into the gut-brain axis. The link between the brain and the gut is therefore partially responsible for the secretion, absorption and motility of poop through the intestines. Another cause of IBS may be a result of decreased healthy bacteria such as lactobacilli and bifido bacteria. These two kinds of bacteria compete with pathogens to take up space and do not stimulate gas production. Studies have found that IBS patients have decreased activity of these bacteria in the colon. IBS is also related to SIBO or small intestinal bacterial overgrowth. This is where there is an overgrowth of bacteria in the small intestine. SIBO damages the intestinal lining and creates a state of mild-severe leaky gut syndrome and resulting food allergies, sensitivities and chronic inflammatory processes. The malnutrition and inflammation this can lead to bouts of diarrhea and constipation. (Source: 16 Ways to Achieve Healthy Poop. Web drjockers.com.)

IBD, including UC and CD, are chronic, disabling, and progressive disorders characterized by lifelong treatment and whose incidences are increasing in Asia [141]. EIMs of IBD occur in up to 55% of patients with CD and 35% of those with UC. Although arthritis/arthralgia is the most common EIM in both disorders, multiple organs may be affected including skin, eye and liver [145]. Approximately 2.5 million–3 million people in Europe are affected by IBD. The highest rates of IBD are reported in Scandinavia and the UK. The incidence and prevalence of UC in the UK is estimated to be 14 cases per 100,000 person-years and 244 cases per 100,000 people, respectively. The incidence and prevalence of CD in the UK is estimated to be 7-11 per 100,000 and 85–145 cases per 100,000 people, respectively [144]. An increasing number of these children are being treated with immunosuppressive and biological medications. Although these medications can improve the short-term outcome and quality of life of children with IBD, they have been associated with opportunistic infections, malignancy, and lymphoproliferative disorders among IBD populations. It is estimated that 15% to 20% of all cases of IBD are diagnosed in the childhood and adolescent period [146]. Patients with IBD have a 2- to 3-fold increased risk of colorectal cancer death; therefore, colorectal cancer surveillance via colonoscopy is recommended for IBD patients [147]. Environmental factors probably have a major role in IBD; antibiotic use, childbirth mode, breastfeeding, air pollution, NSAID use, hypoxia or high altitude, diet and urban environments have been studied [148].

7.2. Rationale of DS and Probiotics in IBD

A recent survey by de Vries et al., 2019, DS were used by 68% of the IBD patients. Although over 71% had received dietary advice mainly by dieticians, 81% stated that the main source of their nutritional knowledge related to IBD was their own experience [137]. Despite recent advancements, Crohn's disease and ulcerative colitis remain chronic and progressive diseases. One of the primary reasons for persistent inflammation and bowel damage is failure of medical therapy. With growing therapeutic options, there is an increased temptation to quickly move to the next therapy and label the prior therapy as a failure; however, this can lead to inadequate optimization of medications and poor control of disease. On the other hand, failure to recognize ongoing mucosal inflammation despite optimized treatment and moving to the next agent can lead to progression of disease and long-term complications [138]. Anti-tumor necrosis factor antibodies have led to a revolution in the treatment of IBD; however, a sizable proportion of patients does not respond to therapy. There is increasing evidence suggesting that treatment failure may be classified as mechanistic (pharmacodynamic), pharmacokinetic, or immune-mediated. Data regarding the contribution of these factors in children with IBD treated with infliximab (IFX) are still incomplete [139]. Endoscopic therapy has been explored and used in the management of strictures, fistulas/abscesses, colitis-associated neoplasia, postsurgical acute or chronic leaks, and obstructions [140]. For several decades, medical treatments for IBD were limited to non-biological therapies (i.e., aminosalicylates, thiopurines, and steroids), which provide symptomatic improvement but do not change the disease course [141]. Anti-TNF agents (infliximab, adalimumab, and certolizumab) have reduced the need for surgery and hospitalization and have improved the quality of life of patients by changing the course of the disease. Thus, guidelines recommend the use of anti-TNF agents initially in moderate-to-severe IBD or if non-biological therapy fails. However, these treatments have not been effective in all patients, and patients who initially responded to treatment have also lost their responsiveness over time. Furthermore, although anti-TNF agents are generally well tolerated, their use is associated with adverse effects, including risks of infection and malignancies [142, 143].

7.3. Use of Herbs and Probiotics

The use of herbal therapy in IBD is increasing worldwide. It can be assumed that the efficacy of herbal therapies in IBD is promising. The most important clinical trials conducted so far refer to the use of mastic gum, tormentil extracts, wormwood herb, triticum aestivum, germinated barley foodstuff, and boswellia serrata. In ulcerative colitis, *Triticum aestivum, Andrographis paniculata* extract and topical Xilei-san were superior to placebo in inducing remission or clinical response, and curcumin was superior to placebo in maintaining remission; boswellia serrata gum resin and plantago ovata seeds were as effective as mesalazine, whereas oenothera biennis had similar relapse rates as ω-3 fatty acids in the treatment of ulcerative colitis. In Crohn's disease, mastic gum, Artemisia absinthium, and Tripterygium wilfordii were superior to placebo in inducing remission and preventing clinical postoperative recurrence, respectively [149].

Altered gut bacteria and bacterial metabolic pathways are two important factors in initiation and progression of IBD. However, efficacy of probiotics in remission of patients with IBD has not been characterized [156]. Among the effects claimed for probiotics are beneficial immunomodulation, reduction of serum cholesterol, improved lactose digestion and protection against colon cancer [157, 158]. Probiotic administration improved the clinical symptoms, histological alterations, and mucus production in most of the evaluated animal studies, but some results suggest that caution should be taken when administering these agents in the relapse stages of IBD [158]. In CD, the entire gastrointestinal tract can be involved and the inflammation can extend through the intestinal wall from mucosa to serosa. Areas of inflammation may be interspersed with relatively normal mucosa. In CD, the predominant symptoms are diarrhea, abdominal pain and weight loss whereas in UC diarrhea is the main symptom, often accompanied by rectal bleeding. Both diseases are common in the industrialized world, with highest incidences in North America and Northern Europe [159].

Exhibit 7. Herbs used for treatment of IBD

Herbal Medicine	Type of Study	Ref No.	Results
Triticum aestivum (Poaceae)	randomized, double-blind, placebo-controlled study	150	Treatment was associated with significant reduction in the overall disease activity index and in the severity of rectal bleeding. Apart from nausea, no other serious side effects were noticed
Andrographis paniculata	Randomized, double-blind multicentre study	151	Compared with Mesalazine (4.5 mg/day), there were no significant differences between the two treated groups when considering the clinical efficacy rates or the safety profile
Boswellia serrata (Burseraceae)	Single Centered study	152	Compared with Sulfasalazine, all parameters tested improved after treatment with Boswellia serrata gum in 82% patients
Artemisia absinthium	Randomized, double-blind multicentre study	153	Compared with placebo, after 8 weeks of treatment with wormwood, there was almost complete remission of symptoms in 65% of the patients,
Tripterygium wilfordii Hook F (TWHF)	Randomized controlled trials	154	Patients receiving mesalazine experienced less adverse events, but no significant difference was found about ADEs resulted withdrawal in the 3 groups. In addition, compared with low-dose TwHF and mesalazine, the authors also detected significant superiority of high-dose TwHF arm in the decrease of CDAI and SESCD
Evening primrose oil *Oenothera biennis*	Randomized controlled trials	155	*Oenothera biennis* had similar relapse rates as omega-3 fatty acids in the treatment of UC

Exhibit 8. Summary of probiotic anti-inflammatory effects in in vitro studies [160]

Cell Type	Probiotic Strain	Type of Study	Main Outcome
human DC	*L. casei* Shirota	In vitro	DC from UC patients samples have an increase of IL-4 production and loss of IL-22 and IFN-γ secretion. *L. casei* Shirota treatment restored the normal stimulatory capacity through a reduction in the TLR-2 and TLR4 expression
IPEC-J2 model	*L. plantarum* strain CGMCC1258	In vitro	*L. plantarum* decreased transcript abundances of IL-8, TNF-α, and negative regulators of TLRs. Moreover, *L. plantarum* treatment decreased the gene and protein expression of occludin
PIE cells	*L. delbrueckii* subsp. *delbrueckii* TUA4408L	In vitro	The activation of MAPK and NF-κB pathways induced by *E. coli* 987P were downregulated through upregulation of TLR negative regulators, principally by TLR2
IEC-6	*E. coli* Nissle 1917 and *L. rhamnosus* GG	In vitro	Pre-treatment with these probiotics could prevent or inhibit enterocyte apoptosis and loss of intestinal barrier function induced by 5-FU
DC	*L. paracasei* CNCM I-4034, *B. breve* CNCM I-4035, and *L. rhamnosus* CNCM I-4036	In vitro	Induction of TLR-9 expression and TGF-β2 secretion. CFS treatment decreased the pro-inflammatory cytokines and chemokines

8. Peptic Ulcer Disease (PUD)

The presenting symptoms of PUD vary depending on the age of the patient. Hematemesis or melena is reported in up to half of patients with PUD. Infants and younger children usually present with feeding difficulty, vomiting, crying episodes, hematemesis, or melena [161]. The major symptom of uncomplicated PUD is upper abdominal dyspepsia such as bloating, early satiety, and nausea. H. pylori infection plays a crucial role in the pathogenesis of PUD. H. pylori infection is involved in various gastroduodenal pathologies, and evokes the production of proinflammatory interleukin-1beta, leading to the reduction of blood flow to the gastroduodenal tract and increasing the risk of peptic ulcers. H. pylori can colonize not only in the stomach, but also in the oral cavity. The oral cavity may be a reservoir for H. pylori and a potential source for infection of the stomach [162]. EGD is most accurate diagnostic test with sensitivity and specificity up to 90% in diagnosing gastric and duodenal ulcers. Surgical treatment is indicated if the patient is unresponsive to medical treatment, noncompliant or at high risk of complications. Surgical options include vagotomy or partial gastrectomy [163]. Factors that increase risk of developing peptic ulcer include smoking, older individuals, O blood type, and stress. Peptic ulcers that tend to heal longer than duodenal ulcer is at higher risk of developing gastritis and gastric malignancy [168]. Classically, patients with duodenal ulcers complain of worsening abdominal pain on an empty stomach and describe hunger or abdominal pain two to three hours after meals or at night. In contrast, patients with gastric ulcers report nausea, vomiting, weight loss and post-prandial abdominal pain. Elderly patients are often minimally symptomatic and some patients with untreated PUD may have intermittent symptoms due to spontaneous healing and then relapse due to persistence of risk factors, such as continued NSAIDs use or H. pylori infection [169].

8.1. Prevalence and Economic Burden of PUD

The prevalence of PUD ranges from 0.12 to 1.5% and increases with age [162]. H. pylorus is a gram-negative bacillus that is found within the gastric epithelial cells. This bacterium is responsible for 90% of duodenal ulcers and 70% to 90% of gastric ulcers, up to 85% of individuals infected with H. pylori are asymptomatic and have no complications [163, 165]. PUD is a global problem with a lifetime risk of development ranging from 5% to 10% [164]. In many studies worldwide (United States, Brazil and China), the prevalence of H. pylori among subjects with dyspepsia was 28.9%, 57%, and 84% respectively [165]. The prevalence differs in the world population between the duodenal and gastric ulcers, and the mean age of people with the disease is between 30 and 60 years, but it can happen in any age [166]. Environmental elements such as alcohol and nicotine can inhibit or reduce secretion of mucus and bicarbonate, increasing acid secretion. Genetic factors can influence, and children of parents with duodenal ulcer are three times more likely to have ulcer than the population [167]. 30% PUD patients are smoker [168]. NSAIDs account for over 90% of all ulcers and approximately 25% of NSAID users will develop peptic ulcer disease [169]. Approximately 500,000 persons develop PU in the United States each year [170]. Peptic ulcers accounted for 301,000 deaths in 2013, which is down from 327,000 deaths in 1990 [174]. Low socioeconomic status and concrete life difficulties are associated with peptic ulcer in the general population cross-sectionally and prospectively after adjustment for major physical risk factors, lending credence to a relationship between psychological stress and peptic ulcer [175].

8.2. Lifestyle Modification for PUD

Exhibit 9. Allowed foods, foods that should be consumed with caution, and foods that must be avoided [172]

Food Groups	Allowed	Use with Caution	Prohibited
Dairy	Milk, low-fat cheeses, yogurt, fermented milk	Fatty cheeses (mascarpone, cream cheese, gorgonzola)	-
Oilseeds	Flaxseed, Brazilian nut, walnuts	-	-
Oils and olive oils	Vegetable oils, olive oil	-	Fried foods
Fruits	Apple, papaya, melon, banana	Orange, pineapple, acerola, passion fruit	Lemon
Vegetables	Leafy dark green vegetables, carrot, beet, green bean, spinach, kale, radish, zucchini, leek	Broccoli, cauliflower, cabbage, cucumber, onion, red pepper	Spicy peppers (black pepper, chilies)
Legumes	Bean soup, lentils, chickpeas, soybean	Beans	-
Meats	Lean meat (beef, pork, chicken, fish)	Fatty meats, organ meats and sausages	-
Sweets	-	Concentrated sweets	Chocolate
Beverages	Natural juices	Citrus/acidic fruit juices	Coffee, black tea, fizzy/cola drinks
Other foods	-	Industrialized seasonings, spices and condiments (Ketchup, mayonnaise, mustard)	Mustard grain

The physicochemical properties of fiber fractions produce different physiological effects in the organism. Soluble fibers, found in apple, oatmeal, and pear are responsible, for instance, for an increased viscosity in the intestinal content. Insoluble fibers (whole grains, granola, flaxseed) increase stool bulk, reduce transit time in the large intestine, and make fecal elimination easier and quicker [171]. Physical activity has numerous health benefits and may also represent a cost-effective approach to the prevention of peptic ulcers. At the levels observed in this study among the moderately active group (walking or jogging <10 miles a week), possible adverse effects—for example, injuries—are minimized. In the general population, only about a third of adults undertake this much physical activity. Strategies to promote safe walking, jogging, and cycling may benefit many aspects of health in addition to the cardiovascular and musculoskeletal systems [173]. Moderate physical activity could have a favorable impact on a number of risk factors for peptic ulceration. It could reduce gastric secretions and enhance immune function, with the latter reducing the risk of Helicobacter pylori infection. Moderate activity might also reduce anxiety and encourage the adoption of a healthy lifestyle, with avoidance of smoking and an excessive consumption of alcohol. However, prolonged endurance exercise seems likely to have a negative impact, suppressing immune function, reducing mucosal blood flow, and calling for frequent administration of NSAIDs [176].

8.3. Herbs and Probiotics for PUD Management

The potential of plants as source of new drugs still offers a large field for scientific research. Even if is observed a large number of known plants, a small percentage has already been phytochemically investigated and only a fraction of them has already been assessed to determine its pharmacological potential.

Exhibit 10. Herbs for PUD management

Plant Name/Family	Description
Acacia arabica (Mimosaceae)	Locally known as babul tree. Aqueous extract of A. arabica gum showed protection against meloxicam-induced intestinal damage and attenuated intestinal enzyme activity. Chemical constituents reported in this plant are gum containing arabic acid combined with calcium, magnesium, and potassium and also small quantity of malic acid, sugar, moisture 14%, and ash 3-4%. As gargle it is useful as wash in haemorrhagic ulcer and wounds [178].
Psidium guajava L., popularly known as guava (Myrtaceae)	The leaves have shown the ability to protect the stomach against ulceration by inhibiting gastric lesions, reducing gastric secretory volume, and acid secretion, and raising the gastric pH. This anti-ulcer activity, resulting from the protection of the mucosa, was related to the flavonoids in the leaves [179]
Aegle marmelos (Rutaceae), Bael Fruit	Ulcers are induced by aspirin plus pylorus ligated gastric ulceration in rats and aqueous extract of leaves is to be administered orally for 21 days, daily dose of 1 gm/kg. The result indicated a significant reduction in the ulcer lesion count compared to control [180]
Allium sativum (Liliaceae) garlic	Chemical constituents in this plant arean acrid volatile oil which is the active principle, starch, mucilage, albumen, and sugar. Seeds yield aromatic oil. The juice, more particularly its oil constituents, is rich in organically bound sulphur, iodine, and salicylic acid combinations, apart from important nutrient and complementary substances containing vitamins [178]. Garlic extract has been also studied to show

Plant Name/Family	Description
	suppressive effect of Helicobacter pylori-induced gastric inflammation in vivo and reduction of gastric cancer incidence in a clinical trial [181]. AGE corrected the histopathological abnormalities in gastric tissue and proved (investigated in an experimental model of indomethacin-induced gastric ulcer) a promising gastroprotective role in gastric ulcer [182].
Azadirachta indica (Meliaceae) Neem	Administration of lyophilized powder of the extract for 10 days at the dose of 30 mg twice daily showed significant decrease (77%) of gastric acid secretion. The bark extract at the dose of 30–60 mg twice daily for 10 weeks almost completely healed the duodenal ulcers and one case of esophageal ulcer and one case of gastric ulcer healed completely when administrated at the dose of 30 mg twice daily for 6 weeks [184]
Bauhinia purpurea L. (Fabaceae)	Chemical constituents reported in this plant are quercetin, rutin, apigenin, and apigenin 7-0-glucoside. Bark contains tannin (tannic acid), glucose, and a brownish gum. The Bauhinia purpurea aqueous extract (BPAE) was prepared in the doses of 100, 500 and 1,000 mg/kg. Antiulcer activity of BPAE was evaluated by absolute ethanol- and indomethacin-induced gastric ulcer, and pyloric ligation models. Acute toxicity was also carried out. The BPAE exhibits antiulcer activity, which could be due to the presence of saponins or sugar-free polyphenols, and, thus, confirmed the traditional uses of Bauhinia purpurea in the treatment of ulcers [185]
T. indica (Caesalpinioideae) Tamarind	The methanolic extract of the seed coat of this plant (100 mg/kg and 200 mg/kg) has been evaluated for determining their antiulcer potential on ibuprofen, alcohol and pyloric ligation-induced gastric lesions using albino Wistar rats [63]. The results of this study showed that the methanolic extract reduced total gastric juice volume and free and total gastric secretion acidity in pylorus ligation-induced ulcer model, while reduced ulcer index (comparable with ranitidine, 50 mg/kg, as control) [186]
Flavonoids	Also known as bioflavonoids, some research suggested that these molecules may be beneficial in stomach ulcers, naturally present in many fruits and vegetables such as apple, soybeans, berries, and broccoli. As a disorder of the GI tract, pathological conditions in peptic ulcer could be alleviated by nutritional factors. Dietary consumption of a significant amount of "natural" protective supplements in early life leads to prevention or delayed peptic ulcer [187]
Deglycyrrhizinated licorice	It is beneficial in H. pylori-associated ulcer. In modern medicine, licorice extract has been used for peptic ulcer and as an alternative to bismuth that has a protective role against acid and pepsin secretions by covering the site of lesion and promoting the mucous secretion [188].
Honey	Natural honey is composed of around 82% carbohydrates, water, phytochemicals, proteins, minerals, and antioxidants. It is also beneficial in H. pylori-associated ulcer because honey is a powerful antibacterial agent. In gastric curative effects of manuka honey in rat model with acetic acid-induced chronic gastric ulcer, manuka honey provided significant gastroprotective effects in acute gastric ulcer animal model [189]

It has been shown that lactobacilli are particularly useful in promoting gastric ulcer healing in rats, when administered as an individual probiotic strain, such as *Lactobacillus rhamnosus* GG, Lactobacillus gasseri OLL2716, or Lactobacillus acidophilus or as a probiotic mixture, VSL#3. *Lactobacillus rhamnosus* GG increases the cellular proliferation to apoptosis ratio and therefore promotes regeneration of epithelial cells, particularly at the ulcer margins. In clinical studies, a probiotic mixture was demonstrated to be better than a single strain for improving the characteristics of indigenous microflora [191].

Promising results for studies exploring both prophylactic and therapeutic effects (Exhibit 11) of probiotics have been obtained. The studies concerning the roles of probiotics in gastric ulcer healing reported in the literature were mainly conducted in rats. These studies were based on the use of either individual probiotic strains, such as *Lactobacillus rhamnosus* GG, *Lactobacillus gasseri* OLL2716, Lactobacillus acidophilus, Escherichia coli Nissle 1917, Bifidobacterium animalis VKL/VKB, *Bifidobacterium bifidum*/brevis and *Saccharomyces boulardii*, or a mixture of probiotic strains, such as VSL#3. A number of studies have reported that probiotics not only inhibit the development of acute gastric mucosal lesions, but also accelerate the process of healing of induced gastric ulcers [191].

Exhibit 11. Summary of studies on the therapeutic effects of probiotics in gastric ulcer [191]

Probiotic Strain(s)	Modeling Method	Lesions	Effects of Probiotics
Lactobacillus spp.	Acetic acid	Gastric ulcer	Enhance healing of a pre-existing gastric ulcer
Lactobacillus rhamnosus GG	Acetic acid	Gastric ulcer	Inhibit cell apoptosis to proliferation ratio, and induce angiogenesis
Lactobacillus gasseri OLL 2716	Acetic acid	Gastric ulcer	Accelerate healing by enhancing generation of gastric mucosal prostaglandin E2
Lactobacillus acilidophilus encapsulated in ginger extract	Stress	Gastric ulcer	Improve healing by restoring all biochemical, physiological and histological changes
Lactobacillus acidophilus and alginate floating beads	Stress	Gastric ulcer	Improve healing by restoring all biochemical, physiological and histological changes
Probiotic mixture (VSL#3) (8 probiotic strains)	Acetic acid	Gastric ulcer	Enhance healing by promoting angiogenesis via upregulation of vascular endothelial growth factor
Saccharomyces boulardii	Ibuprofen	Gastric ulcer	Potential treatment or prevention
Polysaccharides fractions (PSFs) of *Bifidobacterium breve* and *bifidum*	Acetic acid and ethanol	Gastric erosion and ulcer	Repair and protect gastric mucosa by increasing expression of epidermal and fibroblast growth factors and 6-ketoprostaglandin F1
Probiotic mixture (2 bacterial strains) and composite probiotic (3 bacterial strains)	Stress	Gastric erosion and ulcer	Reduce lesions and intensity of bleeding through the restoration of pro- and antioxidant balance
Probiotic mixture (14 bacterial strains)	Stress	Gastric mucosal lesions	Enhance recovery of stress hormones, downregulate pro-inflammatory cytokines and upregulate anti-inflammatory cytokines

Probiotics can also protect the integrity of the gastric mucosal barrier by upregulating prostaglandin, mucous secretion, tight junction protein expression and cell proliferation, and by inhibiting apoptosis (43, 48, 130–132). In rats, the administration of *Bifidobacterium bifidum* BF-1 or *Bifidobacterium animalis* VKL and VKB has been found to protect the gastric mucosa through either preventing the mucous barrier from degradation or increasing gastric mucous production. The probiotic mixture VSL#3 protects the epithelial barrier and upregulates the expression of tight junction proteins (occludin and zonula occludens-1) in vivo and in vitro via the activation of p38 or mitogen-activated protein (MAP) kinase and extracellular signal-regulated kinase (ERK) signaling pathways. Mennigen et al. demonstrated that probiotics can strengthen the gastric mucosal barrier by inhibiting the redistribution and expression of tight junction proteins and blocking apoptosis [135]. The probiotic strains Lactobacillus gasseri OLL2716, Lactobacillus rhamnosus GG and Escherichia coli Nissle 1917 are able to protect the altered gastric mucosal barrier (43, 48, 114). In humans, Gotteland et al. found that pretreatment with Lactobacillus GG protected against indomethacin-induced disruption of the gastric mucosal barrier [191].

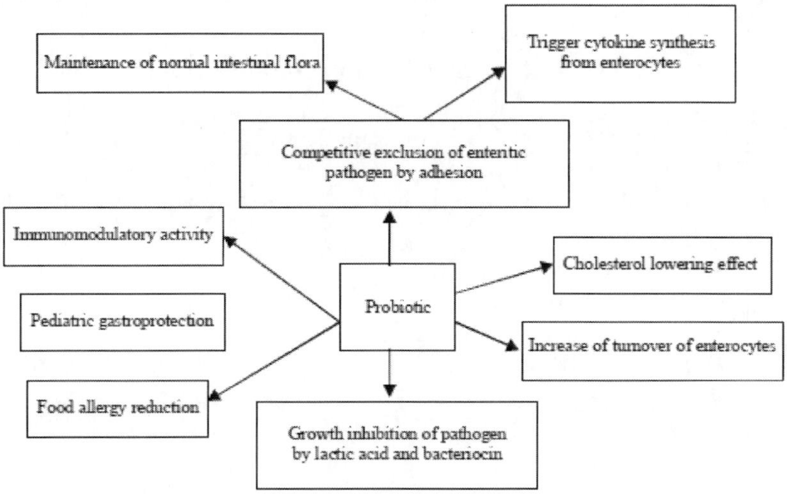

Figure 11. Mechanisms of action of probiotics. Probiotics are engaged to adherence to host epithelial tissue, acid resistance and bile tolerance, elimination of pathogens or reduction in pathogenic adherence production of acids, hydrogen peroxide and bacteriocins antagonistic to pathogen growth, safety, non-pathogenic and non-carcinogenic, and Improvement of intestinal microflora. Prebiotics of proven efficacy are able to modulate the gut microbiota by stimulating indigenous beneficial flora while inhibiting the growth of pathogenic bacteria therein. Preferred target organisms for prebiotics are specific belonging to the Lactobacillus and Bifidobacterium genera. The most efficient prebiotics may also reduce or suppress numbers and activities of organisms seen as pathogenic (Bandyopadhyay B, Mandal NC. Probiotics, Prebiotics and Symbiotic - In Health Improvement by Modulating Gut Microbiota: The Concept Revisited. Int. J. Curr. Microbiol. App. Sci (2014) 3(3): 410-420).

The mode of action of probiotics is not completely understood but they may act as surrogate normal microflora following antibiotic therapy until recovery is achieved. However, probiotic combinations appeared to induce only minor changes in the microbiota. For instance, the mechanisms of action of S. boulardii include luminal action (anti-toxic effect, antimicrobial activity), trophic action (enzymatic activity, increased IgA) and mucosal-anti-inflammatory signaling effects (decreased synthesis of inflammatory cytokines). Short-chain fatty acids (SCFAs) and bacteriocin proteins have been implicated in the inhibition of H. pylori by lactic acid bacteria. SCFAs such as formic, acetic, propionic, butyric and lactic acids are produced as a result of the metabolism of carbohydrates by probiotics and play an important role in decreasing the pH in vitro. Their antimicrobial activity could be due to the inhibition of urease activity by high lactic acid producers, such as *Lactobacillus salivarius* and *Lactobacillus casei* Shirota. *Lactobacillus salivarius* significantly decreased IL-8 production [IL-8 is induced after injection of virulence factor CagA into epithelial cells] upon exposure to H. pylori and led to CagA accumulation in H. pylori cells, presumably as a result of loss of functionality of the Cag secretion system. Alterations in gastrointestinal permeability are an initial step in the development of lesions such as ulcers. Probiotics may stabilize the intestinal barrier by stimulating the expression of gastric mucins, decreasing bacterial overgrowth and stimulating local immune responses and the release of antioxidant substances [192].

Exhibit 12. Selection criteria of probiotic strains [190]

Criterion	Required Properties
Safety	• Human or animal origin. • Isolated from the gastrointestinal tract of healthy individuals. • History of safe use. • Precise diagnostic identification (phenotype and genotype traits). • Absence of data regarding an association with infective disease. • Absence of the ability to cleave bile acid salts. • No adverse effects. • Absence of genes responsible for antibiotic resistance localized in non-stable elements.
Functionality	• Competitiveness with respect to the microbiota inhabiting the intestinal ecosystem. • Ability to survive and maintain the metabolic activity, and to grow in the target site. • Resistance to bile salts and enzymes. • Resistance to low pH in the stomach. • Competitiveness with respect to microbial species inhabiting the intestinal ecosystem (including closely related species). • Antagonistic activity towards pathogens (e.g., *H. pylori*, *Salmonella* sp., *Listeria monocytogenes*, *Clostridium difficile*). • Resistance to bacteriocins and acids produced by the endogenic intestinal microbiota. • Adherence and ability to colonise some particular sites within the host organism, and an appropriate survival rate in the gastrointestinal system.
Technological usability	• Easy production of high biomass amounts and high productivity of cultures. • Viability and stability of the desired properties of probiotic bacteria during the fixing process (freezing, freeze-drying), preparation, and distribution of probiotic products. • High storage survival rate in finished products (in aerobic and micro-aerophilic conditions). • Guarantee of desired sensory properties of finished products (in the case of the food industry). • Genetic stability. • Resistance to bacteriophages.

Conclusion

This review is conducted and correlate the published literature on the effectiveness of herbs and probiotics, for the treatment of FAPDs. Despite its common use, research on the efficacy, safety, and optimal dosage remains limited. Many responsible members of the dietary supplements industry have taken significant steps to regain consumer trust by improving transparency along the supply chain, enhancing traceability of raw botanical materials, and bringing attention to ingredients with potential adulteration concerns, among other efforts. Lifestyle and food habit also found important factor to improve GI related disorders to much extent. Several randomized controlled trials have now shown that microbial modification by probiotics may improve gastrointestinal symptoms and multiorgan inflammation in rheumatoid arthritis, ulcerative colitis, and multiple sclerosis. In the USA, microorganisms used for consumption purposes should have the GRAS status, regulated by the FDA. In Europe, EFSA introduced the term of QPS. The QPS concept involves some additional criteria of the safety assessment of bacterial supplements, including the history of safe usage and absence of the risk of acquired resistance to antibiotics. Future work will need to carefully assess safety issues, selection of optimal strains and combinations, and attempts to prolong the duration of colonization of beneficial microbes. This doesn't mean conventional therapies don't work, it just means that experts haven't studied them enough to know if they do. The most important thing is safe healing and better life. To ensure this, researchers needs to work more on both conventional and complimentary drugs.

References

[1] Sandhu DS, Fass R. Current Trends in the Management of Gastroesophageal Reflux Disease. *Gut Liver.* 2017;12(1):7-16.

[2] Nasrollah L, Maradey-Romero C, Jha LK, Gadam R, Quan SF, Fass R. Naps are associated more commonly with gastroesophageal reflux, compared with nocturnal sleep. *Clin Gastroenterol Hepatol.* 2015;13:94–99. doi: 10.1016/j.cgh.2014.05.017.

[3] Fass R. Non-erosive reflux disease (NERD) and erosive esophagitis: a spectrum of disease or special entities? *Z Gastroenterol.* 2007;45:1156–1163. doi: 10.1055/s-2007-963628.

[4] Poh CH, Navarro-Rodriguez T, Fass R. Review: treatment of gastroesophageal reflux disease in the elderly. *Am J Med.* 2010;123:496–501. doi: 10.1016/j.amjmed.2009.07.036.

[5] Jacobson BC, Somers SC, Fuchs CS, Kelly CP, Camargo CA., Jr Body-mass index and symptoms of gastroesophageal reflux in women. *N Engl J Med.* 2006;354:2340–2348. doi: 10.1056/NEJMoa054391.

[6] Kaltenbach T, Crockett S, Gerson LB. Are lifestyle measures effective in patients with gastroesophageal reflux disease? An evidence-based approach. *Arch Intern Med.* 2006;166:965–971. doi: 10.1001/archinte.166.9.965.

[7] Yamasaki T, O'Neil J, Fass R. Update on Functional Heartburn. *Gastroenterol Hepatol* (N Y). 2017;13(12):725-734.

[8] Fass R. Erosive esophagitis and nonerosive reflux disease (NERD): comparison of epidemiologic, physiologic, and therapeutic characteristics. *J Clin Gastroenterol.* 2007;41(2):131–137.

[9] Alecci U, Bonina F, Bonina A, et al. Efficacy and Safety of a Natural Remedy for the Treatment of Gastroesophageal Reflux: A Double-Blinded Randomized-Controlled Study. *Evid Based Complement Alternat Med.* 2016;2016:2581461.

[10] Henry MA. Diagnosis and management of gastroesophageal reflux disease. *Arq Bras Cir Dig.* 2014;27(3):210-5.

[11] El-Serag H., Becher A., Jones R. Systematic review: persistent reflux symptoms on proton pump inhibitor therapy in primary care and community studies. *Alimentary Pharmacology and Therapeutics.* 2010;32(6):720–737. doi: 10.1111/j.1365-2036.2010.04406.x

[12] Perry K. A., Pham T. H., Spechler S. J., Hunter J. G., Melvin W. S., Velanovich V. 2014 SSAT state-of-the-art conference: advances in diagnosis and management of gastroesophageal reflux disease. *Journal of Gastrointestinal Surgery.* 2015;1 9(3):458–466. doi: 10.1007/s11605-014-2724-9.

[13] Galati E. M., Pergolizzi S., Miceli N., Monforte M. T., Tripodo M. M. Study on the increment of the production of gastric mucus in rats treated with Opuntia ficus indica (L.) Mill. cladodes. *Journal of Ethnopharmacology.* 2002;83(3):229–233. doi: 10.1016/s0378-8741(02)00243-x.

[14] Galati E. M., Mondello M. R., Giuffrida D., et al. Chemical characterization and biological effects of sicilian Opuntia ficus indica (L.) Mill. fruit juice: antioxidant and antiulcerogenic activity. *Journal of Agricultural and Food Chemistry.* 2003;51(17):4903–4908. doi: 10.1021/jf030123d.

[15] Trachtenberg S., Mayer A. M. Biophysical properties of Opuntia ficus-indica mucilage. *Phytochemistry.* 1980;21(12):2835–2843. doi: 10.1016/0031-9422(80)85052-7.

[16] Goulas V., Papoti V. T., Exarchou V., Tsimidou M. Z., Gerothanassis I. P. Contribution of flavonoids to the overall radical scavenging activity of olive (Olea europapaea L.) leaf polar extracts. *Journal of Agricultural and Food Chemistry.* 2010;58(6):3303–3308. doi: 10.1021/jf903823x.

[17] Herbella FA, Patti MG. Gastroesophageal reflux disease: From pathophysiology to treatment. *World J Gastroenterol.* 2010;16(30):3745-9.

[18] Kahrilas PJ, Smith JA, Dicpinigaitis PV. *A causal relationship between cough and gastroesophageal reflux disease* (GERD) has been established: a pro/con debate. Lung. 2013;192(1):39-46.

[19] Ates F, Vaezi MF. Insight Into the Relationship Between Gastroesophageal Reflux Disease and Asthma. *Gastroenterol Hepatol* (N Y). 2014;10(11):729-736.

[20] Kerr M, Nall R. *What Complementary and Alternative Medicines Work for Acid Reflux?* Medically reviewed by Debra Rose Wilson, PhD, MSN, RN, IBCLC, AHN-BC, CHT. Healthline Web January 24, 2019.

[21] Yeh AM, Golianu B. Integrative Treatment of Reflux and Functional Dyspepsia in Children. *Children* (Basel). 2014;1(2):119-33. Published 2014 Aug 18. doi:10.3390/children1020119.

[22] Hosseinkhani A, Lankarani KB, Mohagheghzadeh A, Long C, Pasalar M. An Evidence-based Review of Medicinal Herbs for the Treatment of Gastroesophageal Reflux Disease (GERD). *Curr Drug Discov Technol.* 2018;15(4):305-314. doi: 10.2174/1570163814666171010113517. PubMed PMID: 29032757.

[23] Modlin I. M., Hunt R. H., Malfertheiner P., et al. Diagnosis and management of non-erosive reflux disease—The vevey NERD consensus group. *Digestion.* 2009;80(2):74–88. doi: 10.1159/000219365.

[24] Mone I, Kraja B, Bregu A, Duraj V, Sadiku E, Hyska J, Burazeri G. Adherence to a predominantly Mediterranean diet decreases the risk of gastroesophageal reflux disease: a cross-sectional study in a South Eastern European population. *Dis Esophagus.* 2016 Oct;29(7):794-800. doi: 10.1111/dote.12384. Epub 2015 Jul 14. PubMed PMID: 26175057.

[25] Gawron AJ, French DD, Pandolfino JE, Howden CW. Economic evaluations of gastroesophageal reflux disease medical management. *Pharmacoeconomics.* 2014;32(8):745-58.

[26] Benias PC, D'Souza L, Lan G, et al. Initial experience with a novel resection and plication (RAP) method for acid reflux: a pilot study. *Endosc Int Open.* 2018;6(4): E443-E449.

[27] Gelardi M, Ciprandi G. Focus on gastroesophageal reflux (GER) and laryngopharyngeal reflux (LPR): new pragmatic insights in clinical practice. *J Biol Regul Homeost Agents.* 2018 Jan-Feb;32(1 Suppl. 2):41-47. PubMed PMID: 29436209.

[28] Web Truhealth Medicine (May 16, 2018). *How to naturally treat acid reflux at home?*

[29] Kiefer D, Cherney K. Herbs and Supplements for Acid Reflux (GERD). Reviewed by University of Illinois-Chicago, College of Medicine. *Healthline* March 22, 2016.

[30] Wong C. Remedies for Acid Reflux. Reviewed by Richard N. Fogoros, MD. Web *Verywell Health* March 05, 2018.

[31] Deters A, Zippel J, Hellenbrand N, Pappai D, Possemeyer C, Hensel A. Aqueous extracts and polysaccharides from Marshmallow roots (Althea officinalis L.): cellular internalisation and stimulation of cell physiology of human epithelial cells in vitro. *J Ethnopharmacol.* 2010 Jan 8;127(1):62-9. doi: 10.1016/j.jep.2009.09.050. Epub 2009 Sep 30. PubMed PMID: 19799989.

[32] Jirsa A. *3 Herbs to Heal Heartburn. Mindbodygreen Web.* Available From: https://www.mindbodygreen.com/0-7555/3-herbs-to-heal-heartburn.html.

[33] Di Pierro F, Gatti M, Rapacioli G, Ivaldi L. Outcomes in patients with nonerosive reflux disease treated with a proton pump inhibitor and alginic acid ± glycyrrhetinic acid and anthocyanosides. *Clin Exp Gastroenterol.* 2013;6:27-33.

[34] NaturalON Web. 12 *Best Herbs for Acid Reflux.*

[35] Muss C, Mosgoeller W, Endler T. Papaya preparation (Caricol®) in digestive disorders. *Neuro Endocrinol Lett.* 2013;34(1):38-46. PubMed PMID: 23524622.

[36] Aravind G, Bhowmik D, Duraivel S, Harish G. Traditional and Medicinal Uses of Carica papaya. *Journal of Medicinal Plants Studies* Year: 2013, Volume: 1, Issue: 1, pp 7-15.

[37] DiSilvestro RA, Verbruggen MA, Offutt EJ. Anti-heartburn effects of a fenugreek fiber product. *Phytother Res.* 2011 Jan;25(1):88-91. doi: 10.1002/ptr.3229. PubMed PMID: 20623611.

[38] Pandian RS, Anuradha CV, Viswanathan P. Gastroprotective effect of fenugreek seeds (Trigonella foenum graecum) on experimental gastric ulcer in rats. *J Ethnopharmacol.* 2002 Aug;81(3):393-7. PubMed PMID: 12127242.

[39] Thavorn K, Mamdani MM, Straus SE. Efficacy of turmeric in the treatment of digestive disorders: a systematic review and meta-analysis protocol. *Syst Rev.* 2014;3:71. Published 2014 Jun 28. doi:10.1186/2046-4053-3-71.

[40] Yadav SK, Sah AK, Jha RK, Sah P, Shah DK. Turmeric (curcumin) remedies gastroprotective action. *Pharmacogn Rev.* 2013;7(13):42-6.

[41] von Schoen-Angerer T, Madeleyn R, Kiene H, Kienle GS, Vagedes J. Improvement of Asthma and Gastroesophageal Reflux Disease With Oral Pulvis stomachicus cum Belladonna, a Combination of Matricaria recutita, Atropa belladonna, Bismuth, and Antimonite: A Pediatric Case Report. *Glob Adv Health Med.* 2016;5(1):107-11.

[42] Slikkerveer A, de Wolff FA. Pharmacokinetics and toxicity of bismuth compounds. *Med Toxicol Adverse Drug Exp.* 1989 Sep-Oct;4(5):303-23. Review. PubMed PMID: 2682129.

[43] Mastronarde JG. Is There a Relationship Between GERD and Asthma?. *Gastroenterol Hepatol* (N Y). 2012;8(6):401-3.

[44] Whitfield KL, Shulman RJ. Treatment options for functional gastrointestinal disorders: from empiric to complementary approaches. *Pediatr Ann.* 2009; 38(5):288-90, 292-4.

[45] Lee AL, Goldstein RS. Gastroesophageal reflux disease in COPD: links and risks. *Int J Chron Obstruct Pulmon Dis.* 2015;10:1935-49. Published 2015 Sep 14. doi:10.2147/COPD.S77562.

[46] Panahi Y, Khedmat H, Valizadegan G, Mohtashami R, Sahebkar A. Efficacy and safety of Aloe vera syrup for the treatment of gastroesophageal reflux disease: a pilot randomized positive-controlled trial. *J Tradit Chin Med.* 2015 Dec;35(6):632-6. PubMed PMID: 26742306.

[47] Baradaran A, Nasri H, Nematbakhsh M, Rafieian-Kopaei M. Antioxidant activity and preventive effect of aqueous leaf extract of Aloe Vera on gentamicin-induced nephrotoxicity in male Wistar rats. *Clin Ter.* 2014;165(1):7–11. doi: 10. 7471/CT. 2014. 1653. PubMed PMID.

[48] Guo X, Mei N. Aloe vera: A review of toxicity and adverse clinical effects. *J Environ Sci Health C Environ Carcinog Ecotoxicol Rev.* 2016 Apr 2;34(2):77-96. doi: 10.1080/10590501.2016.1166826. Review. PubMed PMID: 26986231.

[49] Rabe C, Musch A, Schirmacher P, Kruis W, Hoffmann R. Acute hepatitis induced by an Aloe vera preparation: a case report. *World J Gastroenterol.* 2005;11(2): 303-4.

[50] Feld L, Cifu AS. Management of Dyspepsia. *JAMA.* 2018;319(17):1816–1817. doi:10.1001/jama.2018.3435.

[51] Seyedmirzaei SM, Haghdoost AA, Afshari M, Dehghani A. Prevalence of dyspepsia and its associated factors among the adult population in southeast of iran in 2010. *Iran Red Crescent Med J.* 2014;16(11):e14757. Published 2014 Nov 1. doi:10.5812/ircmj.14757.

[52] Madisch A, Andresen V, Enck P, Labenz J, Frieling T, Schemann M. The Diagnosis and Treatment of Functional Dyspepsia. *Dtsch Arztebl Int.* 2018;115(13):222-232.

[53] Ghoshal UC, Singh R, Chang FY, et al. Epidemiology of uninvestigated and functional dyspepsia in Asia: facts and fiction. *J Neurogastroenterol Motil.* 2011;17(3):235-44.

[54] Nwokediuko SC, Ijoma U, Obienu O. Functional dyspepsia: subtypes, risk factors, and overlap with irritable bowel syndrome in a population of african patients. *Gastroenterol Res Pract.* 2012;2012:562393.

[55] Tack J, Talley NJ, Camilleri M, et al. Functional gastroduodenal disorders. *Gastroenterology.* 2006;130(5):1466–1479.

[56] Yamawaki H, Futagami S, Wakabayashi M, et al. Management of functional dyspepsia: state of the art and emerging therapies. *Ther Adv Chronic Dis.* 2017;9(1):23-32.

[57] Haag S, Talley NJ, Holtmann G. Symptom patterns in functional dyspepsia and irritable bowel syndrome: relationship to disturbances in gastric emptying and response to a nutrient challenge in consulters and non-consulters. *Gut* 2004; 53: 1445–1451.

[58] Lacy BE, Weiser KT, Kennedy AT, et al. Functional dyspepsia: the economic impact to patients. *Aliment Pharmacol Ther* 2013; 38: 170–177.

[59] Aro P, Talley NJ, Agreus L, et al. Functional dyspepsia impairs quality of life in the adult population. *Aliment Pharmacol Ther* 2011; 33: 1215–1224.

[60] Moayyedi P, Mason J. Clinical and economic consequences of dyspepsia in the community. *Gut* 2002; 50(Suppl. 4): iv10– iv12.

[61] Talley NJ, Ford AC. Functional dyspepsia. *N Engl J Med* 2015; 373: 1853–1863.

[62] Pittayanon R, Yuan Y, Bollegala NP, Khanna R, Lacy BE, Andrews CN, Leontiadis GI, Moayyedi P. Prokinetics for Functional Dyspepsia: A Systematic Review and Meta-Analysis of Randomized Control Trials. *Am J Gastroenterol.* 2019 Jan 11. doi: 10.1038/s41395-018-0258-6. [Epub ahead of print] PubMed PMID: 30337705.

[63] Kinoshita Y, Ishimura N, Ishihara S. Advantages and Disadvantages of Long-term Proton Pump Inhibitor Use. *J Neurogastroenterol Motil.* 2018;24(2):182-196.

[64] de Bortoli N, Tolone S, Frazzoni M, et al. Gastroesophageal reflux disease, functional dyspepsia and irritable bowel syndrome: common overlapping gastrointestinal disorders. *Ann Gastroenterol.* 2018;31(6):639-648.

[65] Swedish Council on Health Technology Assessment. Dyspepsia and Gastro-oesophageal Reflux: A Systematic Review (Summary and conclusions) [Internet]. *Stockholm: Swedish Council on Health Technology Assessment* (SBU); 2007 Oct. SBU Yellow Report No. 185. Available from: https://www.ncbi.nlm.nih.gov/books/NBK448002/

[66] Simadibrata M. Dyspepsia and gastroesophageal reflux disease (GERD): is there any correlation? *Acta Med Indones.* 2009 Oct;41(4):222-7. Review. PubMed PMID: 20737754.

[67] Chiarioni G, Pesce M, Fantin A, Sarnelli G. Complementary and alternative treatment in functional dyspepsia. *United European Gastroenterol J.* 2017;6(1):5-12.

[68] Jaber N, Oudah M, Kowatli A, et al. Dietary and Lifestyle Factors Associated with Dyspepsia among Pre-clinical Medical Students in Ajman, United Arab Emirates. *Cent Asian J Glob Health.* 2016; 5(1):192. Published 2016 Aug 15. doi:10.5195/cajgh.2016.192.

[69] Piessevaux H, De Winter B, Louis E, et al. Dyspeptic symptoms in the general population: a factor and cluster analysis of symptom groupings. *Neurogastro-enterol Motil* 2009; 21: 378–388.

[70] Welen K, Faresjo A, Faresjo T. Functional dyspepsia affects women more than men in daily life: a case-control study in primary care. *Gened Med* 2008; 5: 62–73.

[71] Raveendra KR, Jayachandra, Srinivasa V, Sushma KR, Allan JJ, Goudar KS, Shivaprasad HN, Venkateshwarlu K, Geetharani P, Sushma G, Agarwal A. An Extract of Glycyrrhiza glabra (GutGard) Alleviates Symptoms of Functional Dyspepsia: A Randomized, Double-Blind, Placebo-Controlled Study. *Evid Based Complement Alternat Med.* 2012;2012:216970. doi: 10.1155/2012/216970. Epub 2011 Jun 16. PubMed PMID: 21747893; PubMed Central PMCID: PMC3123991.

[72] Mohtashami R, Huseini HF, Heydari M, Amini M, Sadeqhi Z, Ghaznavi H, Mehrzadi S. Efficacy and safety of honey based formulation of Nigella sativa seed oil in functional dyspepsia: A double blind randomized controlled clinical trial. *J Ethnopharmacol.* 2015 Dec 4;175:147-52. doi: 10.1016/j.jep.2015.09.022. Epub 2015 Sep 18. PubMed PMID: 26386381.

[73] Piero Sestili, Tariq Ismail, Cinzia Calcabrini, Michele Guescini, Elena Catanzaro, Eleonora Turrini, Anam Layla, Saeed Akhtar & Carmela Fimognari (2018) The potential effects of Ocimum basilicum on health: a review of pharmacological and toxicological studies, *Expert Opinion on Drug Metabolism & Toxicology,* 14:7, 679-692, DOI: 10.1080/17425255.2018.1484450.

[74] Rafieian K, Hosseini-Asl K. Effects of Ocimum basilicum on functional dyspepsia: a double-blind placebo-controlled study. *IJMS.* 2005;30:134–7.

[75] Chawla YK, Dubey P, Singh R, Nundy S, Tandon BN. Treatment of dyspepsia with Amalaki (Emblica officinalis Linn.)--an Ayurvedic drug. *Indian J Med Res.* 1982; 76 Suppl:95–8.

[76] Grover HS, Deswal H, Singh Y, Bhardwaj A. Therapeutic effects of amla in medicine and dentistry: A review. *J Oral Res Rev* 2015;7:65-8.

[77] Usharani P, Fatima N, Muralidhar N. Effects of Phyllanthus emblica extract on endothelial dysfunction and biomarkers of oxidative stress in patients with type 2 diabetes mellitus: a randomized, double-blind, controlled study. *Diabetes Metab Syndr Obes.* 2013;6:275-84. Published 2013 Jul 26. doi:10.2147/DMSO.S46341.

[78] Dabos KJ, Sfika E, Vlatta LJ, Frantzi D, Amygdalos GI, Giannikopoulos G. Is Chios mastic gum effective in the treatment of functional dyspepsia? A prospective randomised double-blind placebo controlled trial. *J Ethnopharmacol.* 2010;127(2) :205–9. doi: 10.1016/j.jep.2009.11.021.

[79] Maliheh Safavi, Mohammadreza Shams-Ardakani & Alireza Foroumadi (2015) Medicinal plants in the treatment of Helicobacter pylori infections, *Pharmaceutical Biology,* 53:7, 939-960, DOI: 10.3109/13880209.2014.952837.

[80] de Lima RMT, Dos Reis AC, de Menezes APM, Santos JVO, Filho JWGO, Ferreira JRO, de Alencar MVOB, da Mata AMOF, Khan IN, Islam A, Uddin SJ, Ali ES, Islam MT, Tripathi S, Mishra SK, Mubarak MS, Melo-Cavalcante AAC. Protective and therapeutic potential of ginger (Zingiber officinale) extract and [6]-gingerol in cancer: A comprehensive review. *Phytother Res.* 2018 Oct;32 (10): 1885-1907. doi: 10.1002/ptr.6134. Epub 2018 Jul 16. Review. PubMed PMID: 30009484.

[81] Haniadka R, Saldanha E, Sunita V, Palatty PL, Fayad R, Baliga MS. A review of the gastroprotective effects of ginger (Zingiber officinale Roscoe). *Food Funct.* 2013 Jun;4(6):845-55. doi: 10.1039/c3fo30337c. Epub 2013 Apr 24. Review. PubMed PMID: 23612703.

[82] Hu ML, Rayner CK, Wu KL, et al. Effect of ginger on gastric motility and symptoms of functional dyspepsia. World J Gastroenterol. 2011;17(1):105-10.

[83] Bode AM, Dong Z. The Amazing and Mighty Ginger. In: Benzie IFF, Wachtel-Galor S, editors. *Herbal Medicine: Biomolecular and Clinical Aspects.* 2nd edition. Boca Raton (FL): CRC Press/Taylor & Francis; 2011. Chapter 7. Available from: https://www.ncbi.nlm.nih.gov/books/NBK92775/

[84] MacFarlane B. Management of gastroesophageal reflux disease in adults: a pharmacist's perspective. *Integr Pharm Res Pract.* 2018;7:41-52. Published 2018 Jun 5. doi:10.2147/IPRP.S142932.

[85] Sanati S, Razavi BM, Hosseinzadeh H. A review of the effects of Capsicum annuum L. and its constituent, capsaicin, in metabolic syndrome. *Iran J Basic Med Sci.* 2018;21(5):439-448.

[86] Pasalar M, Nimrouzi M, Choopani R, et al. Functional dyspepsia: A new approach from traditional Persian medicine. *Avicenna J Phytomed.* 2016;6(2):165-74.

[87] Forootan M, Bagheri N, Darvishi M. *Chronic constipation: A review of literature. Medicine* (Baltimore). 2018;97(20):e10631.

[88] Diaz S, Mendez MD. Constipation. [Updated 2018 Nov 18]. In: *StatPearls [Internet].* Treasure Island (FL): StatPearls Publishing; 2018 Jan-. Available from: https://www.ncbi.nlm.nih.gov/books/NBK513291/

[89] Tack J, Müller-Lissner S, Stanghellini V, et al. Diagnosis and treatment of chronic constipation—a European perspective. *Neurogastroenterol Motil* 2011;23:697–710.

[90] De Giorgio R, Ruggeri E, Stanghellini V, Eusebi LH, Bazzoli F, Chiarioni G. Chronic constipation in the elderly: a primer for the gastroenterologist. *BMC Gastroenterol.* 2015;15:130. Published 2015 Oct 14. doi:10.1186/s12876-015-0366-3.

[91] Higgins PD, Johanson JF. Epidemiology of constipation in North America: a systematic review. *Am J Gastroenterol.* 2004;99:750–9. doi: 10.1111/j.1572-0241.2004.04114.x.

[92] Bharucha AE, Pemberton JH, Locke GR., III American Gastroenterological Association technical review on constipation. *Am Gastroenterol Assoc Gastroenterol.* 2013;144:218–38.

[93] Fragakis A, Zhou J, Mannan H, Ho V. Association between Drug Usage and Constipation in the Elderly Population of Greater Western Sydney Australia. *Int J Environ Res Public Health.* 2018;15(2):226. Published 2018 Jan 29. doi:10.3390/ijerph15020226.

[94] Sandler R, Drossman DA. Bowel habits in young adults not seeking health care. *Dig Dis Sci.* 1987;32:841–5.

[95] Huang L, Jiang H, Zhu M, et al. Prevalence and Risk Factors of Chronic Constipation Among Women Aged 50 Years and Older in Shanghai, China. *Med Sci Monit.* 2017;23:2660-2667. Published 2017 May 31. doi:10.12659/MSM.904040.

[96] Sanchez MI, Bercik P. Epidemiology and burden of chronic constipation. *Can J Gastroenterol.* 2011;25 Suppl B(Suppl B):11B-15B.

[97] Colopast Web. *The Cost of Constipation report.* Available From: https://www.coloplast.co.uk/Global/UK/Continence/Cost_of_Constipation_Report_FINAL.pdf.

[98] WebMD. *Vitamins & Supplements. CASCARA SAGRADA*. Available From: https://www.webmd.com/vitamins/ai/ingredientmono-773/cascara-sagrada.

[99] Portalatin M, Winstead N. Medical management of constipation. *Clin Colon Rectal Surg.* 2012;25(1):12-9.

[100] Liu LW. Chronic constipation: Current treatment options. *Can J Gastroenterol.* 2011;25 Suppl B(Suppl B):22B-28B.

[101] Nguyen NQ, Chapman M, Fraser RJ, et al. Prokinetic therapy for feed intolerance in critical illness: one drug or two? *Crit Care Med* 35: 2561-2567, 2007.

[102] Shimizu K, Kageyama M, Ogura H, Yamada T, Shimazu T. Effects of Rhubarb on Intestinal Dysmotility in Critically Ill Patients. *Intern Med.* 2017;57(4):507-510.

[103] Chen DC, Wang L. Mechanisms of therapeutic effects of rhubarb on gut origin sepsis. *Chin J Traumatol* 12: 365-369, 2009.

[104] Iizuka N, Hamamoto Y. Constipation and herbal medicine. *Front Pharmacol.* 2015;6:73. Published 2015 Apr 8. doi:10.3389/fphar.2015.00073.

[105] McDermott A. 5 *Herbal Remedies for Constipation.* Reviewed by Debra Rose Wilson, PhD, MSN, RN, IBCLC, AHN-BC, CHT. Healthline Web November 21, 2017.

[106] Vilanova-Sanchez A, Gasior AC, Toocheck N, Weaver L, Wood RJ, Reck CA, Wagner A, Hoover E, Gagnon R, Jaggers J, Maloof T, Nash O, Williams C, Levitt MA. Are Senna based laxatives safe when used as long term treatment for constipation in children? *J Pediatr Surg.* 2018 Apr;53(4):722-727. doi: 10.1016/j.jpedsurg.2018.01.002. Epub 2018 Jan 31. Review. PubMed PMID: 29429768.

[107] Trottier M, Erebara A, Bozzo P. Treating constipation during pregnancy. *Can Fam Physician.* 2012;58(8):836-8.

[108] John LJ, Shantakumari N. Herbal Medicines Use During Pregnancy: A Review from the Middle East. *Oman Med J.* 2015;30(4):229-36.

[109] Since herbal medicines are a part of traditional medicine, they are not included in the FDA pregnancy categories giving a false impression of safety. The whole extracts of these herbal drugs contain numerous active molecules that could elicit adverse effects including teratogenicity.

[110] Marcus DM, Snodgrass WR. Do no harm: avoidance of herbal medicines during pregnancy. *Obstet Gynecol* 2005. May;105(5 Pt 1):1119-1122. 10.1097/01.AOG.0000158858.79134.ea.

[111] Cuzzolin L, Benoni G. Safety issues of phytomedicine in pregnancy and pediatrics. In: Ramawat KJ (ed). *Herbal Drugs: Ethnomedicine to Modern Medicine.* Springer-Verlag Berlin Heidelberg 2009: 382.

[112] Tiran D. The use of herbs by pregnant and childbearing women: a risk-benefit assessment. *Complement Ther Nurs Midwifery* 2003. Nov;9(4):176-181. 10.1016/S1353-6117(03)00045-3.

[113] Igarashi M, Nakae H, Matsuoka T, et al. Alteration in the gastric microbiota and its restoration by probiotics in patients with functional dyspepsia. *BMJ Open Gastroenterology* 2017;4:e000144. doi: 10.1136/bmjgast-2017-000144.

[114] Tabbers MM, Dilorenzo C, Berger MY, Faure C, Langendam MW, Nurko S, Staiano A, Vandenplas Y, Benninga MA. Evaluation and treatment of functional constipation in infants and children: evidence-based recommendations from ESPGHAN and NASPGHAN. *J Pediatr Gastroenterol Nutr.* 2014;58:265–281. doi: 10.1097/MPG.0000000000000266.

[115] Alammar N, Stein E. Irritable Bowel Syndrome: What Treatments Really Work. *Med Clin North Am.* 2019 Jan;103(1):137-152. doi: 10.1016/j.mcna.2018.08.006. Review. PubMed PMID: 30466670.

[116] Garcia-Etxebarria K, Zheng T, Bonfiglio F, Bujanda L, Dlugosz A, Lindberg G, Schmidt PT, Karling P, Ohlsson B, Simren M, Walter S, Nardone G, Cuomo R, Usai-Satta P, Galeazzi F, Neri M, Portincasa P, Bellini M, Barbara G, Jonkers D, Eswaran S, Chey WD, Kashyap P, Chang L, Mayer EA, Wouters MM, Boeckxstaens G, Camilleri M, Franke A, D'Amato M. Increased Prevalence of Rare Sucrase-isomaltase Pathogenic Variants in Irritable Bowel Syndrome Patients. *Clin Gastroenterol Hepatol.* 2018 Oct;16(10):1673-1676. doi: 10.1016/j.cgh.2018.01.047. Epub 2018 Feb 21. PubMed PMID: 29408290; PubMed Central PMCID: PMC6103908.

[117] Lacy B, Ayyagari R, Guerin A, Lopez A, Shi S, Luo M. Factors associated with more frequent diagnostic tests and procedures in patients with irritable bowel syndrome. *Therap Adv Gastroenterol.* 2019;12:1756284818818326. Published 2019 Jan 1. doi:10.1177/1756284818818326.

[118] Borghini R, Donato G, Alvaro D, Picarelli A. New insights in IBS-like disorders: Pandora's box has been opened; a review. *Gastroenterol Hepatol Bed Bench.* 2017;10(2):79-89.

[119] Wald A, Talley N, Grover S. *Treatment of irritable bowel syndrome in adults.* Available From: https://www.uptodate.com/contents/treatment-of-irritable-bowel-syndrome-in-adults?source=search_result&search=irritable%20bowel%20 syndrome&selectedTitle=1~150.

[120] IBS Global Impact Report 2018. BS Global Impact Report 2018. *With significant contribution from the Gastrointestinal Society Uncovering the true burden of irritable bowel syndrome (IBS) on people's lives.* Available From: https://www.badgut.org/wp-content/uploads/IBS-Global-Impact-Report.pdf.

[121] Su AM, Shih W, Presson AP, Chang L. Characterization of symptoms in irritable bowel syndrome with mixed bowel habit pattern. *Neurogastroenterol Motil.* 2014 Jan;26(1):36-45. doi: 10.1111/nmo.12220. Epub 2013 Aug 29. PubMed PMID: 23991913; PubMed Central PMCID: PMC3865067.

[122] Cañón M, Ruiz AJ, Rondón M, Alvarado J. Prevalence of irritable bowel syndrome and health-related quality of life in adults aged 18 to 30 years in a Colombian University: an electronic survey. *Ann Gastroenterol.* 2016;30(1):67-75.

[123] Abdul Rani R, Raja Ali RA, Lee YY. Irritable bowel syndrome and inflammatory bowel disease overlap syndrome: pieces of the puzzle are falling into place. *Intest Res.* 2016;14(4):297-304.

[124] Goldbaum E. *IBS patients obtain robust, enduring relief from home-based treatment program.* ScienceDaily Web April 23, 2018.

[125] Bahrami HR, Hamedi S, Salari R, Noras M. Herbal Medicines for the Management of Irritable Bowel Syndrome: A Systematic Review. *Electron Physician.* 2016;8(8):2719-2725. Published 2016 Aug 25. doi:10.19082/2719.

[126] Rahimi R, Abdollahi M. Herbal medicines for the management of irritable bowel syndrome: a comprehensive review. *World J Gastroenterol.* 2012;18(7):589-600.

[127] Grundmann O, Yoon SL. Complementary and alternative medicines in irritable bowel syndrome: an integrative view. *World J Gastroenterol.* 2014;20(2):346-62.

[128] US FDA Admin Web. *Zelnorm (tegaserod maleate) Information.* Available From: https://www.fda.gov/Drugs/DrugSafety/ucm103223.htm.

[129] Key Point. *Tegaserod Withdrawn From U.S. Market.* APhA Drug Info Online Web April 1, 2007.

[130] WHO Web. *Alosetron - withdrawn: severe adverse reactions.* Available From: http://apps.who.int/medicinedocs/en/d/Jh1466e/2.3.html.

[131] National Collaborating Centre for Nursing and Supportive Care (UK). Irritable Bowel Syndrome in Adults: Diagnosis and Management of Irritable Bowel Syndrome in Primary Care [Internet]. London: Royal College of Nursing (UK); 2008 Feb. (NICE Clinical Guidelines, No. 61.) 7, *Diet and lifestyle.* Available from: https://www.ncbi.nlm.nih.gov/books/NBK51960/

[132] Hawrelak JA, Myers SP. Effects of two natural medicine formulations onirritable bowel syndrome symptoms: a pilot study. *J Altern Complement Med.* 2010 Oct;16(10):1065-71. doi: 10.1089/acm.2009.0090. PubMed PMID: 20954962.

[133] Walker AF, Middleton RW, Petrowicz O. Artichoke leaf extract reduces symptomsof irritable bowel syndrome in a post-marketing surveillance study. *PhytotherRes.* 2001 Feb;15(1):58-61. PubMed PMID: 11180525.

[134] Villumsen M, Aznar S, Pakkenberg B, Jess T, Brudek T. Inflammatory bowel disease increases the risk of Parkinson's disease: a Danish nationwide cohort study 1977-2014. *Gut.* 2019 Jan;68(1):18-24. doi: 10.1136/gutjnl-2017-315666. Epub 2018 May 21. PubMed PMID: 29785965.

[135] Kreuter R, Wankell M, Ahlenstiel G, Hebbard L. The role of obesity in inflammatory bowel disease. *Biochim Biophys Acta Mol Basis Dis.* 2019 Jan;1865(1):63-72. doi: 10.1016/j.bbadis.2018.10.020. Epub 2018 Oct 22. Review. PubMed PMID: 30352258.

[136] Christensen B. Inflammatory bowel disease and sexual dysfunction. *Gastroenterol Hepatol* (N Y). 2014;10(1):53-5.

[137] de Vries JHM, Dijkhuizen M, Tap P, Witteman BJM. Patient's Dietary Beliefs and Behaviours in Inflammatory Bowel Disease. *Dig Dis.* 2019;37(2):131-139. doi: 10.1159/000494022. Epub 2018 Nov 2. PubMed PMID: 30391940.

[138] Volk N, Siegel CA. Defining Failure of Medical Therapy for Inflammatory Bowel Disease. *Inflamm Bowel Dis.* 2019 Jan 1;25(1):74-77. doi: 10.1093/ibd/izy238. PubMed PMID: 30016434.

[139] Naviglio S, Lacorte D, Lucafò M, Cifù A, Favretto D, Cuzzoni E, Silvestri T, Pozzi Mucelli M, Radillo O, Decorti G, Fabris M, Bramuzzo M, Taddio A, Stocco G, Alvisi P, Ventura A, Martelossi S. Causes of Treatment Failure in Children With Inflammatory Bowel Disease Treated With Infliximab: A Pharmacokinetic Study. *J Pediatr Gastroenterol Nutr.* 2019 Jan;68(1):37-44. doi: 10.1097/MPG.0000000000002112. PubMed PMID: 30211845.

[140] Shen B, Kochhar G, Navaneethan U, Liu X, Farraye FA, Gonzalez-Lama Y, Bruining D, Pardi DS, Lukas M, Bortlik M, Wu K, Sood A, Schwartz DA, Sandborn WJ; Global Interventional Inflammatory Bowel Disease Group. Role of interventional inflammatory bowel disease in the era of biologic therapy: a position statement from the Global Interventional IBD Group. *Gastrointest Endosc.* 2019 Feb;89(2):215-237. doi: 10.1016/j.gie.2018.09.045. Epub 2018 Oct 24. Review. PubMed PMID: 30365985.

[141] Lee HS, Park SK, Park DI. Novel treatments for inflammatory bowel disease. *Korean J Intern Med.* 2017;33(1):20-27.

[142] Ford AC, Peyrin-Biroulet L. Opportunistic infections with anti-tumor necrosis factor-α therapy in inflammatory bowel disease: meta-analysis of randomized controlled trials. *Am J Gastroenterol.* 2013;108:1268–1276.

[143] Walsh AJ, Weltman M, Burger D, et al. Implementing guidelines on the prevention of opportunistic infections in inflammatory bowel disease. *J Crohns Colitis.* 2013;7:e449–e456.

[144] Wilhelm SM, Love BL. Management of patients with inflammatory bowel disease: current and future treatments. Clinical Pharmacist, Web *The Pharmaceutical Journal* 1 February 2017.

[145] Feagan BG, Sandborn WJ, Colombel JF, et al. Incidence of Arthritis/Arthralgia in Inflammatory Bowel Disease with Long-term Vedolizumab Treatment: Post Hoc Analyses of the GEMINI Trials. *J Crohns Colitis.* 2018;13(1):50-57.

[146] Adamiak T, Walkiewicz-Jedrzejczak D, Fish D, et al. Incidence, clinical characteristics, and natural history of pediatric IBD in Wisconsin: a population-based epidemiological study. *Inflamm Bowel Dis.* 2013;19(6):1218-23.

[147] Burnett-Hartman AN, Hua X, Rue TC, Golchin N, Kessler L, Rowhani-Rahbar A. Risk interval analysis of emergency room visits following colonoscopy in patients with inflammatory bowel disease. *PLoS One.* 2019;14(1):e0210262. Published 2019 Jan 9. doi:10.1371/journal.pone.0210262.

[148] Ananthakrishnan AN, Bernstein CN, Iliopoulos D, Macpherson A, Neurath MF, Ali RAR, Vavricka SR, Fiocchi C. Environmental triggers in IBD: a review of progress and evidence. *Nature Reviews Gastroenterology & Hepatology*. volume 15, pages 39–49 (2018).

[149] Triantafyllidi A, Xanthos T, Papalois A, Triantafillidis JK. Herbal and plant therapy in patients with inflammatory bowel disease. *Ann Gastroenterol.* 2015;28(2):210-220.

[150] Ben-Arye E, Goldin E, Wengrower D, Stamper A, Kohn R, Berry E. Wheat grass juice in the treatment of active distal ulcerative colitis: a randomized double-blind placebo-controlled trial. *Scand J Gastroenterol.* 2002;37:444–449.

[151] Tang T., Targan S. R., Li Z.-S., Xu C., Byers V. S., Sandborn W. J. Randomised clinical trial: herbal extract HMPL-004 in active ulcerative colitis—a double-blind comparison with sustained release mesalazine. *Alimentary Pharmacology and Therapeutics.* 2011;33(2):194–202. doi: 10.1111/j.1365-2036.2010.04515.x.

[152] Gupta I, Parihar A, Malhotra P, et al. Effects of gum resin of Boswellia serrata in patients with chronic colitis. *Planta Med.* 2001;67:391–395.

[153] Omer B., Krebs S., Omer H., Noor T. O. Steroid-sparing effect of wormwood (Artemisia absinthium) in Crohn's disease: a double-blind placebo-controlled study. *Phytomedicine.* 2007;14(2-3):87–95. doi: 10.1016/j.phymed.2007.01.001.

[154] Sun J, Shen X, Dong J, Wang H, Zuo L, Zhao J, Zhu W, Li Y, Gong J, Li J. Tripterygium wilfordii Hook F as Maintenance Treatment for Crohn's Disease. *Am J Med Sci.* 2015 Nov;350(5):345-51. doi: 10.1097/MAJ.0000000000000591. PubMed PMID: 26473333.

[155] Ng SC, Lam YT, Tsoi KK, Chan FK, Sung JJ, Wu JC. Systematic review: the efficacy of herbal therapy in inflammatory bowel disease. *Aliment Pharmacol Ther.* 2013 Oct;38(8):854-63. doi: 10.1111/apt.12464. Epub 2013 Aug 25. Review. PubMed PMID: 23981095.

[156] Athasit Kijmanawat, Panyu Panburana, Sirimon Reutrakul and Chayada Tangshewinsirikul, Effects of probiotic supplements on insulin resistance in

gestational diabetes mellitus: A double-blind randomized controlled trial, J*ournal of Diabetes Investigation,* 10, 1, (163-170), (2018).

[157] Holzapfel WH, Haberer P, Snel J, Schillinger U, Huis in `t Veld JHJ. Overview of gut flora and probiotics. *Int J Food Microbiol* 1998;41: 85-101.

[158] Gorbach SL. Lactic acid bacteria and human health. *Ann Med* 1990;22: 37-41.

[159] Jonkers D, Stockbrügger R. Probiotics and inflammatory bowel disease. *J R Soc Med.* 2003;96(4):167-71.

[160] Plaza-Díaz J, Ruiz-Ojeda FJ, Vilchez-Padial LM, Gil A. Evidence of the Anti-Inflammatory Effects of Probiotics and Synbiotics in Intestinal Chronic Diseases. *Nutrients.* 2017;9(6):555. Published 2017 May 28. doi:10.3390/nu9060555.

[161] Lee EJ, Lee YJ, Park JH. Usefulness of Ultrasonography in the Diagnosis of Peptic Ulcer Disease in Children. *Pediatr Gastroenterol Hepatol Nutr.* 2019;22(1):57-62.

[162] Yu HC, Chen TP, Wei CY, Chang YC. Association between Peptic Ulcer Disease and Periodontitis: A Nationwide Population-Based Case-Control Study in Taiwan. *Int J Environ Res Public Health.* 2018;15(5):912. Published 2018 May 4. doi:10.3390/ijerph15050912.

[163] Malik TF, Singh K. Peptic Ulcer Disease. [Updated 2018 Dec 4]. In: *StatPearls* [Internet]. Treasure Island (FL): StatPearls Publishing; 2018 Jan-. Available from: https://www.ncbi.nlm.nih.gov/books/NBK534792/

[164] Lanas A, Chan FKL. Peptic ulcer disease. *Lancet*. 2017 Aug 05;390(10094):613-624.

[165] Akeel M, Elmakki E, Shehata A, et al. Prevalence and factors associated with H. pylori infection in Saudi patients with dyspepsia. *Electron Physician.* 2018;10(9):7279-7286. Published 2018 Sep 9. doi:10.19082/7279.

[166] Vomero ND, Colpo E. Nutritional care in peptic ulcer. *Arq Bras Cir Dig.* 2014;27(4):298-302.

[167] Lafortuna CL, Agosti F, Marinone PG, Marazzi N, Sartorio A. The relationship between body composition and muscle power output in men and women with obesity. *J Endocrinol Invest.* 2004;27:854–861.

[168] Sayehmiri K, Abangah G, Kalvandi G, Tavan H, Aazami S. Prevalence of peptic ulcer in Iran: Systematic review and meta-analysis methods. *J Res Med Sci.* 2018;23:8. Published 2018 Jan 29. doi:10.4103/jrms.JRMS_1035_16.

[169] Narayanan M, Reddy KM, Marsicano E. Peptic Ulcer Disease and Helicobacter pylori infection. *Mo Med.* 2018;115(3):219-224.

[170] Mayank K, Gunja S, Pratap SM. *Pathophysiological status and nutritional therapy of peptic ulcer*: An update. Year: 2017 | Volume: 2 | Issue Number: 3 | Page: 76-86.

[171] Mattos LL, Martins IS. Dietary fiber consumption in an adult population. *Rev Saude Publica.* 2000 Feb; 34(1):50-5.

[172] Vomero ND, Colpo E. Nutritional care in peptic ulcer. *Arq Bras Cir Dig.* 2014;27(4):298-302.

[173] Cheng Y, Macera CA, Davis DR, Blair SN. Physical activity and peptic ulcers. Does physical activity reduce the risk of developing peptic ulcers?. *West J Med.* 2000;173(2):101-7.

[174] Albaqawi ASB, El-Fetoh NMA, Alanazi RFA, et al. Profile of peptic ulcer disease and its risk factors in Arar, Northern Saudi Arabia. *Electron Physician.* 2017;9(11):5740-5745. Published 2017 Nov 25. doi:10.19082/5740.

[175] Levenstein S, Kaplan GA, Smith M. Sociodemographic characteristics, lifestressors, and peptic ulcer. A prospective study. *J Clin Gastroenterol.* 1995Oct; 21(3):185-92. PubMed PMID: 8648050.

[176] Shephard RJ. Peptic Ulcer and Exercise. *Sports Med.* 2017 Jan;47(1):33-40. doi: 10.1007/s40279-016-0563-4. Review. PubMed PMID: 27282926.

[177] Vimala G, Gricilda Shoba F. A review on antiulcer activity of few Indian medicinal plants. *Int J Microbiol.* 2014;2014:519590.

[178] Nadkarni's KM. *Indian Materia Medica,* Volume 1. Mumbai, India: Popular Prakashan; 1976.

[179] Díaz-de-Cerio E, Verardo V, Gómez-Caravaca AM, Fernández-Gutiérrez A, Segura-Carretero A. Health Effects of Psidium guajava L. Leaves: An Overview of the Last Decade. *Int J Mol Sci.* 2017;18(4):897. Published 2017 Apr 24. doi:10.3390/ijms18040897.

[180] Ilavarasan JR, Monideen S, Vijayalakshmi M. Antiulcer activity of Aegle marmelos. *Ancient Science of Life.* 2002;21(4):23–26.

[181] Park JJ. The Garlic Preparation as an Alternative Way for Gastroprotection: From Bench to Clinic. *Gut Liver.* 2016;10(3):321-2.

[182] El-Ashmawy NE, Khedr EG, El-Bahrawy HA, Selim HM. Gastroprotective effect of garlic in indomethacin induced gastric ulcer in rats. *Nutrition.* 2016 Jul-Aug;32(7-8):849-54. doi: 10.1016/j.nut.2016.01.010. Epub 2016 Jan 21. PubMed PMID: 27158056.

[183] Gadekar R, Singour PK, Chaurasiya PK, Pawar RS, Patil UK. A potential of some medicinal plants as an antiulcer agents. *Pharmacogn Rev.* 2010;4(8):136-46.

[184] Alzohairy MA. Therapeutics Role of Azadirachta indica (Neem) and Their Active Constituents in Diseases Prevention and Treatment. *Evid Based Complement Alternat Med.* 2016;2016:7382506.

[185] Zakaria ZA, Abdul Hisam EE, Rofiee MS, Norhafizah M, Somchit MN, Teh LK, Salleh MZ. In vivo antiulcer activity of the aqueous extract of Bauhinia purpurea leaf. *J Ethnopharmacol.* 2011 Sep 2;137(2):1047-54. doi: 10.1016/j.jep.2011.07.038. Epub 2011 Jul 23. PubMed PMID: 21802502.

[186] Sharifi-Rad M, Fokou PVT, Sharopov F, et al. Antiulcer Agents: From Plant Extracts to Phytochemicals in Healing Promotion. *Molecules.* 2018;23(7):1751. Published 2018 Jul 17. doi:10.3390/molecules23071751.

[187] Farzaei MH, Abdollahi M, Rahimi R. Role of dietary polyphenols in the management of peptic ulcer. *World J Gastroenterol.* 2015;21(21):6499-517.

[188] Rahnama M, Mehrabani D, Japoni S, Edjtehadi M, Saberi Firoozi M. The healing effect of licorice (Glycyrrhiza glabra) on Helicobacter pylori infected peptic ulcers. *J Res Med Sci.* 2013;18(6):532-3.

[189] Almasaudi SB, Abbas AT, Al-Hindi RR, et al. Manuka Honey Exerts Antioxidant and Anti-Inflammatory Activities That Promote Healing of Acetic Acid-Induced Gastric Ulcer in Rats. *Evid Based Complement Alternat Med*. 2017;2017:5413917.

[190] Markowiak P, Śliżewska K. Effects of Probiotics, Prebiotics, and Synbiotics on Human Health. *Nutrients.* 2017;9(9):1021. Published 2017 Sep 15. doi: 10.3390/nu9091021.

[191] Khoder G, Al-Menhali AA, Al-Yassir F, Karam SM. Potential role of probiotics in the management of gastric ulcer. *Exp Ther Med.* 2016;12(1):3-17.

[192] Jorge M.B. Vítor, Filipa F. Vale; Alternative therapies for Helicobacter pylori: probiotics and phytomedicine, *FEMS Immunology & Medical Microbiology,* Volume 63, Issue 2, 1 November 2011, Pages 153–164, https://doi.org/10.1111/j.1574-695X.2011.00865.x.

Chapter 5

INDIAN HERBS AND HERBAL DRUGS USED FOR THE TREATMENT OF DIABETES

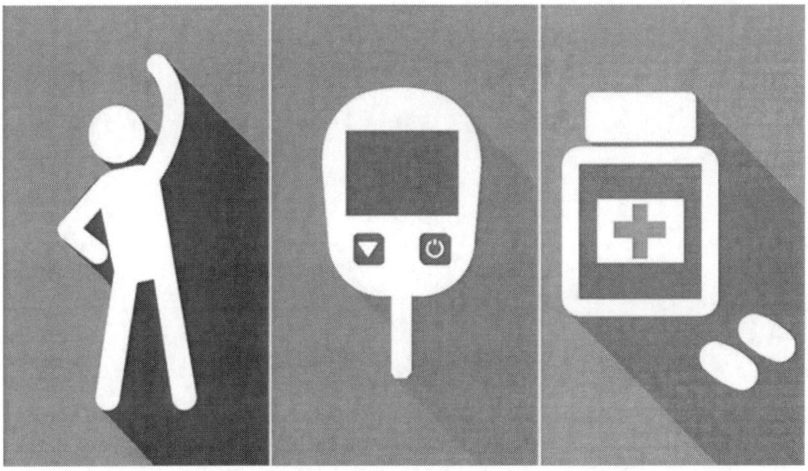

1. ABSTRACT

Traditional Medicines derived from medicinal plants are used by about 60% of the world's population. This review focuses on Indian Herbal drugs and plants used in the treatment of diabetes, especially in India. Diabetes is an important human ailment afflicting many from various walks of life in different countries. In India it is proving to be a major health problem, especially in the urban areas. Though there are various approaches to reduce the ill effects of diabetes and its secondary complications, herbal formulations are preferred due to lesser side effects and low cost. A list of medicinal plants with proven antidiabetic and related beneficial effects and of herbal drugs used in treatment of diabetes is compiled. These include, *Allium sativum*, *Eugenia jambolana*, *Momordica charantia*, *Ocimum sanctum, Phyllanthus amarus*, *Pterocarpus marsupium*, *Tinospora cordifolia*, *Trigonella foenum* graecum and *Withania somnifera*. One of the etiologic factors implicated in the development of diabetes and its complications is the damage induced by free radicals and hence an antidiabetic compound with antioxidant properties would be more beneficial. Therefore, information on antioxidant effects of these medicinal plants is also included.

Keywords: medicinal plant, India, antidiabetic, antioxidant, diabetes

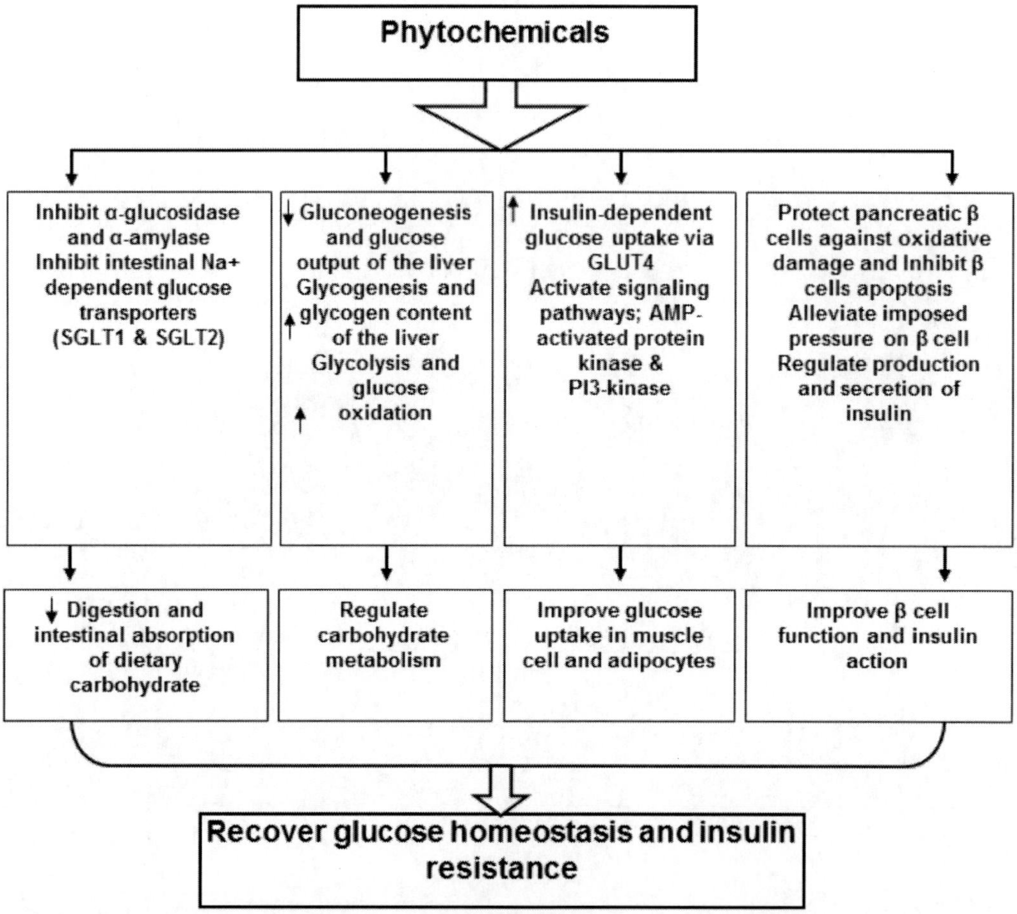

Figure 1. Phytochemicals for diabetes prevention. The hypoglycemic effects of phytochemicals are chiefly ascribed to lower the uptake of carbohydrates in intestine affecting the glucose metabolism by applying an alteration in the enzyme activities, β-cell function betterment and insulin action improvement, insulin release initiation and antioxidant as well as anti-inflammatory characteristic of these components. SGLT: Sodium-Glucose Linked Transporter. (Source: Sayem ASM, Arya A et al. Action of Phytochemicals on Insulin Signaling Pathways Accelerating Glucose Transporter (GLUT4) Protein Translocation. Molecules 2018, 23(2), 258; doi:10.3390/molecules23020258.)

2. INTRODUCTION

In the last few years there has been an exponential growth in the field of herbal medicine and these drugs are gaining popularity both in developing and developed countries because of their natural origin and less side effects. Many traditional medicines in use are derived from medicinal plants, minerals and organic matter [1]. A number of medicinal plants, traditionally used for over 1000 years named rasayana are present in herbal preparations of Indian traditional health care systems [2]. In Indian systems of medicine most practitioners formulate and dispense their own recipes [3]. The WHO has listed 21,000 plants, which are used for medicinal purposes around the world. Among these 2500 species are in India, out of which 150 species are used commercially on a fairly large scale. India is the largest producer of medicinal herbs and is called as botanical garden of the world [3]. The current review focuses on herbal drug preparations and plants used in the treatment of diabetes mellitus, a major crippling disease in the world.

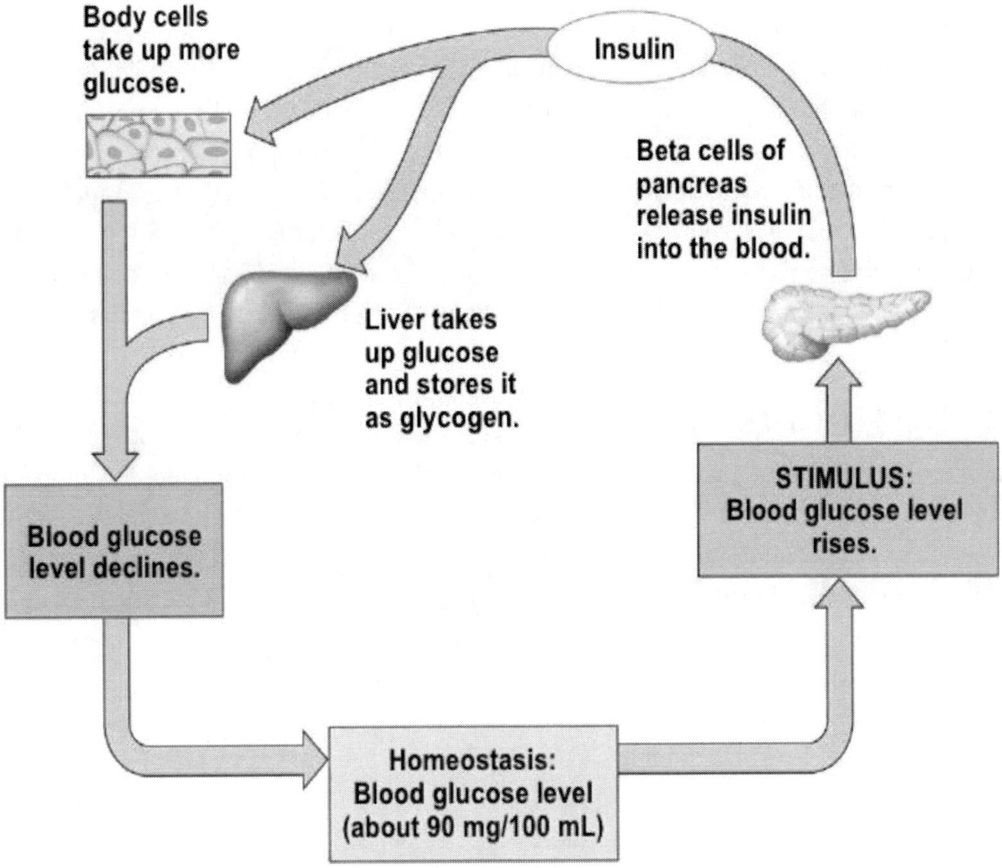

Figure 2. Control of blood glucose by insulin. Insulin is normally secreted by the beta cells (a type of islet cell) of the pancreas. The stimulus for insulin secretion is a high blood glucose. Although there is always a low level of insulin secreted by the pancreas, the amount secreted into the blood increases as the blood glucose rises. Similarly, as blood glucose falls, the amount of insulin secreted by the the pancreatic islets goes down. As can be seen in the picture, insulin has an effect on a number of cells, including muscle, red blood cells, and fat cells. In response to insulin, these cells absorb glucose out of the blood, having the net effect of lowering the high blood glucose levels into the normal range.

3. Diabetes and Significance

Diabetes is a chronic disorder of carbohydrate, fat and protein metabolism characterized by increased fasting and post prandial blood sugar levels. The global prevalence of diabetes is estimated to increase, from 4% in 1995 to 5.4% by the year 2025. WHO has predicted that the major burden will occur in developing countries. Studies conducted in India in the last decade have highlighted that not only is the prevalence of diabetes high but also that it is increasing rapidly in the urban population [4]. It is estimated that there are approximately 33 million adults with diabetes in India. This number is likely to increase to 57.2 million by the year 2025. Diabetes mellitus is a complex metabolic disorder resulting from either insulin insufficiency or insulin dysfunction. Type I diabetes (insulin dependent) is caused due to insulin insufficiency because of lack of functional beta cells. Patients suffering from this are therefore totally dependent on exogenous source of insulin while patients suffering from Type II diabetes (insulin independent) are unable to respond to insulin and can be treated with dietary changes, exercise and medication. Type II diabetes is the more common form of diabetes constituting 90% of the diabetic population. Symptoms for both diabetic conditions may include: (i) high levels of sugar in the blood; (ii) unusual thirst; (iii) frequent urination; (iv) extreme hunger and loss of weight; (v) blurred vision; (vi) nausea and vomiting; (vii) extreme weakness and tiredness; (viii) irritability, mood changes etc. Though pathophysiology of diabetes remains to be fully understood, experimental evidences suggest the involvement of free radicals in the pathogenesis of diabetes [5] and more importantly in the development of diabetic complications [6– 8]. Free radicals are capable of damaging cellular molecules, DNA, proteins and lipids leading to altered cellular functions. Many recent studies reveal that antioxidants capable of neutralizing free radicals are effective in preventing experimentally induced diabetes in animal models [9, 10] as well as reducing the severity of diabetic complications [8].

For the development of diabetic complications, the abnormalities produced in lipids and proteins are the major etiologic factors. In diabetic patients, extra-cellular and long-lived proteins, such as elastin, laminin, collagen are the major targets of free radicals. These proteins are modified to form glycoproteins due to hyperglycemia. The modification of these proteins presents in tissues such as lens, vascular wall and basement membranes are associated with the development of complications of diabetes such as cataracts, microangiopathy, atherosclerosis and nephropathy [11]. During diabetes, lipoproteins are oxidized by free radicals. There are also multiple abnormalities of lipoprotein metabolism in very low-density lipoprotein (VLDL), low density lipoprotein (LDL), and high-density lipoprotein (HDL) in diabetes. Lipid peroxidation is enhanced due to increased oxidative stress in diabetic condition. Apart from this, advanced glycation end products (AGEs) are formed by non-enzymatic glycosylation of proteins. AGEs tend to accumulate on long-lived molecules in tissues and generate abnormalities in cell and tissue functions [12, 13].

In addition, AGEs also contribute to increased vascular permeability in both micro and macrovascular structures by binding to specific macrophage receptors. This results in formation of free radicals and endothelial dysfunction. AGEs are also formed on nucleic acids and histones and may cause mutations and altered gene expression. As diabetes is a multifactorial disease leading to several complications, and therefore demands a multiple therapeutic approach.

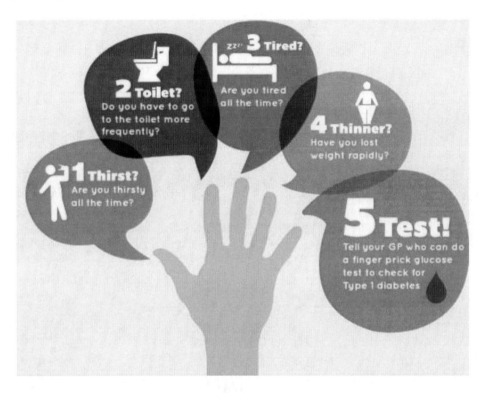

Figure 3. Diabetes symptoms. Low levels of insulin to achieve adequate response and/or insulin resistance of target tissues, mainly skeletal muscles, adipose tissue, and to a lesser extent, liver, at the level of insulin receptors, signal transduction system, and/or effector enzymes or genes are responsible for these metabolic abnormalities. The severity of symptoms is due to the type and duration of diabetes. Some of the diabetes patients are asymptomatic especially those with type 2 diabetes during the early years of the disease, others with marked hyperglycemia and especially in children with absolute insulin deficiency may suffer from polyuria, polydipsia, polyphagia, weight loss, and blurred vision. Uncontrolled diabetes may lead to stupor, coma and if not treated death, due to ketoacidosis or rare from nonketotic hyperosmolar syndrome. (Source: Kharroubi AT, Darwish HM. Diabetes mellitus: The epidemic of the century. World J Diabetes. 2015;6(6):850-67.)

Patients of diabetes either do not make enough insulin or their cells do not respond to insulin. In case of total lack of insulin, patients are given insulin injections. Whereas in case of those where cells do not respond to insulin many different drugs are developed taking into consideration possible disturbances in carbohydrate-metabolism. For example, to manage post-prandial hyper-glycaemia at digestive level, glucosidase inhibitors such as acarbose, miglitol and voglibose are used. These inhibit degradation of carbohydrates thereby reducing the glucose absorption by the cells. To enhance glucose uptake by peripheral cells biguanide such as metphormine is used. Sulphonylureas like glibenclamide is insulinotropic and works as secretogogue for pancreatic cells. Although several therapies are in use for treatment, there are certain limitations due to high cost and side effects such as development of hypoglycemia, weight gain, gastrointestinal disturbances, liver toxicity etc [14]. Based on recent advances and involvement of oxidative stress in complicating diabetes mellitus, efforts are on to find suitable antidiabetic and antioxidant therapy.

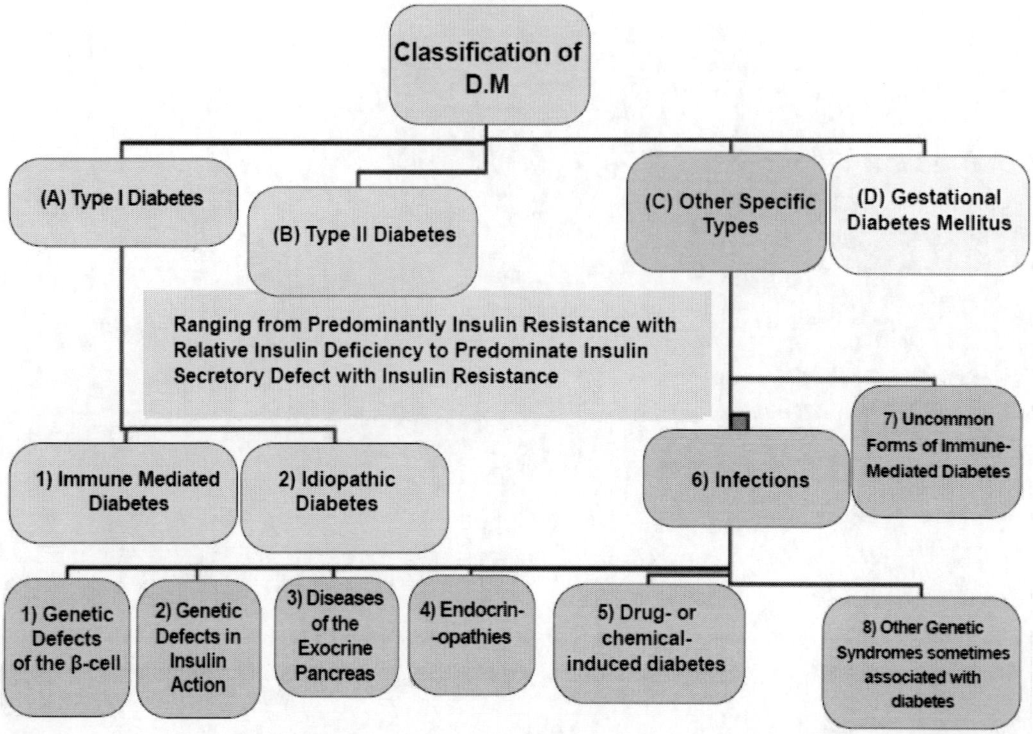

Figure 4. Classification of diabetes mellitus. Diabetes is a heterogeneous, complex metabolic disorder characterized by elevated blood glucose concentrations secondary to either resistance to the action of insulin, insufficient insulin secretion, or both. The most common classifications include Type 1 diabetes mellitus, Type 2 diabetes mellitus, and gestational diabetes. Type 2 diabetes (T2DM) is characterized by insulin resistance and a relative deficiency of insulin secretion. The absolute plasma insulin concentration (both fasting and meal-stimulated) usually is increased, although "relative" to the severity of insulin resistance, the plasma insulin concentration is insufficient to maintain normal glucose homeostasis. Insulin secretion capacity progressively worsens over time in most patients with T2DM. Type 1 DM results in an absolute deficiency in beta-cell function in most. Autoimmune destruction of beta-cells is a common origin, though cases continue to be classified as idiopathic. Gestational diabetes mellitus (GDM) is defined as glucose intolerance which is first recognized during pregnancy. In most women who develop GDM, the disorder has its onset in the third trimester of pregnancy and patients with GDM have a high risk of developing T2DM later in life. Other causes of diabetes include genetic disorders, diseases that cause damage to the pancreas, as well as an excess of certain hormones such as growth hormone and glucocorticoids. Diabetes mellitus may also be due to drugs, chemicals, or infections. Proper classification of the type of diabetes often helps determine appropriate therapy. (Source: Solis-Herrera C, Triplitt C, Reasner C, et al. Classification of Diabetes Mellitus. [Updated 2018 Feb 24]. In: Feingold KR, Anawalt B, Boyce A, et al., editors. Endotext South Dartmouth (MA): MDText.com, Inc.; 2000-. Available from: https://www.ncbi.nlm.nih.gov/books/NBK279119/.)

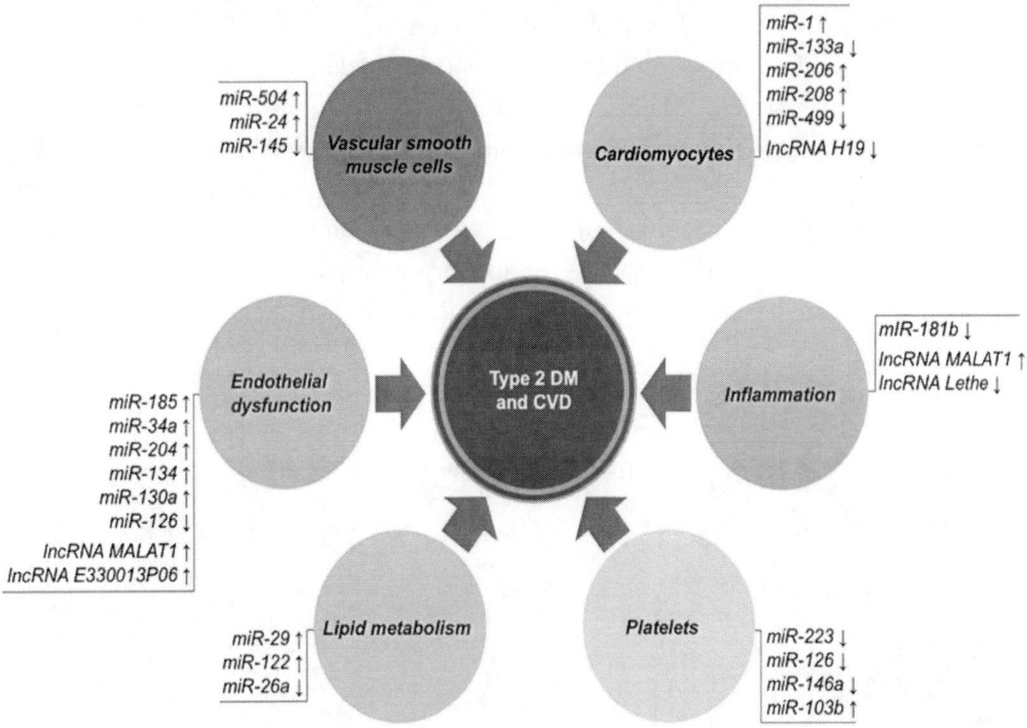

Figure 5. Non-coding RNAs associated with both type 2 diabetes mellitus (DM) and cardiovascular disease (CVD). MicroRNAs (miRNAs) and long non-coding RNAs (lncRNAs) are grouped according to their main biological mechanism involved in atherosclerotic CVD. Arrows indicate overexpression (↑) or underexpression (↓). An important issue is the link between lipid metabolism and miRNAs in diabetic CVD. Several important genes implicated in lipid synthesis or processing, like FoxA2, Ppargcla, Hmgcs2, and Abdhd5 have been shown to be dysregulated by miR-29 in Zucker diabetic fatty rats, while HNF-4 alpha was found to be raised by increased levels of miR-122 in diabetic mice and insulin-resistant HepG2 cells. Both miR-122 and HNF-4 alpha were able to upregulate the expression of SREBP-1 and FAAS genes, causing abnormal cholesterol homeostasis and high levels of fatty acid and triglyceride synthesis. Finally, decreased levels of miR-26a have been reported in obese mice, in which they contribute to increased fatty acid synthesis, and to obesity-related metabolic complications. (Source: Rosa SD, Arcidiacono B et al. Type 2 Diabetes Mellitus and Cardiovascular Disease: Genetic and Epigenetic Links. Front. Endocrinol., 17 January 2018 | https://doi.org/10.3389/fendo.2018.00002.)

Medicinal plants are being looked up once again for the treatment of diabetes. Many conventional drugs have been derived from prototypic molecules in medicinal plants. Metformin exemplifies an efficacious oral glucose-lowering agent. Its development was based on the use of Galega officinalis to treat diabetes. Galega officinalis is rich in guanidine, the hypoglycemic component. Because guanidine is too toxic for clinical use, the alkyl biguanides synthalin A and synthalin B were introduced as oral anti-diabetic agents in Europe in the 1920s but were discontinued after insulin became more widely available. However, experience with guanidine and biguanides prompted the development of metformin. To date, over 400 traditional plant treatments for diabetes have been reported, although only a small number of these have received scientific and medical evaluation to assess their efficacy. The hypoglycemic effect of some herbal extracts has been confirmed in human and animal models of type 2 diabetes. The World Health Organization Expert Committee on diabetes has recommended that traditional medicinal herbs be further investigated. Major hindrance in amalgamation of herbal medicine in modern medical practices is lack of scientific and clinical data proving their efficacy and safety. There is a need for conducting clinical research in herbal drugs, developing simple bioassays for biological standardization, pharmacological and toxicological evaluation, and developing various animal models for toxicity and safety evaluation. It is also important to establish the active component/s from these plant extracts.

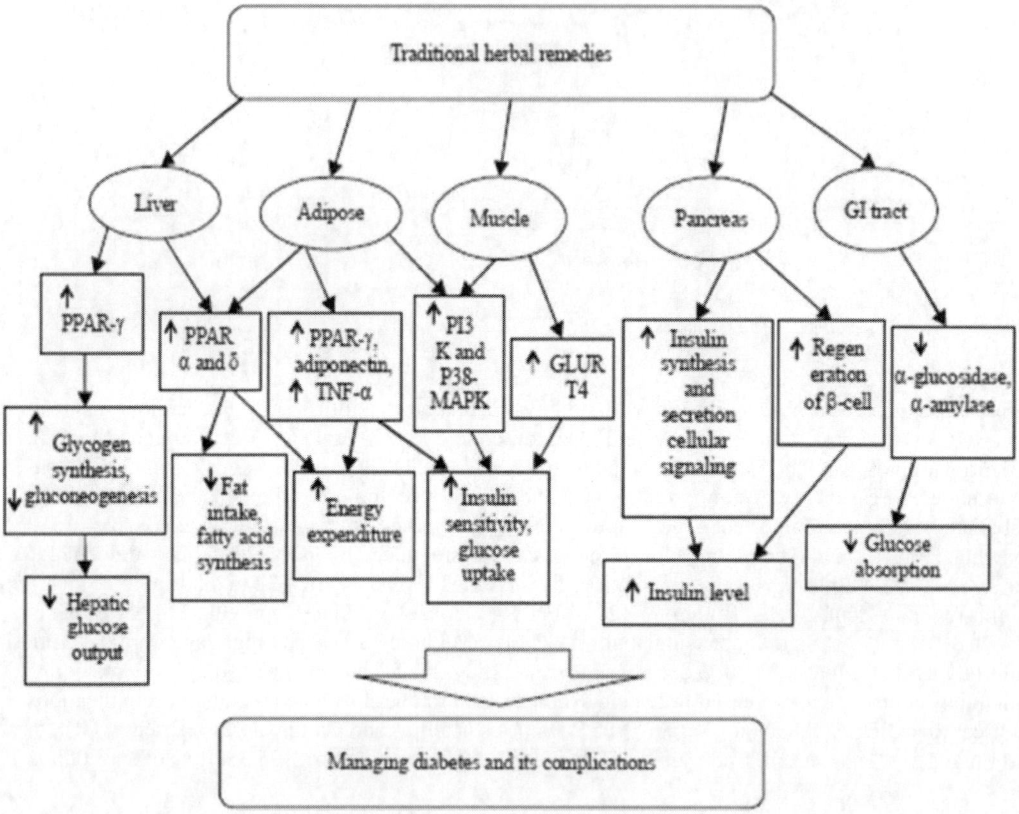

Figure 6. Molecular and cellular mechanisms for the efficacy of traditional herbal remedies and their phytochemicals in diabetes mellitus and its relevant complications. Plants remain as an important source of therapeutic material for maintaining human health with unparalleled diversity and they have improved the quality of human life through disease prevention and treatment for centuries. Moreover, medicinal plants are an abundant source of biologically active molecules that play an important role in past and modern medicine, which act as a "Stepping stone" for the discovery of novel pharmacologically active ligands. This has prompted much interest in the use of traditional medicines for the treatment of diabetes. (Source: Mohammad Hosein Farzaei, Roja Rahimi, Fatemeh Farzaei and Mohammad Abdollahi, 2015. Traditional Medicinal Herbs for the Management of Diabetes and its Complications: An Evidence-Based Review. International Journal of Pharmacology, 11: 874-887. DOI: 10.3923/ijp.2015.874.887.)

4. Indian Medicinal Plants with Antidiabetic and Related Beneficial Effects

There are many herbal remedies suggested for diabetes and diabetic complications. Medicinal plants form the main ingredients of these formulations. A list of medicinal plants with antidiabetic and related beneficial effects is given in Table 1 [15]. A list of such formulations is given in Table 2.

4.1. *Acacia arabica (*Babhul*)*

It is found all over India mainly in the wild habitat. The plant extract acts as an antidiabetic agent by acting as secretagouge to release insulin. It induces hypoglycemia in control rats but not in alloxanized animals. Powdered seeds of Acacia arabica when administered (2,3 and 4 g/kg body weight) to normal rabbits induced hypoglycemic effect by initiating release of insulin from pancreatic beta cells [16].

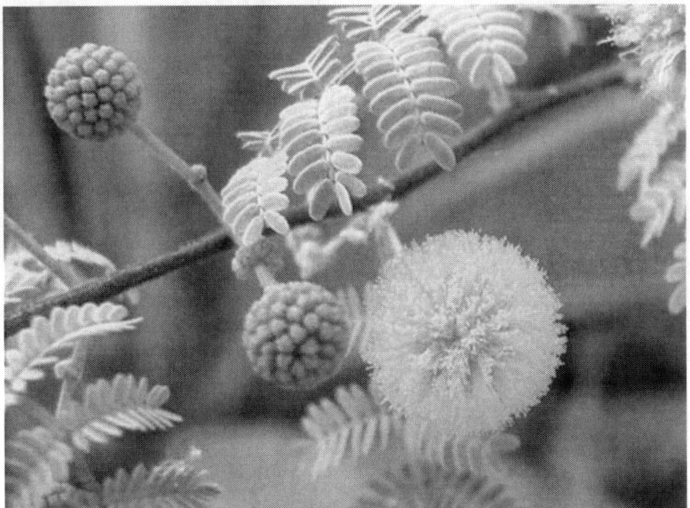

Figure 7. *Acacia arabica*. There is a strong association between cardiometabolic risk and adipose tissue dysfunction with great consequences on type 2 diabetic patients. Visceral Adiposity Index (VAI) is an indirect clinical marker of adipose tissue dysfunction. Gum Arabic (GA) is a safe dietary fiber, an exudate of Acacia Senegal. Gum Arabic had shown lipid lowering effect in both humans and animals. (Source: Babiker R, Elmusharaf K, Keogh MB, Saeed AM. Effect of Gum Arabic (Acacia Senegal) supplementation on visceral adiposity index (VAI) and blood pressure in patients with type 2 diabetes mellitus as indicators of cardiovascular disease (CVD): a randomized and placebo-controlled clinical trial. Lipids Health Dis. 2018;17(1):56. Published 2018 Mar 20. doi:10.1186/s12944-018-0711-y.)

4.2. *Aegle marmelos* (Bengal Quince, Bel or Bilva)

Administration of aqueous extract of leaves improves digestion and reduces blood sugar and urea, serum cholesterol in alloxanized rats as compared to control. Along with exhibiting hypoglycemic activity, this extract also prevented peak rise in blood sugar at 1h in oral glucose tolerance test [17].

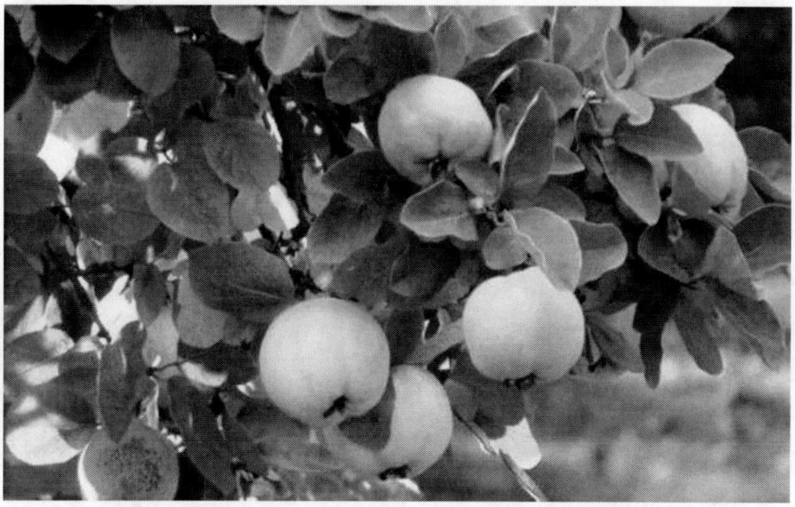

Figure 8. Aegle marmelos/Bilva. The plant is found in all over India and also called as Indian Quince, holy fruit (According to Hindu mythology it is holy plant) anti-diabetic activity of Umbelliferone β-D-galactopyranoside isolated from the stem bark of *Aegle marmelos* Correa. It is established that Umbelliferone is a potent free radical scavenger and works as antioxidant. The antioxidant activity of Umbelliferone β-D-galactopyranoside and the major root cause of diabetes mellitus is the development of free radicals which destroys the β-cells of the pancreatic islets is also reported, responsible for the secretion of insulin in experimental animal. (Source: Kumar V, Ahmed D, Verma A, Anwar F, Ali M, Mujeeb M. Umbelliferone β-D-galactopyranoside from Aegle marmelos (L.) corr. an ethnomedicinal plant with antidiabetic, antihyperlipidemic and antioxidative activity. BMC Complement Altern Med. 2013;13:273. Published 2013 Oct 20. doi:10.1186/1472-6882-13-273.)

4.3. *Allium cepa* (Onion)

Various ether soluble fractions as well as insoluble fractions of dried onion powder show anti-hyperglycemic activity in diabetic rabbits. *Allium cepa* is also known to have antioxidant and hypolipidaemic activity. Administration of a sulfur containing amino acid from Allium cepa, S-methyl cysteine sulphoxide (SMCS) (200 mg/kg for 45 days) to alloxan induced diabetic rats significantly controlled blood glucose as well as lipids in serum and tissues and normalized the activities of liver hexokinase, glucose 6-phosphatase and HMG Co A reductase [18, 19]. When diabetic patients were given single oral dose of 50 g of onion juice, it significantly controlled post-prandial glucose levels [20].

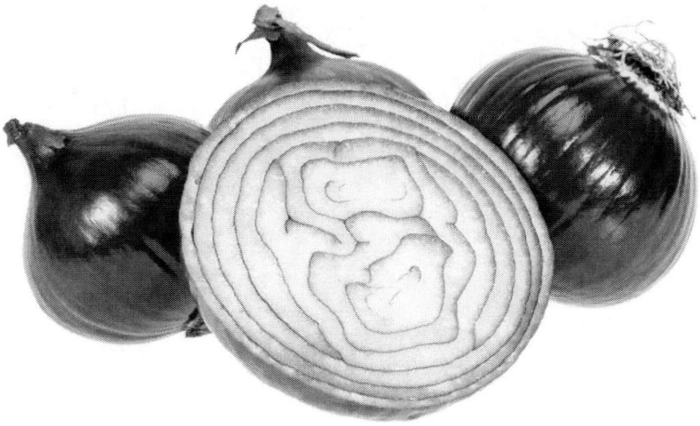

Figure 9. *Allium cepa*. *Allium cepa* has a bulb that lies underground as part of the stem, and is often used as household vegetable. For hundreds of years, Allium has been used medicinally. Its most popular application is to lower blood pressure; besides it acts antiseptic, hypoglycemic, hypocholesterolemic, and inhibits oxidative stress. Allium cepa's active ingredient is allyl propyl disulfide (APDS); it also has active sulfurous compounds, such as S-methyl cysteine sulphoxide (SMCS), which act in an antidiabetic and hypolipidemic manner. (Source: El-Refaei MF, Abduljawad SH, Alghamdi AH. Alternative Medicine in Diabetes - Role of Angiogenesis, Oxidative Stress, and Chronic Inflammation. Rev Diabet Stud. 2015;11(3-4):231-44.)

4.4. *Allium sativum* (Garlic)

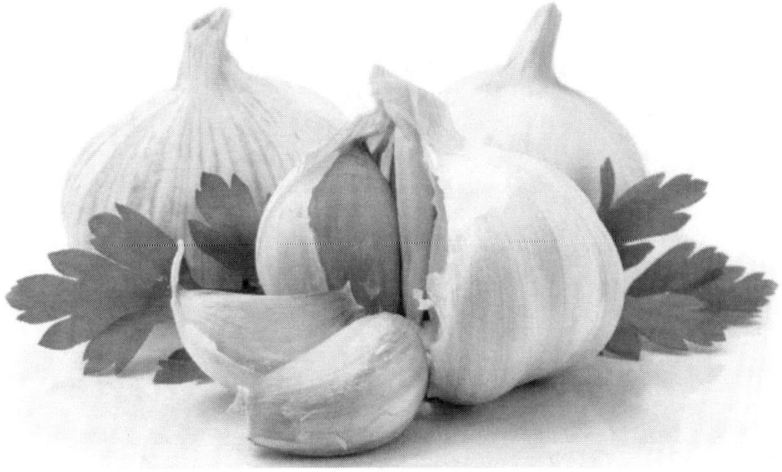

Figure 10. *Allium sativum*. As a promising traditional food and medicine, together with its potential advantages of multiple targets, wide distribution, low cost, and rare complications, garlic would have a very important and significant influence on T2DM. Additional garlic contributes to improved blood glucose control in 1–2 weeks as well as in 24 weeks in T2DM, and plays positive roles in total cholesterol and high/low density lipoprotein regulation in 12 weeks (Wang J, Zhang X, Lan H, Wang W. Effect of garlic supplement in the management of type 2 diabetes mellitus (T2DM): a meta-analysis of randomized controlled trials. Food Nutr Res. 2017;61(1):1377571. Published 2017 Sep 27. doi:10.1080/16546628.2017.1377571).

This is a perennial herb cultivated throughout India. Allicin, a sulfur-containing compound is responsible for its pungent odour and it has been shown to have significant hypoglycemic activity [21]. This effect is thought to be due to increased hepatic metabolism, increased insulin release from pancreatic beta cells and/or insulin sparing effect [22]. Aqueous homogenate of garlic (10 ml/kg/day) administered orally to sucrose fed rabbits (10 g/kg/day in water for two months) significantly increased hepatic glycogen and free amino acid content, decreased fasting blood glucose, and triglyceride levels in serum in comparison to sucrose controls [23]. S-allyl cystein sulfoxide (SACS), the precursor of allicin and garlic oil, is a sulfur containing amino acid, which controlled lipid peroxidation better than glibenclamide and insulin. It also improved diabetic conditions. SACS also stimulated in vitro insulin secretion from beta cells isolated from normal rats [24]. Apart from this, Allium sativum exhibits antimicrobial, anticancer and cardioprotective activities.

4.5. *Aloe vera* and *Aloe barbadensis*

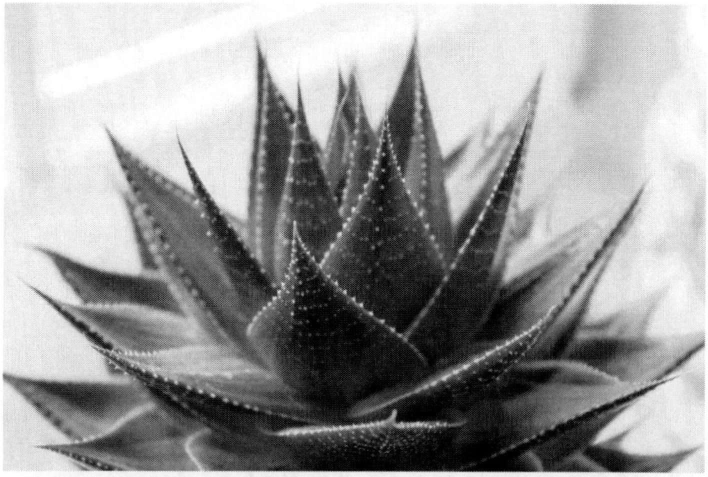

Figure 11. *Aloe vera*. *Aloe vera*, a succulent species, produces gel and latex, plays a therapeutic role in health management through antioxidant, antitumor, and anti-inflammatory activities, and also offers a suitable alternative approach for the treatment of various types of diseases. *Aloe* gels appear to be promising candidates for the treatment of diabetic ulcers. *Aloe vera* and its constituents such as aloe emodin (AE), aloin (barbaloin), anthracene, and emodin are relevant to cancer prevention owing to the activation and inactivation of molecular pathways associated with them. *Aloe vera* also appears to function as an antioxidant through free radical- and superoxide radical-scavenging activities and anti-inflammatory activities via inhibition of prostaglandin E2 production from arachidonic acid and also inhibition of various transcription factors and the activities of enzymes including lypoxygenase and cyclooxygenase. Aloe vera shows antimicrobial activity by rupturing bacterial cell walls. (Source: Rahmani AH, Aldebasi YH, Srikar S, Khan AA, Aly SM. Aloe vera: Potential candidate in health management via modulation of biological activities. Pharmacogn Rev. 2015;9(18):120-6.)

Aloe, a popular houseplant, has a long history as a multipurpose folk remedy. The plant can be separated into two basic products: gel and latex. Aloe vera gel is the leaf pulp or mucilage, aloe latex, commonly referred to as "aloe juice," is a bitter yellow exudate from the pericyclic tubules just beneath the outer skin of the leaves. Extracts of aloe gum effectively increases glucose tolerance in both normal and diabetic rats [25]. Treatment of chronic but not single dose of exudates of Aloe barbadensis leaves showed hypoglycemic effect in alloxanized diabetic rats. Single as well as chronic doses of bitter principle of the same plant also showed hypoglycemic effect in diabetic rats. This action of Aloe vera and its bitter principle is through stimulation of synthesis and/or release of insulin from pancreatic beta cells [26]. This plant also has an anti-inflammatory activity in a dose dependent manner and improves wound healing in diabetic mice [27].

4.6. *Azadirachta indica* (Neem)

Hydroalcoholic extracts of this plant showed antihyperglycemic activity in streptozotocin treated rats and this effect is because of increase in glucose uptake and glycogen deposition in isolated rat hemidiaphragm [28, 29]. Apart from having anti-diabetic activity, this plant also has anti-bacterial, antimalarial, antifertility, hepatoprotective and antioxidant effects [30].

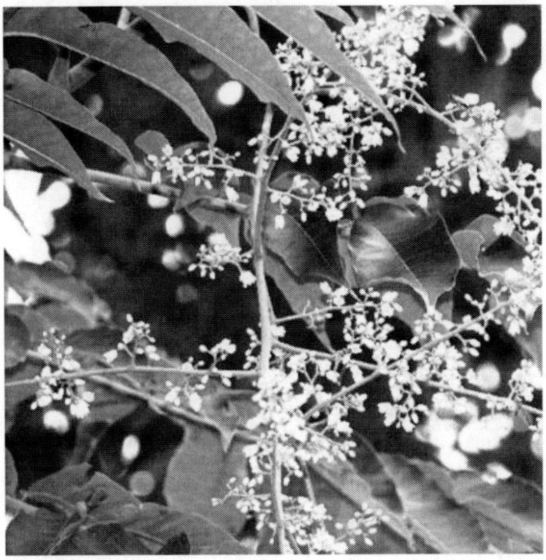

Figure 12. *Azadirachta indica*. An ethanolic extract (400 mg/kg) obtained from neem leaves demonstrated several effects, such as anti-lipid peroxidation, anti-hyperglycaemic and anti-hypercholesterolaemic activities as well as a reduction in serum triglyceride levels in alloxan-induced diabetic rats. The main mechanism of action of azadirachtins (e.g., azadirachtolide, azadiradione, gedunin and meliacinolin) is the inhibition of α-amylase and α-glucosidase. (Source: Governa P, Baini G, Borgonetti V, et al. Phytotherapy in the Management of Diabetes: A Review. Molecules. 2018;23(1):105. Published 2018 Jan 4. doi:10.3390/molecules23010105.)

Table 1. Indian medicinal plants with antidiabetic and related beneficial properties

Plant Name	Ayurvedic/Common Name/Herbal Formulation	Antidiabetic and Other Beneficial Effects in Traditional Medicine	References
Annona squamosa	Sugar apple	Hypoglycemic and antihyperglycemic activities of ethanolic leaf-extract, Increased plasma insulin level	[61–63]
Artemisia pallens	Davana	Hypoglycemic, increases peripheral glucose utilization or inhibits glucose reabsorption	[64]
Areca catechu	Supari	Hypoglycemic	[65]
Beta vulgaris	Chukkander	Increases glucose tolerance in OGTT	[66]
Boerhavia diffusa	punarnava	Increase in hexokinase activity,decrease in glucose-6-phosphatase and fructose bis-phosphatase activity, increase plasma insulin level, antioxidant	[67–69]
Bombax ceiba	Semul	Hypoglycemic	[70]
Butea monosperma	palasa	Antihyperglycemic	[71]
Camellia sinensis	Tea	Anti-hyperglycemic activity, antioxidant	[72, 73]
Capparis decidua	Karir or Pinju	Hypoglycemic, antioxidant, hypolipidaemic	[35]
Caesalpinia bonducella	Sagarghota, Fevernut	Hypoglycemic, insulin secretagogue, hypolipidemic	[74, 31, 32]
Coccinia indica	Bimb or Kanturi	Hypoglycemic	[36]
Emblica officinalis	Amla, Dhatriphala, a constituent of herbal formulation, "Triphala"	Decreases lipid peroxidation, antioxidant, hypoglycemic	[75–77]
Eugenia uniflora	Pitanga	Hypoglycemic, inhibits lipase activity	[78]
Enicostema littorale	krimihrita	Increase hexokinase activity, Decrease glucose 6-phosphatase and fructose 1,6 bisphosphatase activity. Dose dependent hypoglycemic activity	[79, 80]
Ficus bengalenesis	Bur	Hypoglycemic, antioxidant	[81]
Gymnema sylvestre	Gudmar or Merasingi	Anti-hyperglycemic effect, hypolipidemic	[82, 83]
Hemidesmus indicus	Anantamul	Anti snake venom activity, anti-inflammatory	[84]
Hibiscus rosa-sinesis	Gudhal or Jasson	Initiates insulin release from pancreatic beta cells	[85]
Ipomoea batatas	Sakkargand	Reduces insulin resistance	[86]
Momordica cymbalaria	Kadavanchi	Hypoglycemic, hypolipidemic	[87, 88]
Murraya koenigii	Curry patta	Hypoglycemic, increases glycogenesis and decreases gluconeogenesis and glycogenolysis	[89]
Musa sapientum	Banana	Antihyperglycemic, antioxidant	[90–92].
Phaseolus vulgaris	Hulga, white kidney bean	Hypoglycemic, hypolipidemic, inhibit alpha amylase activity, antioxidant. Altered level of insulin receptor and GLUT-4 mRNA in skeletal muscle	[93–95]
Punica granatum	Anar	Antioxidant, anti-hyperglycemic effect	[96]
Salacia reticulata	Vairi	inhibitotory activity against sucrase, α-glucosidase inhibitor	[97]
Scoparia dulcis	Sweet broomweed	Insulin-secretagogue activity, antihyperlipidemic, hypoglycemic, antioxidant	[98–100]
Swertia chirayita	Chirata	Stimulates insulin release from islets	[101]
Syzygium alternifolium	Shahajire	Hypoglycemic and antihyperglycemic	[102]
Terminalia belerica	Behada, a constituent of "Triphala"	Antibacterial, hypoglycemic	[103]
Terminalia chebula	Hirda	Antibacterial, hypoglycemic	[103]
Tinospora crispa		Anti-hyperglycemic, stimulates insulin release from islets	[104]
Vinca rosea	Sadabahar	Anti-hyperglycemic	[105]
Withania somnifera	Ashvagandha, winter cherry	Hypoglycemic, diuretic and hypocholesterolemic	[106]

4.7. *Caesalpinia bonducella*

Caesalpinia bonducella is widely distributed throughout the coastal region of India and used ethnically by the tribal people of India for controlling blood sugar. Both the aqueous and ethanolic extracts showed potent hypoglycemic activity in chronic type II diabetic models. These extracts also increased glycogenesis thereby increasing liver glycogen content [31]. Two fractions BM 169 and BM 170 B could increase secretion of insulin from isolated islets. The aqueous and 50% ethanolic extracts of *Caesalpinia bonducella* seeds showed antihyperglycemic and hypolipidemic activities in streptozotocin (STZ)-diabetic rats [32]. The antihyperglycemic action of the seed extracts may be due to the blocking of glucose absorption. The drug has the potential to act as antidiabetic as well as antihyperlipidemic [33].

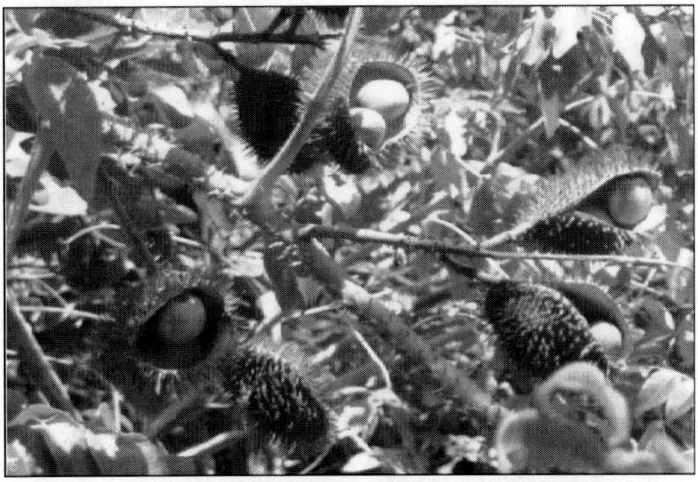

Figure 13. *Caesalpinia bonducella.* Hypoglycemic activities of aqueous extract was examined in normal and STZ diabetic rats. Administration of 100 mg/kg doses showed hypoglycemic activity and the effects of aqueous extract was longer than ethanolic extracts. After the fifth day, both extracts caused a remarkable hypoglycemic activity in diabetic rats (Kooti W, Farokhipour M, Asadzadeh Z, Ashtary-Larky D, Asadi-Samani M. The role of medicinal plants in the treatment of diabetes: a systematic review. Electron Physician. 2016;8(1):1832-42. Published 2016 Jan 15. doi:10.19082/1832).

4.8. *Capparis spinosa*

Capparis spinosa L. (CS) (Capparidaceae) was reported to have a number of potentially pharmacological activities including anti-inflammatory, anti-allergic, antidia--betic, hypolipidemic, hepatoprotective, antimicrobial, antiviral, immunomodulatory, antioxidant, anti-apoptotic, melanogenesis stimulating, antimutagenic, antiparasitic, antihypertensive, antiproliferative, antifungal, anti-HIV, anti-Helicobacter pylori, anti-complement and cardioprotective effects [34, 35].

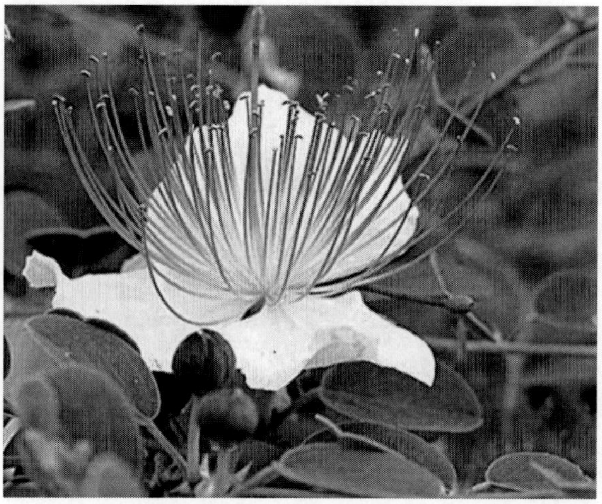

Figure 14. *Capparis spinosa*. Ancient Egypt and Arab consumed the roots of C. spinosa to treat liver and kidney diseases; Ancient Romans used C. spinosa for the treatment of paralysis; Moroccans used C. spinosa to treat diabetes. In the Northern areas of Pakistan, the root barks of C. spinosa have been used to treat splenomegaly, mental disorders and tubercular glands. In China, C. spinosa has been used in traditional Uighur Medicine for the treatment of rheumatoid arthritis and gout. In Iran, C. spinosa is used to treat hemorrhoids and gout. Studies revealed an improvement in hypertriglyceridemia and hyperglycemia in diabetic patients. In addition, no renal and hepatic adverse events were reported in the patients. The possible mechanism is that C. spinosa decreases the rate of carbohydrate absorption and exert its postprandial hypoglycemic effect in the gastrointestinal tract. Therefore, the consumption of C. spinosa may be beneficial and safe for controlling and treating blood glucose levels in diabetic patients. (Source: Kazemian M, Abad M, Haeri MR, Ebrahimi M, Heidari R. Anti-diabetic effect of Capparis spinosa L. root extract in diabetic rats. Avicenna J Phytomed. 2015;5(4):325-32.)

4.9. *Coccinia indica*

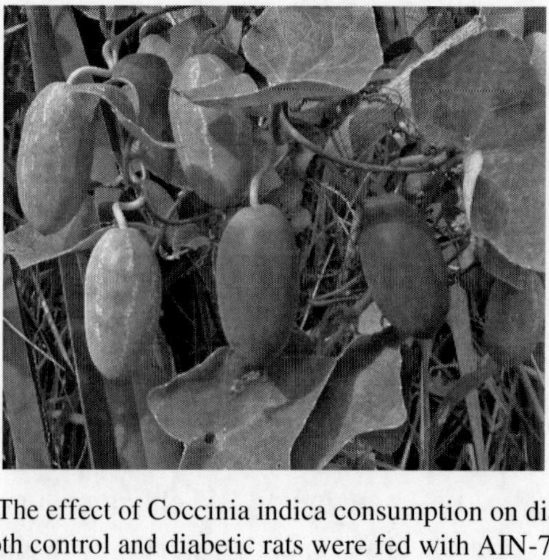

Figure 15. Coccinia indica. The effect of Coccinia indica consumption on diabetes-mediated kidney damage was determined. Both control and diabetic rats were fed with AIN-76 diet supplemented with C. indica fruits and leaves individually at 10% and 5%, respectively, for a period of 2 months. Various parameters, such as fasting blood glucose, urine sugar, albumin excretion, kidney index, and glomerular filtration rate, were ameliorated to various extents by the supplementation of C. indica in the diet. (Gurukar MS, Mahadevamma S, Chilkunda ND. Renoprotective effect of Coccinia indica fruits and leaves in experimentally induced diabetic rats. J Med Food. 2013;16(9):839-46.)

Dried extracts of Coccinia indica (C. indica) (500 mg/kg body weight) were administered to diabetic patients for 6 weeks. These extracts restored the activities of enzyme lipoprotein lipase (LPL) that was reduced and glucose-6phosphatase and lactate dehydrogenase, which were raised in untreated diabetics [36]. Oral administration of 500 mg/kg of C. indica leaves showed significant hypoglycemia in alloxanized diabetic dogs and increased glucose tolerance in normal and diabetic dogs.

Table 2. Formulated herbal drugs with antidiabetic properties

Drug	Company	Ingredients
Diabecon	Himalaya	*Gymnema sylvestre, Pterocarpus marsupium, Glycyrrhiza glabra, Casearia esculenta, Syzygium cumini, Asparagus racemosus, Boerhavia diffusa, Sphaeranthus indicus, Tinospora cordifolia, Swertia chirata, Tribulus terrestris, Phyllanthus amarus, Gmelina arborea, Gossypium herbaceum, Berberis aristata, Aloe vera, Triphala, Commiphora wightii, shilajeet, Momordica charantia, Piper nigrum, Ocimum sanctum, Abutilon indicum, Curcuma longa, Rumex maritimus*
Diasulin		*Cassia auriculata, Coccinia indica, Curcuma longa, Emblica officinalis, Gymnema sylvestre, Momordica charantia, Scoparia dulcis, Syzygium cumini, Tinospora cordifolia, Trigonella foenum graecum*
Pancreatic tonic 180 cp	ayurvedic herbal supplement	*Pterocarpus marsupium, Gymnema sylvestre, Momordica charantia, Syzygium cumini, Trigonella foenum graceum, Azadirachta indica, Ficus racemosa, Aegle marmelos, Cinnamomum tamala*
Ayurveda alternative herbal formula to Diabetes:	Chakrapani Ayurveda	Gurmar (Gymnema sylvestre) Karela (Momordica charantia) Pushkarmool (Inula racemosa) Jamun Gutli (Syzygium cumini) Neem (Azadirachta indica) Methika (Trigonella foenum gracecum) Guduchi (Tinospora cordifolia)
Bitter gourd Powder	Garry and Sun natural Remedies	Bitter gourd (*Momordica charantia*)
Dia-care	Admark Herbals Limited	Sanjeevan Mool; Himej, Jambu beej, Kadu, Namejav, Neem chal.
Diabetes-Daily Care	Nature's Health Supply	Alpha Lipoic Acid, Cinnamon 4% Extract, Chromax, Vanadium, Fenugreek 50% extract, *Gymnema sylvestre* 25% extract Momordica 7% extract, Licorice Root 20% extract
Gurmar powder	Garry and Sun natural Remedies	Gurmar (*Gymnema sylvestre)*
Epinsulin	Swastik Formulations	vijaysar (*Pterocarpus marsupium*)
Diabecure	Nature beaute sante	*Juglans regia, Berberis vulgaris, Erytherea centaurium,* Millefolium, Taraxacum
Diabeta	Ayurvedic cure Ayurvedic Herbal Health Products	*Gymnema sylvestre, Vinca rosea* (Periwinkle), *Curcuma longa* (Turmeric), *Azadirachta indica* (Neem), *Pterocarpus marsupium* (Kino Tree), *Momordica charantia* (Bitter Gourd), *Syzygium cumini* (Black Plum), *Acacia arabica* (Black Babhul), *Tinospora cordifolia, Zingiber officinale* (Ginger)
Syndrex	Plethico Laboretaries	Germinated Fenugreek seed extract

4.10. *Eugenia jambolana* (Indian Gooseberry, Jamun)

In India decoction of kernels of Eugenia jambolana is used as household remedy for diabetes. This also forms a major constituent of many herbal formulations for diabetes. Antihyperglycemic effect of aqueous and alcoholic extract as well as lyophilized powder shows reduction in blood glucose level. This varies with different level of diabetes. In mild diabetes (plasma sugar >180 mg/dl) it shows 73.51% reduction, whereas in moderate (plasma sugar >280 mg/dl) and severe diabetes (plasma sugar >400 mg/dl) it is reduced to 55.62% and 17.72% respectively [21]. The extract of jamun pulp showed the hypoglycemic activity in streptozotocin induced diabetic mice within 30 min of administration while the seed of the same fruit required 24 h. The oral administration of the extract resulted in increase in serum insulin levels in diabetic rats. Insulin secretion was found to be stimulated on incubation of plant extract with isolated islets of Langerhans from normal as well as diabetic animals. These extracts also inhibited insulinase activity from liver and kidney [37].

4.11. *Mangifera indica* (Mango)

The leaves of this plant are used as an antidiabetic agent in Nigerian folk medicine, although when aqueous extract given orally did not alter blood glucose level in either normoglycemic or streptozotocin induced diabetic rats. However, antidiabetic activity was seen when the extract and glucose were administered simultaneously and also when the extract was given to the rats 60 min before the glucose. The results indicate that aqueous extract of Mangifera indica possess hypoglycemic activity. This may be due to an intestinal reduction of the absorption of glucose [38].

4.12. *Momordica charantia* (Bitter Gourd)

Momordica charantia is commonly used as an antidiabetic and antihyperglycemic agent in India as well as other Asian countries. Extracts of fruit pulp, seed, leaves and whole plant was shown to have hypoglycemic effect in various animal models. Polypeptide p, isolated from fruit, seeds and tissues of M. charantia showed significant hypoglycemic effect when administered subcutaneously to langurs and humans [39]. Ethanolic extracts of M. charantia (200 mg/kg) showed an antihyperglycemic and also hypoglycemic effect in normal and STZ diabetic rats. This may be because of inhibition of glucose-6-phosphatase besides fructose-1, 6biphosphatase in the liver and stimulation of hepatic glucose6-phosphate dehydrogenase activities [40].

4.13. *Ocimum sanctum* (Holy Basil)

Table 3. Medicinal plants used by the Marakh sect of Garo tribal practitioners for treatment of diabetes

Serial Number	Scientific Name	Family Name	Local Name	Utilized Part	Formulation
1	*Lannea coromandelica* (Houtt.) Merr.	Anacardiaceae	Jiol bondi	Bark, root	Barks or roots are soaked in water overnight followed by taking the water the following morning on an empty stomach.
2	*Alstonia scholaris* (L.) R.Br.	Apocynaceae	Chaitan	Leaf	Green leaves are chewed before meals.
3	*Catharanthus roseus* (L.) G. Don	Apocynaceae	Noyon tara	Leaf	Leaves of *Catharanthus roseus* and *Clerodendrum viscosum* are crushed in water. One teaspoonful of the water is taken daily before meals.
4	*Enhydra fluctuans* Lour.	Asteraceae	Helencha	Leaf, stem	One cup of juice obtained from crushed leaves and stems is taken orally before meals.
5	*Terminalia chebula* Retz.	Combretaceae	Hortoki	Fruit	Fresh fruits are taken daily when in season. Fresh fruits are also dried when available and when not available, dried fruits are soaked in water overnight followed by drinking the water in the morning.
6	*Coccinia grandis* (L.) J. Voigt	Cucurbitaceae	Telamon	Leaf, root	Juice obtained from a crushed mixture of leaves and roots is taken daily in the morning.
7	*Momordica charantia* L.	Cucurbitaceae	Usta, Korola	Leaf, fruit	Half cup of juice obtained from squeezed leaves is taken in the morning on an empty stomach. Fruits are cooked and eaten as vegetable during afternoon and evening meals.
8	*Cuscuta reflexa* Roxb.	Cuscutaceae	Alo lota	Stem	Half cup of juice obtained from crushed stems is taken in the morning on an empty stomach.
9	*Phyllanthus emblica* L.	Euphorbiaceae	Amloki	Leaf, fruit	One teaspoonful of juice obtained from squeezed leaves is taken in the morning on an empty stomach. Fruits are chewed and taken as much as possible. When fresh fruits are not available, dried fruits are soaked in water and the water is taken orally with the fruit.
10	*Syzygium aqueum* (Burm.f.) Alston	Myrtaceae	Jamrul	Fruit	Fruits are taken orally when in season. They can be taken any time before or after meals.
11	*Drynaria quercifolia* (L.) J. Smith	Polypodiaceae	Bandor shoal	Stem	Two teaspoonful of juice obtained from crushed stem is taken daily.
12	*Clerodendrum viscosum* Vent.	Verbenaceae	Baik pata	Leaf	Leaves of *Catharanthus roseus* and *Clerodendrum viscosum* are crushed in water. One teaspoonful of the water is taken daily before meals.

It is commonly known as Tulsi. Since ancient times, this plant is known for its medicinal properties. The aqueous extract of leaves of Ocimum sanctum showed the significant reduction in blood sugar level in both normal and alloxan induced diabetic rats [41]. Significant reduction in fasting blood glucose, uronic acid, total amino acid, total cholesterol, triglyceride and total lipid indicated the hypoglycemic and hypolipidemic effects of tulsi in diabetic rats [42]. Oral administration of plant extract (200 mg/kg) for 30 days led to decrease in the plasma glucose level by approximately 9.06 and 26.4% on 15 and 30 days of the experiment respectively. Renal glycogen content increased 10 fold while skeletal muscle and hepatic glycogen levels decreased by 68 and 75% respectively in diabetic rats as compared to control [43]. This plant also showed antiasthemitic, antistress, antibacterial, antifungal, antiviral, antitumor, gastric antiulcer activity, antioxidant, antimutagenic and immunostimulant activities.

4.14. *Phyllanthus urinaria*

P. urinaria is used in folk medicine as a cure to treat jaundice, diabetes, malaria, and liver diseases. Phytochemical investigations reveal that the plant is a rich source of lignans, tannins, flavonoids, phenolics, terpenoids, and other secondary metabolites. Pharmacological activities include anticancer, hepatoprotective, antidiabetic, antimicrobial, and cardioprotective effects [44].

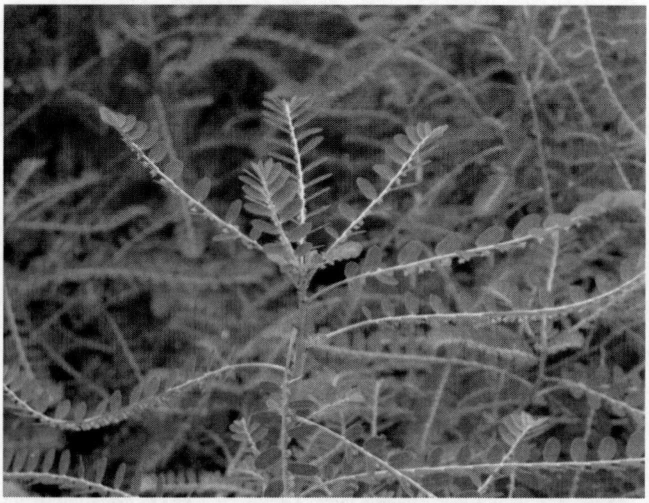

Figure 16. *Phyllanthus urinaria*. Oral administration (30 mg/kg) decreased the blood glucose levels. Ethanol and water extracts obtained from whole plant of P. urinaria inhibit α-glucosidase with IC50 values of 39.7 ± 9.7 and 14.6 ± 4.6 μg/mL, respectively. The use of natural products as α-glucosidase inhibitors has gained interest because they do not induce toxicity or negative symptoms for the liver, kidney, and gastrointestinal system. (Source: Trinh B. T. D., Staerk D., Jager A. K. (2016). Screening for potential α-glucosidase and α-amylase inhibitory constituents from selected Vietnamese plants used to treat type 2 diabetes. J. Ethnopharmacol. 186, 189–195. 10.1016/j.jep.2016.03.060.)

4.15. *Pterocarpus marsupium*

It is a deciduous moderate to large tree found in India mainly in hilly region. Pterostilbene, a constituent derived from wood of this plant caused hypoglycemia in dogs [45, 46] showed that the hypoglycemic activity of this extract is because of presence of tannates in the extract. Flavonoid fraction from Pterocarpus marsupium has been shown to cause pancreatic beta cell regranulation [47]. *Marsupin, pterosupin* and liquiritigenin obtained from this plant showed antihyperlipidemic activity [48]. (−) Epicatechin, its active principle, has been found to be insulinogenic, enhancing insulin release and conversion of proinsulin to insulin in vitro. Like insulin, (−) epicatechin stimulates oxygen uptake in fat cells and tissue slices of various organs, increases glycogen content of rat diaphragm in a dose-dependent manner [49].

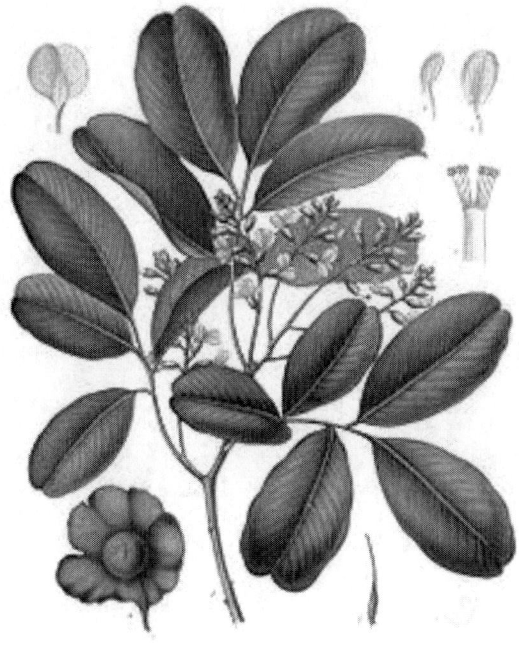

Figure 17. *Pterocarpus marsupium*. The blood sugar-lowering activity has been endorsed to be due to the presence of tannates in the extract of the plant. (−) Epicatechin has been shown to have insulinogenic property by enhancing insulin release and conversion of proinsulin to insulin. (−) Epicatechin has also been shown to possess insulin-like activity. Epicatechin has also been shown to strengthen the insulin signaling by activating key proteins of that pathway and regulating glucose production through AKT and AMPK modulation in HepG2 cells. *Pterocarpus marsupium* is reported to have not only hypoglycemic property but also β-cell protective and regenerative properties, effects which have been attributed to the flavonoid content in the plant. (Source: Rizvi SI, Mishra N. Traditional Indian medicines used for the management of diabetes mellitus. J Diabetes Res. 2013;2013:712092.)

4.16. *Trigonella foenum* graecum (Fenugreek)

It is found all over India and the fenugreek seeds are usually used as one of the major constituents of Indian spices. 4-hydroxyleucine, a novel amino acid from fenugreek seeds increased glucose stimulated insulin release by isolated islet cells in both rats and humans [50]. Oral administration of 2 and 8 g/kg of plant extract produced dose dependent decrease in the blood glucose levels in both normal as well as diabetic rats [51]. Administration of fenugreek seeds also improved glucose metabolism and normalized creatinine kinase activity in heart, skeletal muscle and liver of diabetic rats. It also reduced hepatic and renal glucose-6-phosphatase and fructose –1,6-biphosphatase activity [52]. This plant also shows antioxidant activity [53, 54].

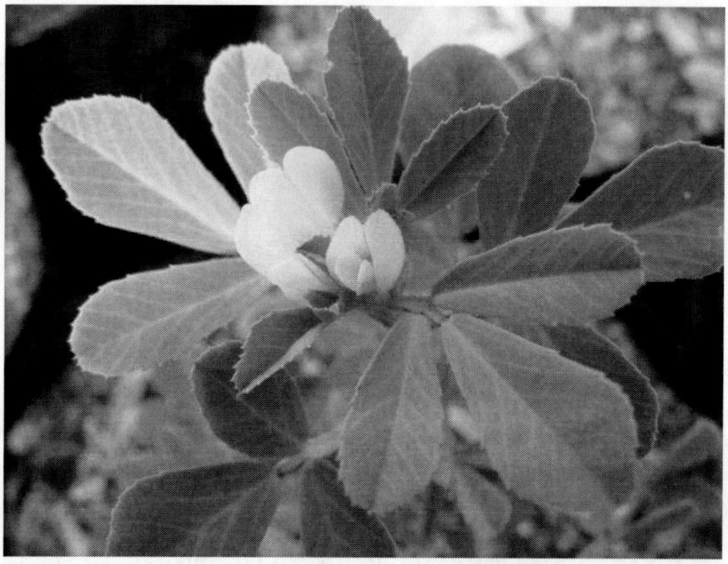

Figure 18. *Trigonella foenum*. It has been commonly used as herbal preparation for diabetes treatment. Multiple mechanisms are suggested for its efficacy in diabetes population. Soluble fibers in fenugreek including glucomannan fiber delays intestinal absorption of ingested sugars and alkaloids such as fenugrecin and trigonelline have demonstrated to possess hypoglycemic action, and 4 hydroxyisoleucine (4-OH Ile) amino acids act on pancreas to release insulin. (Source: Ranade M, Mudgalkar N. A simple dietary addition of fenugreek seed leads to the reduction in blood glucose levels: A parallel group, randomized single-blind trial. Ayu. 2017;38(1-2):24-27.)

4.17. *Tinospora cordifolia* (Guduchi)

It is a large, glabrous, deciduous climbing shrub belonging to the family Menispermaceae. It is widely distributed throughout India and commonly known as Guduchi. Oral administration of the extract of *Tinospora cordifolia* (T. cordifolia) roots for 6 weeks resulted in a significant reduction in blood and urine glucose and in lipids in serum and tissues in alloxan diabetic rats. The extract also prevented a decrease in body weight.

[55] T. *cordifolia* is widely used in Indian ayurvedic medicine for treating diabetes mellitus [56–58]. Oral administration of an aqueous T. *cordifolia* root extract to alloxan diabetic rats caused a significant reduction in blood glucose and brain lipids. Though the aqueous extract at a dose of 400 mg/kg could elicit significant antihyperglycemic effect in different animal models, its effect was equivalent to only one unit/kg of insulin [59]. It is reported that the daily administration of either alcoholic or aqueous extract of T. cordifolia decreases the blood glucose level and increases glucose tolerance in rodents [60].

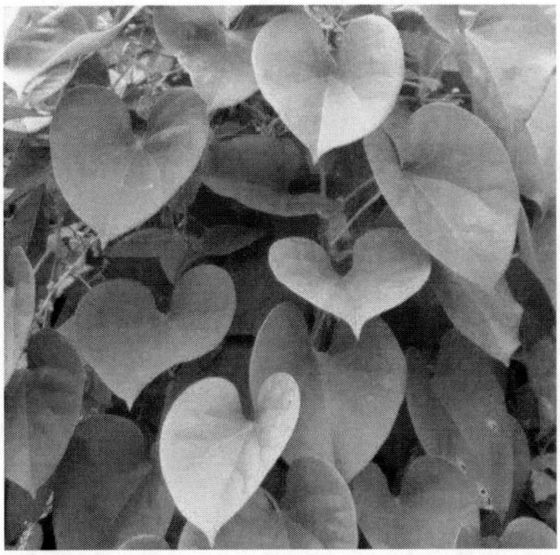

Figure 19. *Tinospora cordifolia*. T. cordifolia has been shown to be effective against diabetes mellitus. The isoquinoline alkaloid rich fraction from stem, including, palmatine, jatrorrhizine, and magnoflorine have been reported for insulin-mimicking and insulin-releasing effect both in vitro and in vivo. Oral treatments of root extracts have been reported to regulate blood glucose levels, enhance insulin secretion and suppress OS markers. Initiation and restoration of cellular defence anti-oxidant markers including superoxide dismutase (SOD), glutathione peroxidase (GPx) and glutathione (GSH), inhibition of glucose 6-phosphatase and fructose 1, 6-diphosphatase, restoration of glycogen content in liver was reported in in vitro studies. The crude stem ethyl acetate, dichloromethane (DCM), chloroforms and hexane extracts of Tinospora cordifolia inhibited the enzyme's salivary and pancreatic amylase and glucosidase thus increasing the post-prandial glucose level and finds potential application in treatment of diabetes mellitus. (Source: Saha S, Ghosh S. Tinospora cordifolia: One plant, many roles. Anc Sci Life. 2012;31(4):151-9.)

5. HERBAL DRUG FORMULATIONS

Many formulations (see Table 2) are in the market and are used regularly by diabetic patients on the advice of the physicians.

Diabecon manufactured by 'Himalaya' is reported to increase peripheral utilization of glucose, increase hepatic and muscle glucagon contents, promote B cells repair and regeneration and increase c peptide level. It has antioxidant properties and protects B cells from oxidative stress. It exerts an insulin like action by reducing the glycated haemoglobin levels, normalizing the microalbuminurea and modulating the lipid profile. It minimizes long term diabetic complications.

Epinsulin marketed by Swastik formulations, contains epicatechin, a benzopyran, as an active principle. Epicatechin increases the cAMP content of the islet, which is associated with increased insulin release. It plays a role in the conversion of proinsulin to insulin by increasing cathepsin activity. Additionally it has an insulin-mimetic effect on osmotic fragility of human erythrocytes and it inhibits Na/K ATPase activity from patient's erythrocytes. It corrects the neuropathy, retinopathy and disturbed metabolism of glucose and lipids. It maintains the integrity of all organ systems affected by the disease. It is reported to be a curative for diabetes, Non Insulin Dependant Diabetes Mellitus (NIDDM) and a good adjuvant for Insulin Dependant Diabetes Mellitus (IDDM), in order to reduce the amount of needed insulin. It is advised along with existing oral hypoglycemic drugs. And is known to prevent diabetic complication. It has gentle hypoglycemic activity and hence induces no risk of being hypoglycemic.

Pancreatic Tonic (ayurvedic herbal supplement): Pancreas Tonic is a botanical mixture of traditional Indian Ayurvedic herbs currently available as a dietary supplement.

Bitter gourd powder marketed by Garry and Sun. It lowers blood & urine sugar levels. It increases body's resistance against infections and purifies blood. Bitter Gourd has excellent medicinal virtues. It is antidotal, antipyretic tonic, appetizing, stomachic, antibilious and laxative. The bitter Gourd is also used in native medicines of Asia and Africa. The Bitter gourd is specifically used as a folk medicine for diabetes. It contains compounds like bitter glycosides, saponins, alkaloids, reducing sugars, phenolics, oils, free acids, polypeptides, sterols, 17-amino acids including methionine and a crystalline product named p-insulin. It is reported to have hypoglycemic activity in addition to being antihaemorrhoidal, astringent, stomachic, emmenagogue, hepatic stimulant, anthelmintic and blood purifier.

Dia-Care manufactured by Admark Herbals Ltd. is claimed to be effective for both Type 1, Type 2 diabetes within 90 days of treatment and cures within 18 months. Persons taking insulin will eventually be liberated from the dependence on it. The whole treatment completes in 6 phases, each phase being of 90 days. Approx. 5 grams (1 tea spoon) powder is mixed with 1/2 glass of water, stirred properly and kept overnight. Only the water and not the sediment must be taken in the morning on empty stomach. To the remaining medicine fresh water is added and kept for the whole day and is consumed half an hour before dinner. The taste of the drug is very bitter. It is a pure herbal formula without any side effects.

Diabetes-Daily Care manufactured by Nature's Health Supply is a Unique, Natural Formula, which effectively and safely Improves Sugar Metabolism. Diabetes Daily Care™ was formulated for type 2 diabetics and contains all natural ingredients listed in Table 2 in the proportion optimal for the body's use.

Gurmar powder manufactured by Garry and Sun is an anti-diabetic drug, which suppresses the intestinal absorption of sacharides, which prevents blood sugar fluctuations. It also correlates the metabolic activities of liver, kidney and muscles. Gurmar stimulates insulin secretion and has blood sugar reducing properties. It blocks sweet taste receptors when applied to tongue in diabetes to remove glycosuria. It deadens taste of sweets and bitter things like quinine (effects lasts for 1 to 2 hours). Besides having these properties, it is a cardiac stimulant and diuretic and corrects metabolic activities of liver, kidney and muscles.

Table 4. Medicinal plants used to manage diabetes mellitus type II: parts used and informant consensus [108]

Sr.	English Name	Scientific Name	Plant Part(S) Used
1.	Aloevera	*Aloe vera var.*	Leaves
2.	Bitter Berries	*Solanum indicum*	Fruits
3.	Bitter leaf	*Vernonia amygydalina*	Leaves
4.	Pumpkin	*Cucurbita maxima*	Fruits
5.	Graviola	*Anonamuricata*	Fruits and leaves
6.	Natal Plum	*Carissa macrocarpa*	Fruits
7.	Albizia tree	*Albiziachinensis*	Leaves
8.	Wild Date Palm	*Phoenix reclinata*	Seeds
9.	White's Ginger	*Mondiawhytei*	Roots
10.	Egg plant	*Solanum melongena*	Fruits and leaves
11.	Java plum	*Syzygium cumini*	Seeds and fruits
12.	Goats' Weed	*Ageratum conyzoides*	Leaves
13.	*Natal Indigo*	*Indigofera arrecta*	Leaves
14.	Lion's ear	*Leonatis mollisima*	Leaves
15.	Garden egg	*Solanum gilo*	Fruits
16.	Ovacado	*Persea Americana*	Seeds
17.	Jack fruit	*Artocarpus heterophyllus*	Seeds
18.	-	*Crassocephalum vitellinum*	Leaves

Diabeta, a formulation of Ayurvedic Cure, available in the capsule form is an anti-diabetic with combination of proven anti-diabetic fortified with potent immunomodulators, antihyperlipidemics, anti-stress and hepatoprotective of plant origin. The formulation of Diabeta is based on ancient ayurvedic references, further corroborated through modern research and clinical trials. Diabeta acts on different sites in differing ways to effectively control factors and pathways leading to diabetes mellitus. It attacks the various factors, which precipitate the diabetic condition, and corrects the degenerative complications, which result because of diabetes. Diabeta is safe and effective in managing Diabetes Mellitus as a single agent supplement to synthetic anti-diabetic drugs. Diabeta helps overcome resistance to oral hypoglycemic drugs when used as adjuvant to cases of uncontrolled diabetes. Diabeta confers a sense of well -being in patients and promotes symptomatic relief of complaints like weakness giddiness, pain in legs, body ache, polyuria and pruritis.

Syndrex manufactured by Plethico Laboratory contains extracts of germinated fenugreek seed. Fenugreek is used as an ingredient of traditional formulations over 1000 years. We are currently studying the mechanism of this antidiabetic drug using animal model on one hand and cultured islet cells on the other.

Conclusion

Many different plants have been used individually or in formulations for treatment of diabetes and its complications. One of the major problems with this herbal formulation is that the active ingredients are not well defined. It is important to know the active component and their molecular interaction, which will help to analyze therapeutic efficacy of the product and also to standardize the product. Efforts are now being made to investigate mechanism of action of some of these plants using model systems.

References

[1] Grover, J.K., Yadav, S., and Vats, V.: Medicinal plants of India with antidiabetic potential. *J. Ethnopharmacol.,* 81, 81–100, 2002.

[2] Scartezzini, P. and Sproni, E.: Review on some plants of Indian traditional medicine with antioxidant activity. *J. Ethnopharmacol.,* 71, 23–43, 2000.

[3] Seth, S.D. and Sharma, B.: Medicinal plants of India. *Indian J. Med. Res.,* 120, 9–11, 2004.

[4] Ramachandran, A., Snehalatha, C., and Viswanathan, V.: Burden of type 2 diabetes and its complications- the Indian scenario. *Curr. Sci.,* 83, 1471–1476, 2002.

[5] Matteucci, E. and Giampietro, O.: Oxidative stress in families of type 1 diabetic patients. *Diabetes Care,* 23, 1182–1186, 2000.

[6] Oberlay, L.W.: Free radicals and diabetes. *Free Radic. Biol. Med.,* 5, 113–124, 1988.

[7] Baynes, J.W. and Thorpe, S.R.: The role of oxidative stress in diabetic complications. *Curr. Opin. Endocrinol.,* 3, 277– 284, 1997.

[8] Lipinski, B.: Pathophysiology of oxidative stress in diabetes mellitus. *J. Diabet. Complications,* 15, 203–210, 2001.

[9] Kubish, H.M., Vang, J., Bray, T.M., and Phillips, J.P.: Targeted over expression of Cu/Zn superoxide dismutase protects pancreatic beta cells against oxidative stress. *Diabetes,* 46, 1563–1566, 1997.

[10] Naziroglu, M. and Cay, M.: Protective role of intraperitoneally administered vitamin E and selenium on the oxidative defense mechanisms in rats with diabetes induced by streptozotocin. *Biol. Stress Elem. Res.,* 47, 475–488, 2001.

[11] Glugliano. D., Ceriello, A., and Paolisso, G.: Oxidative stress and diabetic vascular complications. *Diabet. Care,* 19, 257–267, 1996.

[12] Brownlee, M.: Advanced protein glycosylation in diabetes in diabetes and ageing. *Ann. Rev. Med.,* 46, 223–234, 1996.

[13] Elgawish, A., Glomb, M., Friendlander, M., and Monnier, V.M.: Involvement of hydrogen peroxide in collagen crosslinking by high glucose in vitro and in vivo. *J. Biol. Chem.,* 271, 12964–12971, 1999.

[14] Dey, L., Anoja, S.A., and Yuan, C-S.: Alternative therapies for type 2 diabetes. *Alternative Med. Rev.,* 7, 45–58, 2002.

[15] Dixit, P.P., Londhe, J.S., Ghaskadbi, S.S., and Devasagayam, T.P.A.: Antidiabetic and related beneficial properties of Indian medicinal plants, in *Herbal Drug Research- A twenty first century perspective,* eds. By Sharma, R.K. and Arora, R., Jaypee brothers medical publishers (New Delhi, India) Limited, pp. 377–386, 2006.

[16] Wadood, A., Wadood, N., and Shah, S.A.: Effects of Acacia arabica and Caralluma edulis on blood glucose levels on normal and alloxan diabetic rabbits. *J. Pakistan Med. Assoc.,* 39, 208–212, 1989.

[17] Karunanayake, E.H., Welihinda, J., Sirimanne, S.R., and Sinnadorai, G.: Oral hypoglycemic activity of some medicinal plants of Sri Lanka. *J. Ethnopharmacol.,* 11, 223–231, 1984.

[18] Roman-Ramos, R., Flores-Saenz, J.L., and Alaricon-Aguilar, F.J.: Anti-hyperglycemic effect of some edible plants. *J. Ethnopharmacol.,* 48, 25–32, 1995.

[19] Kumari, K., Mathew, B.C., and Augusti, K.T.: Antidiabetic and hypolipidaemic effects of S-methyl cysteine sulfoxide, isolated from Allium cepa Linn. *Ind. J. Biochem. Biophys.,* 32, 49–54, 1995.

[20] Mathew, P.T. and Augusti, K.T.: Hypoglycemic effects of onion, Allium cepa Linn. on diabetes mellitus- a preliminary report. *Ind. J. Physiol. Pharmacol.,* 19, 213–217, 1975.

[21] Sheela, C.G. and Augusti, K.T.: Antidiabetic effects of S-allyl cysteine sulphoxide isolated from garlic Allium sativum Linn. *Indian J. Exp. Biol.,* 30, 523–526, 1992.

[22] Bever, B.O. and Zahnd, G.R.: Plants with oral hypoglycemic action. *Quart. J. Crude Drug Res.,* 17, 139–146, 1979.

[23] Zacharias, N.T., Sebastian, K.L., Philip, B., and Augusti, K.T.: Hypoglycemic and hypolipidaemic effects of garlic in sucrose fed rabbits. *Ind. J. Physiol. Pharmacol.,* 24, 151– 154, 1980.

[24] Augusti, K.T. and Shella, C.G.: Antiperoxide effect of S-allyl cysteine sulfoxide, an insulin secretagogue in diabetic rats. *Experientia,* 52, 115–120, 1996.

[25] Al-Awadi, F.M. and Gumaa, K.A.: Studies on the activity of individual plants of an antidiabetic plant mixture. *Acta Diabetologica,* 24, 37–41, 1987.

[26] Ajabnoor, M.A.: Effect of aloes on blood glucose levels in normal and alloxan diabetic mice. *J. Ethnopharmacol.,* 28, 215–220, 1990.

[27] Davis, R.H. and Maro, N.P.: Aloe vera and gibberellins, Anti-inflammatory activity in diabetes. *J. Am. Pediat. Med. Assoc.,* 79, 24–26, 1989.

[28] Chattopadhyay, R.R., Chattopadhyay, R.N., Nandy, A.K., Poddar, G., and Maitra, S.K.: Preliminary report on antihyperglycemic effect of fraction of fresh leaves of Azadiracta indica (Beng neem). *Bull. Calcutta. Sch. Trop. Med.,* 35, 29–33, 1987.

[29] Chattopadhyay, R.R., Chattopadhyay, R.N., Nandy, A.K., Poddar, G., and Maitra, S.K.: The effect of fresh leaves of Azadiracta indica on glucose uptake and glycogen content in the isolated rat hemidiaphragm. *Bull. Calcutta. Sch. Trop. Med.,* 35, 8–12, 1987.

[30] Biswas, K., Chattopadhyay, I., Banerjee, R.K., and Bandyopadhyay, U.: Biological activities and medicinal properties of neem (Azadiracta indica). *Curr. Sci.,* 82, 1336–1345, 2002.

[31] Chakrabarti, S., Biswas, T.K., Rokeya, B., Ali, L., Mosihuzzaman, M., Nahar, N., Khan, A.K., and Mukherjee, B.: Advanced studies on the hypoglycemic effect of Caesalpinia bonducella F. in type 1 and 2 diabetes in Long Evans rats. *J. Ethnopharmacol.,* 84, 41–46, 2003.

[32] Sharma, S.R., Dwivedi, S.K., and Swarup, D.: Hypoglycemic, antihyperglycemic and hypolipidemic activities of Caesalpinia bonducella seeds in rats. *J. Ethnopharmacol.,* 58, 39–44, 1997.

[33] Kannur, D.M., Hukkeri, V.I., and Akki, K.S.: Antidiabetic activity of Caesalpinia bonducella seed extracts in rats. *Fitoterapia.* In press.

[34] Eddouks M, Lemhadri A, Hebi M, et al. Capparis spinosa L. aqueous extract evokes antidiabetic effect in streptozotocin-induced diabetic mice. *Avicenna J Phytomed.* 2017;7(2):191-198..

[35] Zhang H, Ma ZF. Phytochemical and Pharmacological Properties of Capparis spinosa as a Medicinal Plant. *Nutrients.* 2018;10(2):116. Published 2018 Jan 24. doi:10.3390/nu10020116.

[36] Kamble, S.M., Kamlakar, P.L., Vaidya, S., and Bambole, V.D.: Influence of Coccinia indica on certain enzymes in glycolytic and lipolytic pathway in human diabetes. *Indian J. Med. Sci.,* 52, 143–146, 1998.

[37] Acherekar, S., Kaklij, G.S, Pote, M.S., and Kelkar, S.M.: Hypoglycemic activity of Eugenia jambolana and ficus bengalensis: mechanism of action. *In vivo,* 5, 143–147, 1991.

[38] Aderibigbe, A.O., Emudianughe, T.S., and Lawal, B.A.: Antihyperglycemic effect of Mangifera indica in rat. *Phytother Res.,* 13, 504–507, 1999.

[39] Khanna, P., Jain, S.C., Panagariya, A., and Dixit, V.P.: Hypoglycemic activity of polypeptide- p from a plant source. *J. Nat. Prod.,* 44, 648–655, 1981.

[40] Shibib, B.A., Khan, L.A., and Rahman, R.: Hypoglycemic activity of Coccinia indica and Momordica charantia in diabetic rats: depression of the hepatic gluconeogenic enzymes glucose-6-phosphatase and fructose-1, 6biphosphatase and elevation of liver and red-cell shunt enzyme glucose-6-phosphate dehydrogenase. *Biochem. J.,* 292, 267–270, 1993.

[41] Vats, V., Grover, J.K., and Rathi, S.S.: Evaluation of antihyperglycemic and hypoglycemic effect of Trigonella foenumgraecum Linn, Ocimum sanctum Linn and Pterocarpus marsupium Linn in normal and alloxanized diabetic rats. *J. Ethnopharmacol.,* 79, 95–100, 2002.

[42] Rai, V., Iyer, U., and Mani, U.V.: Effect of Tulasi (Ocimum sanctum) leaf powder supplementation on blood sugar levels, serum lipids and tissue lipid in diabetic rats. *Plant Food for Human Nutrition,* 50, 9–16, 1997.

[43] Vats, V. and Yadav, S.P.: Grover, Ethanolic extract of Ocimum sanctum leaves partially attenuates streptozotocin induced alteration in glycogen content and carbohydrate metabolism in rats. *J. Ethnopharmacol.,* 90, 155–160, 2004.

[44] Geethangili M, Ding ST. A Review of the Phytochemistry and Pharmacology of Phyllanthus urinaria L. *Front Pharmacol.* 2018;9:1109. Published 2018 Oct 1. doi:10.3389/fphar.2018.01109.

[45] Haranath, P.S.R.K., Ranganathrao, K., Anjaneyulu, C.R., and Ramnathan, J.D.: Studies on the hypoglycemic and pharmacological actions of some stilbenes. *Ind. J. Medl. Sci.,* 12, 85–89, 1958.

[46] Joglekar, G.V., Chaudhary, N.Y., and Aiaman, R.: Effect of Indian medicinal plants on glucose absorption in mice. *Indian J. Physiol. Pharmacol.,* 3, 76–77, 1959.

[47] Chakravarty, B.K., Gupta, S., Gambhir, S.S., and Gode, K.D.: Pancreatic beta cell regeneration. A novel antidiabetic mechanism of Pterocarpus marsupium Roxb. *Ind. J. Pharmacol.,* 12, 123–127, 1980.

[48] Jahromi, M.A., Ray, A.B., and Chansouria, J.P.N.: Antihyperlipidemic effect of flavonoids from Pterocarpus marsupium. *J. Nat. Prod.,* 56, 989–994, 1993.

[49] Ahmad, F., Khalid, P., Khan, M.M., Rastogi, A.K., and Kidwai, J.R.: Insulin like activity in (−) epicatechin. *Acta. Diabetol. Lat.*, 26, 291–300, 1989.

[50] Sauvaire, Y., Petit, P., Broca, C., Manteghetti, M., Baissac, Y., Fernandez-Alvarez, J., Gross, R., Roy, M., Leconte, A., Gomis, R., and Ribes, G.: 4-hydroxyisoleucine: a novel amino acid potentiator of insulin secretion. *Diabetes,* 47, 206–210, 1998.

[51] Khosla, P., Gupta, D.D., and Nagpal, R.K.: Effect of Trigonella foenum graecum (fenugreek) on blood glucose in normal and diabetic rats. *Indian J. Physiol. Pharmacol.,* 39, 173–174, 1995.

[52] Gupta, D., Raju, J., and Baquer, N.Z.: Modulation of some gluconeogenic enzyme activities in diabetic rat liver and kidney: effect of antidiabetic compounds. *Indian J. Expt. Biol.,* 37, 196–199, 1999.

[53] Ravikumar, P. and Anuradha, C.V.: Effect of fenugreek seeds on blood lipid peroxidation and antioxidants in diabetic rats. *Phytother. Res.,* 13, 197–201, 1999.

[54] Dixit, P.P., Ghaskadbi, S.S., Hari M., and Devasagayam, T.P.A.: Antioxidant properties of germinated fenugreek seeds. *Phytother. Res.,* 19, 977–983, 2005.

[55] Stanely, P., Prince, M., and Menon, V.P.: Hypoglycemic and hypolipidemic action of alcohol extract of Tinospora cordifolia roots in chemical induced diabetes in rats. *Phytother. Res.,* 17, 410–413, 2003.

[56] Stanely, M., Prince, P., and Menon, V.P.: Antioxidant action of Tinospora cordifolia root extract in alloxan diabetic rats. *Phytother. Res.,* 15, 213–218, 2001.

[57] Price, P.S. and Menon, V.P.: Antioxidant activity of Tinospora cordifolia roots in experimental diabetes. *J. Ethnopharmacol.,* 65, 277–281, 1999.

[58] Mathew, S. and Kuttan, G.: Antioxidant activity of Tinospora cordifolia and its usefulness in the amelioration of cyclophosphamide-induced toxicity. *J. Exp. Clin. Cancer. Res.,* 16, 407–411, 1997.

[59] Dhaliwal, K.S.: *Method and composition for treatment of diabetes.* US Patent 5886029, 1999.

[60] Gupta, S.S., Varma, S.C.L., Garg, V.P., and Rai, M.: Antidiabetic effect of Tinospora cordifolia. I. Effect on fasting blood sugar level, glucose tolerence and adrenaline induced hyperglycemia. *Indian J. Exp. Biol.,* 55, 733–745, 1967.

[61] Kaleem, M., Asif, M., Ahmed, Q.U., and Bano, B.: Antidiabetic and antioxidant activity of Annona squamosa extract in streptozotocin-induced diabetic rats. *Singapore Med. J.,* 47, 670–675, 2006.

[62] Gupta, R.K., Kesari, A.N., Murthy, P.S., Chandra, R., Tandon, V., and Watal, G.: Hypoglycemic and antidiabetic effect of ethanolic extract of leaves of Annona squamosa L. in experimental animals. *J. Ethnopharmacol.,* 99, 75–81, 2005.

[63] Gupta, R.K., Kesari, A.N., Watal, G., Murthy, P.S., Chandra, R., and Tandon, V.: Nutritional and hypoglycemic effect of fruit pulp of Annona squamosa in normal healthy and alloxan-induced diabetic rabbits. *Ann. Nutr. Metab.,* 49, 407–413, 2005.

[64] Subramonium, A., Pushpangadan, P., Rajasekharan, A., Evans, D.A., Latha, P.G., and Valsaraj, R.: Effects of Artemisia pallens Wall. On blood glucose levels in normal and alloxan-induced diabetic rats. *J. Ethnopharmacol.,* 50, 13–17, 1996.

[65] Chempakam, B.: Hypoglycemic activity of arecoline in betel nut Areca catechu L. *Ind. J. Exp. Biol.,* 31, 474–475, 1993.

[66] Yoshikawa, M., Murakami, T., Kadoya, M., Matsuda, H., Muraoka, O., Yamahara, J., and Murakami, N.: Medicinal foodstuff. III. Sugar beet. Hypoglycemic oleanolic acid oligoglycosides, betavulgarosides I, II, III and IV, from the root of Beta vulgaris L. *Chemical and Pharmaceutical Bulletin,* 44, 1212–1217, 1996.

[67] Pari, L. and Amarnath Satheesh, M.: Antidiabetic activity of Boerhavia diffusa L. effect on hepatic key enzymes in experimental diabetes. *J. Ethnopharmacol.,* 91, 109–113, 2004.

[68] Satheesh, M.A. and Pari, L.: Antioxidant effect of Boerhavia diffusa L. in tissues of alloxan induced diabetic rats. *Indian J. Exp. Biol.,* 42, 989–992, 2004.

[69] Pari, L. and Amarnath Satheesh, M.: Antidiabetic effect of Boerhavia diffusa: effect on serum and tissue lipids in experimental diabetes. *J. Med. Food.,* 7, 472–476, 2004.

[70] Saleem, R., Ahmad, M., Hussain, S.A., Qazi, A.M., Ahmad, S.I., Qazi, H.M., Ali, M., Faizi, S., Akhtar, S., and Hussain, S.N.: Hypotensive, hypoglycemic and toxicological studies on the flavonol C-glycoside shamimin from Bombax ceiba. *Planta Medica,* 5, 331–334, 1999.

[71] Somani, R., Kasture, S., and Singhai, A.K.: Antidiabetic potential of Butea monosperma in rats. *Fitoterapia.,* 77, 86– 90, 2006.

[72] Gomes, A., Vedasiromoni, J.R., Das, M., Sharma, R.M., and Ganguly, D.K.: Antihyperglycemic effect of black tea (Camellia sinensis) in rats. *J. Ethnopharmacol.*, 45, 223– 226, 1995.

[73] Devasagayam, T.P.A., Kamat, J.P., Mohan, H., and Kesavan, P.C.: Caffeine as an antioxidant: Inhibition of lipid peroxidation induced by reactive oxygen species in rat liver microsomes. *Biochim. Biophys. Acta.,* 1282, 63–70, 1996.

[74] Chakrabarti, S., Biswas, T.K., Seal, T., Rokeya, B., Ali, L., Azad Khan, A.K., Nahar, N., Mosihuzzaman, M., and Mukherjee, B.: Antidiabetic activity of Caesalpinia bonducella F. in chronic type 2 diabetic model in Long-Evans rats and evaluation of insulin secretagogue property of its fractions on isolated islets. *J. Ethnopharmacol.,* 97, 117–122, 2005.

[75] Bhattacharya, A., Chatterjee, A., Ghosal, S., and Bhattacharya, S.K.: Antioxidant activity of active tannoid principles of Emblica officinalis (amla). *Indian J. Exp. Biol.,* 37, 676– 680, 1999.

[76] Kumar, K.C.S. and Muller, K.: Medicinal plants from Nepal, II. Evaluation as inhibitors of lipid peroxidation in biological membranes. *J. Ethnopharmacol.,* 64, 135–139, 1999.

[77] Devasagayam, T.P.A., Subramanian, M., Singh, B.B., Ramanathan, R., and Das, N.P.: Protection of plasmid pBR322 DNA by flavonoids against single-strand breaks induced by singlet molecular oxygen. *J. Photochem. Photobiol.,* 30, 97–103, 1995.

[78] Arai, I., Amagaya, S., Komatzu, Y., Okada, M., Hayashi, T., Kasai, M., Arisawa, M., and Momose, Y.: Improving effects of the extracts from Eugenia uniflora on

hyperglycemia and hypertriglyceridemia in mice. *J. Ethnopharmacol,* 68, 307– 314, 1999.

[79] Maroo, J., Vasu, V.T., and Gupta, S.: Dose dependent hypoglycemic effect of aqueous extract of Enicostema littorale blume in alloxan induced diabetic rats. *Phytomedicine.,* 10, 196–199, 2003.

[80] Vijayvargia, R., Kumar, M., and Gupta, S.: Hypoglycemic effect of aqueous extract of Enicostema littorale Blume (chhota chirayata) on alloxan induced diabetes mellitus in rats. *Indian J. Exp. Biol.,* 38, 781–784, 2000.

[81] Augusti, K.T., Daniel, R.S., Cherian, S., Sheela, C.G., and Nair, C.R.: Effect of Leucoperalgonin derivative from Ficus bengalensis Linn. on diabetic dogs. *Indian J. Med. Res.,* 99, 82–86, 1994.

[82] Chattopadhyay, R.R.: A comparative evaluation of some blood sugar lowering agents of plant origin. *J. Ethnopharmacol.,* 67, 367–372, 1999.

[83] Preuss, H.G., Jarrell, S.T., Scheckenbach, R., Lieberman, S., and Anderson, R.A.: Comparative effects of chromium, vanadium and Gymnema sylvestre on sugar-induced blood pressure elevations in SHR. *J. Am. Coll. Nutr.,* 17, 116–123, 1998.

[84] Alam, M.I. and Gomes, A.: Viper venom-induced inflammation and inhibition of free radical formation by pure compound (2-hydroxy-4-methoxy benzoic acid) isolated and purified from anantamul (Hemidesmus indicus R. BR) root extract. *Toxicon.,* 36, 207–215, 1998.

[85] Sachadeva, A. and Khemani, L.D.: A preliminary investigation of the possible hypoglycemic activity of Hibiscus rosasinensis. *Biomed. Environ. Sci.,* 12, 222–226, 1999.

[86] Kusano, S. and Abe, H.: Antidiabetic activity of whites skinned potato (Ipomoea batatas) in obese Zucker fatty rats. *Biolog. Pharmaceut. Bull.,* 23, 23–26, 2000.

[87] Nagaraju, N.: *Biochemical studies on some medicinal plants of Rayalaseema region.* PhD thesis. S.V. University, Tirupathi, 1992.

[88] Rao, B.K., Kessavulu, M.M., Giri, R., and Apparao, C.: Antidiabetic and hypolipidemic effects of Momordica cymbalaria Hook fruit powder in alloxan-diabetic rats. *J. Ethnopharmacol.,* 67, 103–109, 1999.

[89] Khan, B.A., Abraham, A., and Leelamma, S.: Hypoglycemic action of Murraya koenigii (curry leaf) and Brassica juncea (mustard) mechanism of action. *Ind. J. Biochem. Biophys.,* 32, 106–108, 1995.

[90] Dhanabal, S.P., Sureshkumar, M., Ramanathan, M., and Suresh, B.: Hypoglycemic effect of ethanolic extract of Musa sapientum on alloxan induced diabetes mellitus in rats and its relation with antioxidant potential. *J. Herb. Pharmacother.,* 5, 7–19, 2005.

[91] Pari, L. and Umamaheswari, J.: Antihyperglycaemic activity of Musa sapientum flowers: effect on lipid peroxidation in alloxan diabetic rats. *Phytother. Res.,* 14, 136–138, 2000.

[92] Pari, L. and Maheswari, J.U.: Hypoglycemic effect of Musa sapientum L. in alloxan-induced diabetic rats. *J. Ethnopharmacol.,* 68, 321–325, 1999.

[93] Tormo, M.A., Gil-Exojo, I., Romero de Tejada, A., and Campillo, J.E.: Hypoglycemic and anorexigenic activities of an alpha-amylase inhibitor from white kidney beans (Phaseolus vulgaris) in Wistar rats. *Br. J. Nutr.,* 92, 785– 790, 2004.

[94] Pari, L. and Venkateswaran, S.: Protective role of Phaseolus vulgaris on changes in the fatty acid composition in experimental diabetes. *J. Med. Food.,* 7, 204–209, 2004.

[95] Knott, R.M., Grant, G., Bardocz, S., Pusztai, A., de, Carvalho, A.F., and Hesketh, J.E.: Alterations in the level of insulin receptor and GLUT-4 mRNA in skeletal muscle from rats fed a kidney bean (Phaseolus vulgaris) diet. *Int. J. Biochem.,* 24, 897–902, 1992.

[96] Jafri, M.A., Aslam, M., Javed, K., and Singh, S.: Effect of Punica granatum Linn. (flowers) on blood glucose level in normal and alloxan induced diabetic rats. *J. Ethnopharmacol.,* 70, 309–314, 2000.

[97] Yoshikawa, M., Murakami, T., Yashiro, K., and Matsuda, H.: Kotalanol, a potent α-glucosidase inhibitor with thiosugar sulfonium sulphate structure, from antidiabetic Ayurvedic medicine Salacia reticulata. *Chem. Pharma. Bulletin,* 46, 1339–1340, 1998.

[98] Pari, L. and Latha, M.: Antidiabetic effect of Scoparia dulcis: effect on lipid peroxidation in streptozotocin diabetes. *Gen. Physiol. Biophys.,* 24, 13–26, 2005.

[99] Pari, L. and Latha, M.: Antihyperlipidemic effect of Scoparia dulcis (sweet broomweed) in streptozotocin diabetic rats. *J. Med. Food.,* 9, 102–107, 2006.

[100] Latha, M., Pari, L., Sitasawad, S., and Bhonde, R.: Insulinsecretagogue activity and cytoprotective role of the traditional antidiabetic plant Scoparia dulcis (Sweet Broomweed). *Life Sci.,* 75, 2003–2014, 2004.

[101] Saxena, A.M., Bajpai, M.B., Murthy, P.S., and Mukherjee, S.K.: Mechanism of blood sugar lowcring by a Swcrchirincontaining hexane fraction (SWI) of Swertia chirayita. *Ind. J. Exp. Biol.,* 31, 178–181, 1993.

[102] Rao, B.K. and Rao, C.H.: Hypoglycemic and antihyperglycemic activity of Syzygium alternifolium (Wt.) Walp. seed extracts in normal and diabetic rats. *Phytomedicine.,* 8, 88–93, 2001.

[103] Sabu, M.C. and Kuttan, R.: Antidiabetic activity of medicinal plants and its relationship with their antioxidant property. *J. Ethnopharmacol.,* 81, 155–160, 2002.

[104] Noor, H. and Ashcroft, S.J.: Pharmacological characterization of the anti-hyperglycemic properties of Tinospora crispa extract. *J. Ethnopharmacol.,* 62, 7–13, 1998.

[105] Chattopadhyay, S.R., Sarkar, S.K., Ganguly, S., Banerjee, R.N., and Basu T.K.: Hypoglycemic and anti-hyperglycemic effect of Vinca rosea Linn. *Ind. J. Physiol. Pharmacol.,* 35, 145–151, 1991.

[106] Adallu, B. and Radhika, B.: Hypoglycemic, diuretic and hypocholesterolemic effect of winter cherry (Withania somnifera, Dunal) root. *Indian J. Exp. Biol.,* 38, 607–609, 2000.

[107] Rahmatullah M, Azam NMK et al. Medicinal Plants Used For Treatment Of Diabetes By The Marakh Sect Of The Garo Tribe Living In Mymensingh District, Bangladesh. *Altern Med*. (2012) 9(3):380-385.

[108] Ssenyange CW, Namulindwa A, Oyik B, Ssebuliba J. Plants used to manage type II diabetes mellitus in selected districts of central Uganda. *Afr Health Sci.* 2015;15(2):496-502.

Chapter 6

Plant Secondary Metabolites as Anticancer Agents in Clinical Trials and Therapeutic Application

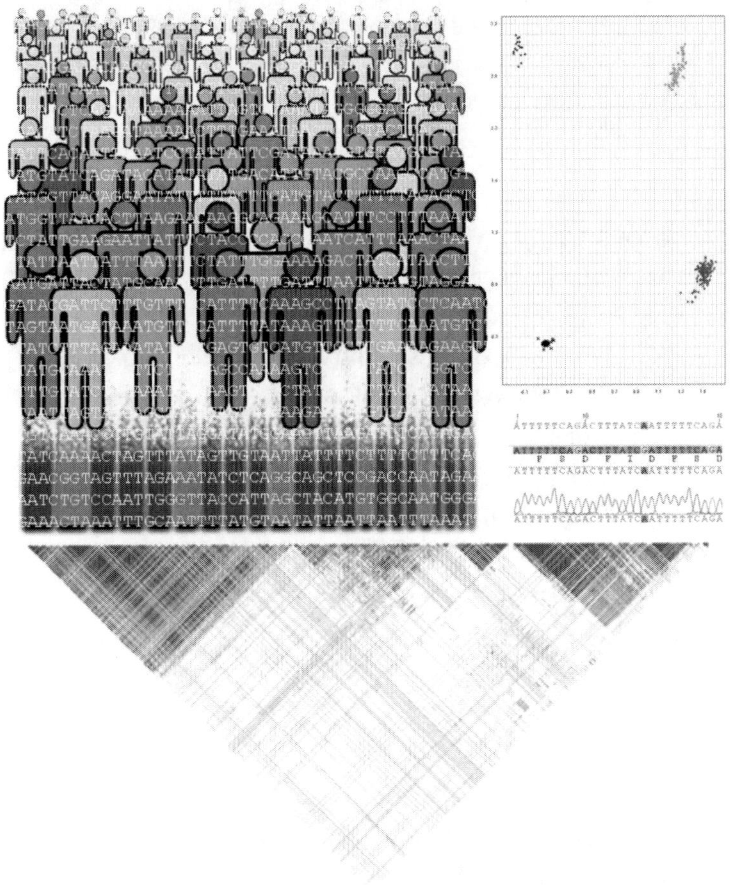

Figure. Genomic epidemiology (Theme for cancer research).

1. ABSTRACT

Cancer is a multistage process resulting in an uncontrolled and abrupt division of cells and is one of the leading causes of mortality. The cases reported and the predictions for the near future are unthinkable. Food and Drug Administration data showed that 40% of the approved molecules are natural compounds or inspired by them, from which, 74% are used in anticancer therapy. In fact, natural products are viewed as more biologically friendly, that is less toxic to normal cells. In this review, the most recent and successful cases of secondary metabolites, including alkaloid, diterpene, triterpene and polyphenolic type compounds, with great anticancer potential are discussed. Focusing on the ones that are in clinical trial development or already used in anticancer therapy, therefore successful cases such as paclitaxel and homoharringtonine (in clinical use), curcumin and *ingenol mebutate* (in clinical trials) will be addressed. Each compound's natural source, the most important steps in their discovery, their therapeutic targets, as well as the main structural modifications that can improve anticancer properties will be discussed in order to show the role of plants as a source of effective and safe anticancer drugs.

Keywords: secondary metabolites, clinical trial, anticancer therapy, vincristine, paclitaxel, homoharringtonine, ingenol mebutate, curcumin, betulinic acid

ABBREVIATIONS

5-FU	5-fluorouracil
A2780	human ovarian carcinoma cell line
ABCB1	ATP binding cassette subfamily B member 1
ABCC10	ATP binding cassette subfamily C member 10
Akt	serine/threonine-specific protein kinase
b.w.	body weight
Bak	pro-apoptotic Bcl-2 protein
Bax	bcl-2-like protein 4
Bcl-2	B-cell lymphoma 2 protein
BCR-ABL1	breakpoint cluster region protein-Abelson murine leukemia viral oncogene homolog 1
CDKI	cyclin-dependent kinase inhibitors
colon 205	human Caucasian colon adenocarcinoma cell line
CoMFA	comparative molecular field analysis
CoMSIA	comparative molecular similarity index analysis
CYP	cytochrome P450
DNA	deoxyribonucleic acid
EMA	European Medicines Agency
ERK	extracellular signal-regulated kinases
FAO	Food and Agriculture Organization

FDA	Food and Drug Administration
FGF	fibroblast growth factor
FLT3-ITD	fms-related tyrosine kinase 3 internal tandem duplication
HIF-1α	hypoxia-inducible factor 1-alpha
HMGB1	high mobility group box 1 protein
IC50	half maximal inhibitory concentration
MAPK	mitogen-activated protein kinase
Mcl-1	induced myeloid leukemia cell differentiation protein
MDR	multidrug resistance
miRNA	micro-ribonucleic acid
MMP	matrix metalloproteinase
mRNA	messenger ribonucleic acid
Myc	proto-oncogene
nab-paclitaxel	nanoparticle albumin-bound paclitaxel
NF-κB	nuclear factor kappa B cells
Nrf2	nuclear factor (erythroid-derived 2)-like 2
P-388	bipotential murine pre-B cell lymphoma
PEP005	ingenol mebutate
PGDF	platelet-derived growth factor
P-gp	p-glycoprotein
PI3K	phosphatidylinositol-4,5-bisphosphate 3-kinase
PICN	paclitaxel injection concentrate for nanodispersion
PKC	protein kinase C
PKCα	protein kinase C-α
PKCδ	protein kinase C-δ
QSAR	quantitative structure activity relationship
RAID	rapid access to intervention in development
SAR	structure activity relationship
SCD-1	stearoyl-CoA- desaturase 1
SCLC	small-cell lung cancer
SIRT1	NAD-dependent protein deacetylase sirtuin-1
SM/Chol	sphingomyelin/cholesterol
smad3	mothers against decapentaplegic homolog 3
Sp1	specificity protein 1
STAT3	signal transducer and activator of transcription 3
T315I	mutation resulting in an amino acid substitution at position 315 in BCR-ABL1, from a threonine (T) to an isoleucine (I).
TGF-β	transforming growth factor beta
TRAIL	tumor necrosis factor-related apoptosis-inducing ligand
tRNA	transfer ribonucleic acid

uPAR	urokinase receptor
VEGF	vascular endothelial growth factor
WHO	World Health Organization

2. INTRODUCTION

Although cancer is the most devastating disease, causing more deaths than all coronary heart diseases or all strokes, with 14.1 million new cases and 8.2 million deaths in 2012 [1], there is a register of a continuous decline in cancer death rates that has resulted in an overall drop of 23% since 1991 [2]. Despite this progress, there is a register of 8.8 million deaths globally in 2015, and cancer is now the leading cause of death in 21 states of the United States of America [2]. The total annual economic cost of cancer in 2010 was approximately $1.16 trillion [3]. This burden is further expected to rise, with over the predicted 20 million new cancer cases expected globally by 2025 [4]. Moreover, incidence and death rates are increasing for several cancer types, for example liver and pancreas [2]. In the low- and middle-income countries, the picture is even darker, where approximately 70% of deaths are due to cancer diseases and where only one in five countries have the necessary data to drive cancer policy [3, 5]. Advancing the fight against cancer requires both increased investment in cancer pathology research and in new safe, effective, inexpensive and minimal side effect anticancer agents.

For millennia, indigenous cultures around the world have used traditional herbal medicine to treat a myriad of maladies. Plants constitute a common alternative for cancer treatment in many countries, and more than 3000 plants worldwide have been reported to have anticancer properties [6, 7]. Although a recent study suggests that nowadays, the traditional medicines are less used, even in populous middle-income countries [8], herbal medicine use is still common in oncology therapy worldwide [6, 7, 9–11]. In the last two decades, the use of herbal remedies has also been widely embraced in many developed countries as complementary and alternative medicine, but following tight legislation and under surveillance [12]. Natural products have garnered increasing attention in cancer chemotherapy because they are viewed as more biologically friendly and consequently more co-evolved with their target sites and less toxic to normal cells [13]. Moreover, there is evidence that natural product-derived anticancer drugs have alternative modes of promoting cell death [14, 15]. Based on these facts, many researchers are now centering their investigations on the plants' potential to deliver natural products that can become useful to the pharmaceutical industry [16–18]. In fact, the utilization of natural products as the background to discover and develop a drug entity is still a research hot point. From small molecules approved for cancer chemotherapy between 1940 and 2014, around 49% are natural products [19].

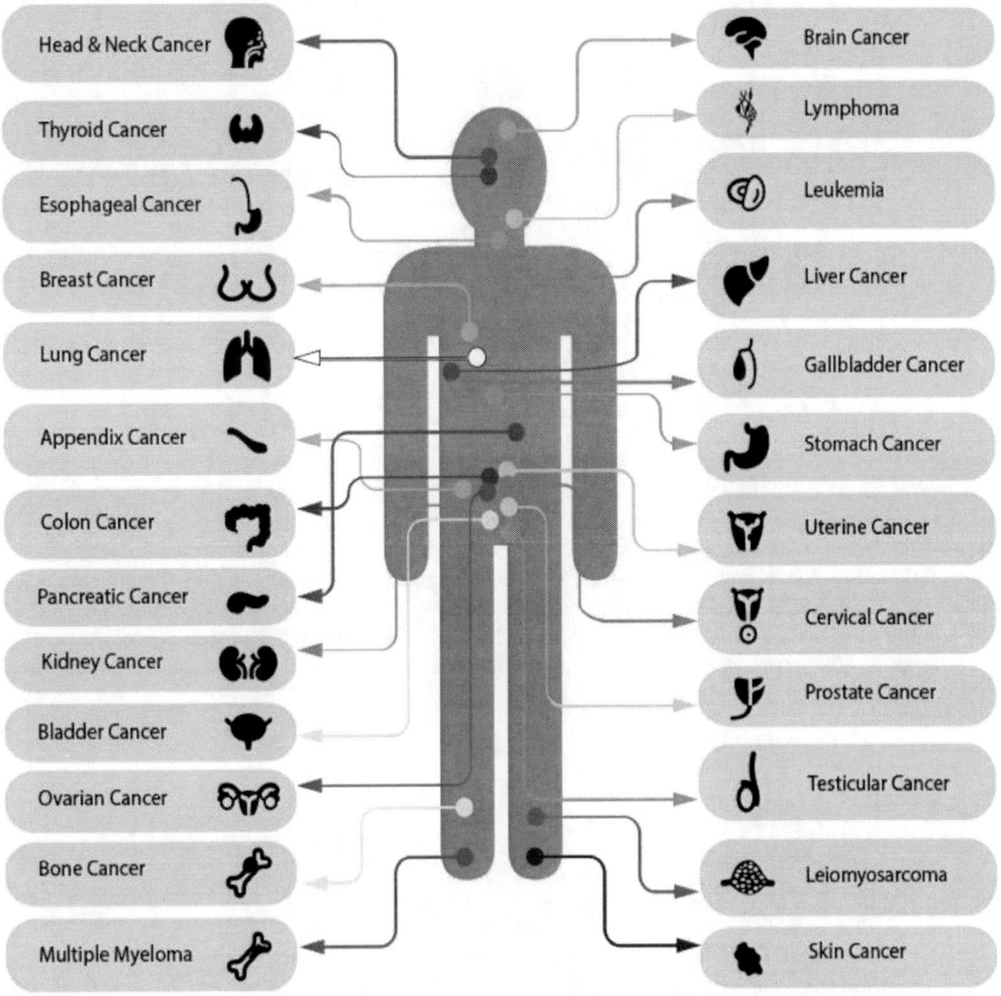

Figure 1. Immunotherapy cancer treatments. When cancer appears some of the body's cells begin to divide without stopping and spread into surrounding tissues, generating abnormal cell growth. These extra cells can divide without stopping and may form growths called tumors. Cancer can start almost anywhere in the human body, which is made up of trillions of cells. Normally, human cells grow and divide to form new cells as and when the body needs them. In the normal process when cells grow old or become damaged, they die, and new cells take their place. When cancer develops, however, this orderly process breaks down. As cells become more and more abnormal, old or damaged cells survive when they should die, and new cells form when they are not needed. Recent years' success of cancer immunotherapy including monoclonal antibodies (mAbs), cancer vaccines, adoptive cancer therapy and the immune checkpoint therapy has revolutionized traditional cancer treatment. However, challenges still exist in this field. Personalized combination therapies via new techniques will be the next promising strategies for the future cancer treatment direction. (Source: Zhang H, Chen J. Current status and future directions of cancer immunotherapy. J Cancer. 2018;9(10):1773-1781. Published 2018 Apr 19. doi:10.7150/jca.24577.)

In spite of all the beneficial potential of medicinal plants and consequently of their products, many continue without adequate monitoring to guarantee their effectiveness and safety [20, 21].

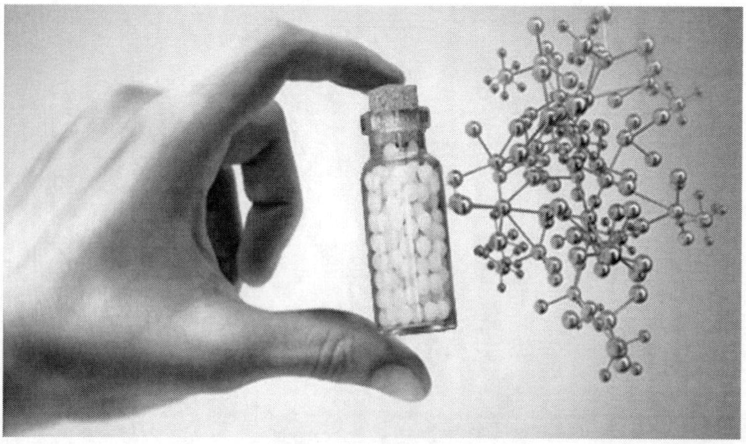

Figure 2. Non-surgical, natural cancer treatment. Cancer pain is one of the physical component has tremendous impact on the QoL of the patient. Cancer pain is multifaceted and complex to understand and managing cancer pain involves a tool box full of pharmacological and non pharmacological interventions but still there are 50-70% of cancer patients who suffer from uncontrolled pain and they fear pain more than death. Aggressive surgeries, radiotherapy and chemotherapy focus more on prolonging the survival of the patient failing to realize that the QoL lived also matters equally. (Source: Singh P, Chaturvedi A. Complementary and alternative medicine in cancer pain management: a systematic review. Indian J Palliat Care. 2015;21(1):105-15.)

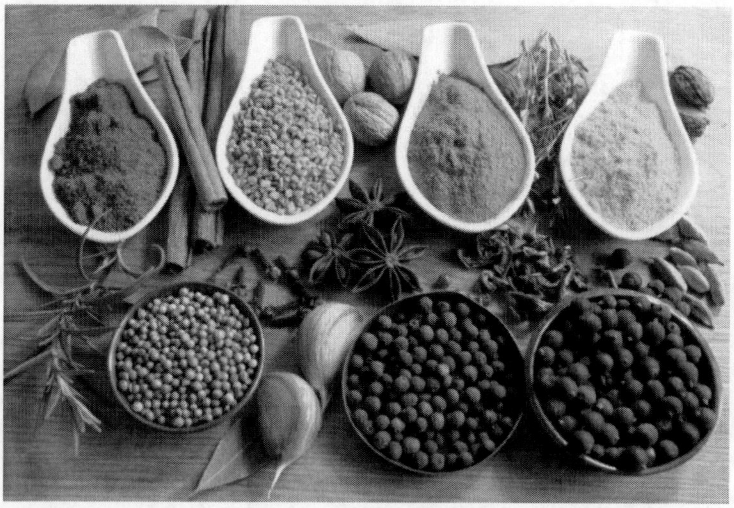

Figure 3. Powerful cancer fighting spices. Spices have been widely used as food flavorings and folk medicines for thousands of years. Numerous studies have documented the antioxidant, anti-inflammatory and immunomodulatory effects of spices, which might be related to prevention and treatment of several cancers, including lung, liver, breast, stomach, colorectum, cervix, and prostate cancers. Several spices are potential sources for prevention and treatment of cancers, such as Curcuma longa (tumeric), Nigella sativa (black cumin), *Zingiber officinale* (ginger), *Allium sativum* (garlic), *Crocus sativus* (saffron), *Piper nigrum* (black pepper) and *Capsicum annum* (chili pepper), which contained several important bioactive compounds, such as curcumin, thymoquinone, piperine and capsaicin. The main mechanisms of action include inducing apoptosis, inhibiting proliferation, migration and invasion of tumors, and sensitizing tumors to radiotherapy and chemotherapy. (Source: Zheng J, Zhou Y, Li Y, Xu DP, Li S, Li HB. Spices for Prevention and Treatment of Cancers. Nutrients. 2016;8(8):495. Published 2016 Aug 12. doi:10.3390/nu8080495.)

The following sections offer an overview of compounds from plants that have been found to exhibit activity against different types of cancer and are now on the market as anticancer drugs or are involved in clinic trials, which means they are involved in the last stage of the development of a clinical drug. Therefore, these compounds, which constitute successful cases in cancer therapy, will be briefly discussed.

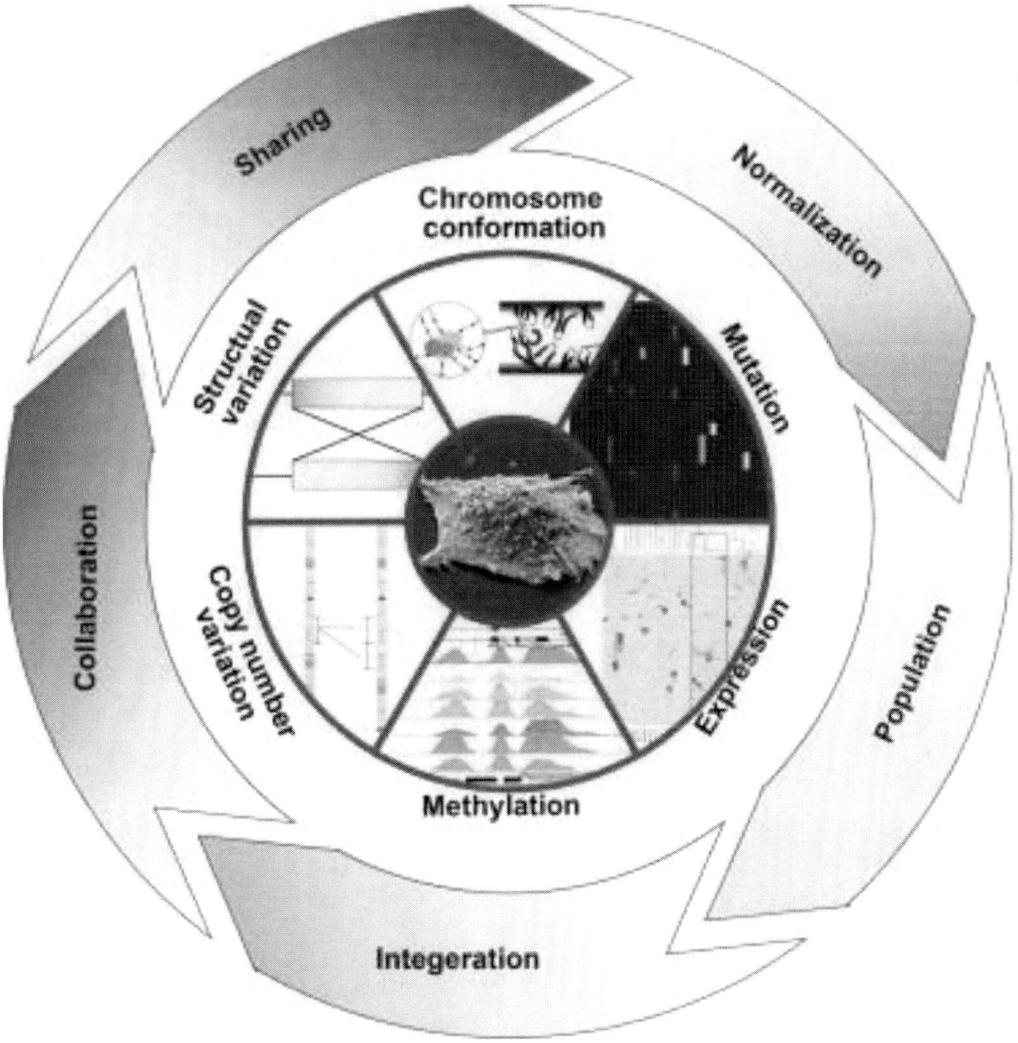

Figure 4. The future of cancer research. In the era of big data, one of the major challenges is to make full use of multi-dimensional data from heterogeneous sources, including different omics data and a variety of medical data from bedside. The success in the battle against cancer will largely depend on population-sized information from both genomic and clinical resources, advanced algorithms for data mining, open and sharing circumstances. (Source: Yang Y, Dong X et al. Databases and Web Tools for Cancer Genomics Study Genomics, Proteomics & Bioinformatics Volume 13, Issue 1, February 2015, Pages 46-50.)

3. SECONDARY METABOLITES FROM PLANTS AS ANTICANCER AGENTS

Throughout history, plants have been a rich source of affordable natural compounds, explicitly the secondary metabolites, that possess sufficient structural complexity so that their synthesis is difficult or at this time not yet accomplished and exhibit a broad spectrum of bioactivities including antitumor activity [22, 23]. Secondary metabolites are mostly small organic molecules, produced by an organism, that are not essential for its growth, development and reproduction. They can be classified based on the pathway by which they are synthesized [24]. Additionally, a simple classification includes three main groups: terpenoids (polymeric isoprene derivatives and biosynthesized from acetate via the mevalonic acid pathway), phenolics (biosynthesized from shikimate pathways, containing one or more hydroxylated aromatic rings) and the extremely diverse alkaloids (non-protein nitrogen-containing compounds, biosynthesized from amino acids such as tyrosine, with a long history in medication) [24, 25]. Several new cytotoxic secondary metabolites are isolated from plants each year and constitute a source of new possibilities to explore in order to fight against cancerous diseases. Although some natural compounds have unique anticancer effects, their use in clinical practice is not possible due to their physico-chemical properties (e.g., limited bioavailability) and/or their toxicity. On the other hand, plant occurring secondary metabolites often can be excellent leads for drug development. Thus, modifying the chemical structure of these more promising compounds is one strategic way to increase their anticancer action and selectivity, improve their absorption, distribution, metabolism and excretion properties and decrease their toxicity and side effects [26, 27]. Herein we will present the most significant achievements in the area of plant secondary metabolites, some already in clinical use and others in clinical trials as anticancer agents, as well as their most efficient derivatives obtained by structural modifications.

3.1. Metabolites Used in Cancer Therapy

During the last few decades, a wide range of cytotoxic agents was discovered from plants, but very few of these managed to reach clinical use after successfully running through the entire long, selective, expensive and bureaucratic process from their chemical identification to their effectiveness in therapeutic cancer treatment. Each of these compounds has their histories of success and limitations, which has been told by many authors and which are hereinafter counted in a historical, molecular, pharmaceutical and clinical point of view.

3.1.1. Vincristine

Vincristine (**1**) has a non-symmetrical dimeric structure, composed of a two indole-type nucleus linked by a carbon–carbon bond, the vindoline portion and the catharanthine type portion (Figure 1). In 1963, the Food and Drug Administration (FDA) approved its clinical use to treat cancer. In fact, it was one of the first plant-derived anticancer agents approved by this agency [19]. It is a naturally-occurring alkaloid extracted from the leaves of *Catharanthus roseus* (L.) G.Don (formerly *Vinca rosea* L.) and has been used in chemotherapy in adult, but mainly in pediatric oncology practice against acute lymphoblastic leukemia. Its incorporation in the treatment regimen increases the survival rate to eighty percent [28]. It is also used to treat rhabdomyosarcoma, neuroblastoma, lymphomas and nephroblastoma [29, 30].

The large interest in vincristine contrasts with its low natural occurrence, and consequently, its extraction is very expensive. This situation has stimulated an intense research effort aiming to find promising strategies to increase vincristine (and other vinca alkaloids) production. Selected enzymes' manipulation by genetic engineering to raise the metabolic flow rate toward vincristine and the use of elicitors to activate genes involved in vincristine metabolic pathways are effective strategies to increase the biotechnological production of this compound [30, 31]. However, some improvements are needed before these processes become economically viable. Another possibility to obtain more vincristine is the application/optimization of high yield extraction methodologies like negative-pressure cavitation extraction [32]. Vincristine, in a concentration-dependent manner, can affect cells' division. However, the most well-known mechanism of vincristine antitumor activity involves interaction with tubulin, the basic constituent of mitotic spindle microtubules, inhibiting its polymerization and resulting in the suppression of mitosis. Therefore, it disrupts the assembly of the mitotic spindle, which in turn leads to the demise of actively-dividing cells [33]. Some authors report that at the lowest effective concentration, the anti-proliferative effect is due to a subtly change in the addition and loss of tubulins at the mitotic spindle microtubule and thus stabilizes the mitotic spindle assembly and disassembly processes that lead to metaphase arrest [30]. Once microtubule dynamics, and therefore cell division, can be perturbed by blocking the polymerization or depolymerization of tubulin in microtubules and thus impairing the mitotic spindle assembly, it seems that vincristine can act by both mechanisms depending on the concentration level. Moreover, a molecular docking study showed some evidence suggesting each part of the vincristine dimeric structure exhibits a specific role on its anticancer activity once the vindoline nucleus binds tubulin heterodimers, while the catharanthine nucleus provides a cytotoxic effect [34]. Despite the long history of vincristine clinical application in fighting cancer, there are three factors that diminish its impact in therapeutics: (i) its antitumor mechanism is cell-cycle-specific, and the duration of its exposure to tumor cells can significantly affect its antitumor activity; (ii) the pharmacokinetic behavior of vincristine in human blood is described by a bi-exponential elimination pattern with a very fast initial distribution half-life followed by a longer elimination half-life, and it has a large volume of distribution, suggesting diffuse distribution and tissue binding [35]; (iii) it may cause temporary or permanent peripheral neuropathy, which is a dose-dependent side effect influenced by several variables such as age, race, genetic profile and administration method, and older children, in particular Caucasian, seem to be more susceptible [36]. Some of these factors could be mitigated by encapsulation of vincristine into liposomes, which is intended to increase the circulation time, optimize delivery to target tissues and facilitate dose intensification without increasing toxicity [35].

In 2012, the FDA approved the use of sphingomyelin/cholesterol (SM/Chol) liposomal vincristine (Marqibo®) to treat adults with relapsed acute lymphoblastic leukemia (New Drug Application: 202497). Vincristine can be loaded into conventional liposomes like SM/Chol liposomes, but other types of liposomes, for example PEGylated liposomes, were already tested, although SM/Chol liposomal vincristine displays a relatively long circulation time, a reduced leakage rate from liposomes and an improved antitumor effect compared to PEGylated liposomal vincristine [33]. Clinical trials involving Marqibo® are underway to pediatric patients with relapsed or chemotherapy-refractory solid tumors and leukemia (ClinicalTrials.gov Identifier: NCT01222780). Moreover, other vincristine encapsulated formulations are involved in clinical studies in which they are tested against other types of cancer such as small-cell lung cancer (ClinicalTrials.gov Identifier: NCT02566993), advanced cervical cancer (ClinicalTrials.gov Identifier: NCT02471027) and liver cancer (ClinicalTrials.gov Identifier: NCT00980460).

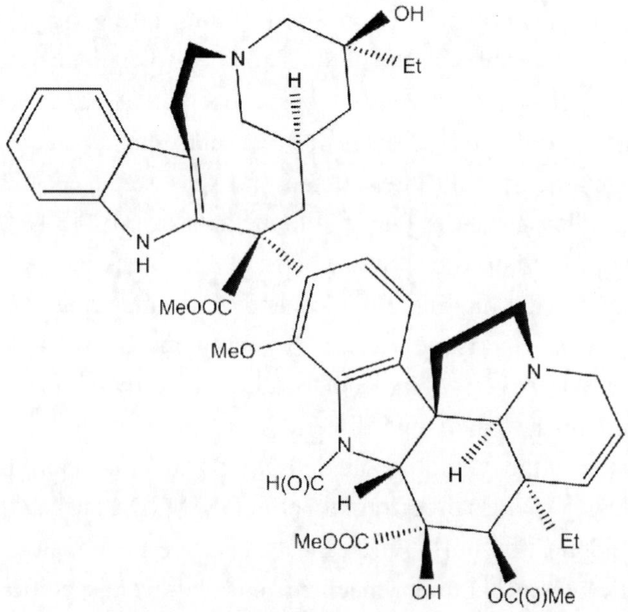

Figure 5. Chemical structure of the vinca alkaloid vincristine (1), an anticancer natural agent that repress cell growth by altering the microtubular dynamics.

Vincristine generally exhibits better efficacy when administered in combination with other antitumor agents. In fact, combined chemotherapy can not only enhance the destruction of tumor cells, but also decrease toxicity and drug resistance with drugs exhibiting different mechanisms of action. Therefore, open clinical trials are in progress involving combined vincristine therapy (e.g., NCT02879643; NCT01527149). Very recently, a case report was done of infantile fibrosarcoma treated by adjuvant therapy after excision, using vincristine and dactinomycin, where the duration of chemotherapy was determined according to tumor response. At the end, there was no functional impairment and no evidence of recurrence at 18 months after therapy [37].

3.1.2. Paclitaxel

The discovery of novel natural structures with significant biological relevance and with new action mechanisms have tremendous impact on the pharmaceutical industry. The discovery of (**2**) is an excellent example. Its high activity and its novel mechanism of action, tubulin-assembly promotion, is a milestone of a new era in anticancer drug discovery. Paclitaxel, isolated from the bark of *Taxus brevifolia* Nutt. (Pacific Yew) and sold under the brand name Taxol® since 1993, is a complex molecule that has become one of the most active cancer chemotherapeutic drugs known [38, 39]. It is a tricyclic diterpenoid, occasionally considered as a pseudo alkaloid, that contains a complex 6,8,6-tri-cycle-fused skeleton, named the "taxane" ring system, linked to a four-member oxetane ring and having alcohol, ester, ketone and amide functions (Figure 2).

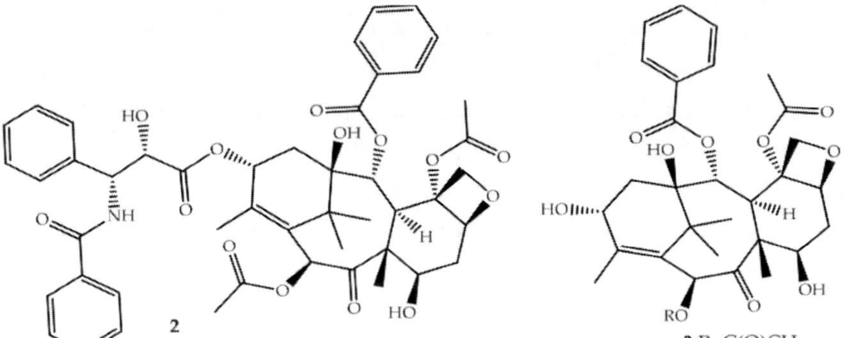

2

3 R=C(O)CH_3
4 R=H

Figure 6. Chemical structure of paclitaxel 920, a natural microtubule inhibitor, and of it's precursors baccatin III (3) and 10-deacetylbaccatin III (4).

Paclitaxel is a non-ionic molecule with high lipophilicity (log P = 3.20) that is practically insoluble in aqueous medium (aqueous solubility ~0.3–0.5 μg/mL) [40]. Due to this hydrophobicity its administration is performed in a solution containing alcohol and polyoxyethylated castor oil to enhance its delivery. The biosynthetic pathway of paclitaxel is a complex process that starts with precursor geranylgeranyl diphosphate and involves 19 steps regulated by several enzymes, and some were already characterized, but the process is not yet fully understood [41]. Although the medicinal use of paclitaxel has been achieved exclusively with purified compound from the bark of Pacific Yew, the plant's low content and the ecological impact of its harvesting have prompted extensive searches for alternative sources. The total synthesis of paclitaxel was not successful until 1994 [42], and even after several improvements [43, 44], it remains a laborious work that prevents its industrial viability. More sustainable alternatives are being used: (i) the fermentation technology with microbes or plant cell culture [45]; (ii) protein engineering to elevate catalytic fitness for paclitaxel production [46]; (iii) semisynthesis from baccatin III (**3**, Figure 2) [47] or 10-deacetylbaccatin III (**4**, Figure 2) [48], two paclitaxel precursor molecules, which are non-cytotoxic and are found in much higher quantities and readily available from the needles of *Taxus baccata*, *Taxus brevifolia* and other *Taxus* species [49]. The last approach is the one employed by the pharmaceutical industry.

The introduction of paclitaxel in the last few decades has expanded the therapeutic options, mainly due to its powerful anticancer activity, and great successes in the treatment of breast, ovarian and lung cancers have been achieved [39]. Moreover, its success is also due to effectiveness on both solid and disseminated tumors and a broad spectrum of antitumor activity predicted by its unique mechanism of action, which targets the very basic elements of the cancer phenotype like cell proliferation and DNA repair [38]. In fact, paclitaxel skeleton functional groups are at special positions and ensure that β-tubulin is targeted in order to prevent the dynamic microtubule disassembly process required for proper mitotic spindle assembly and chromosome segregation during cell division. Consequently, cell death is caused in a time- and concentration-dependent manner [38]. The continuous research on the mechanism of action of paclitaxel together with the structure activity relationship (SARs) and quantitative SAR (QSAR) revealed and assigned the pharmacophores, as well as structural parts that should not be modified (Figure 3). This allowed the design of novel derivatives with the best efficacy and fewer side effects [26, 50]. Based on this knowledge, two semi-synthetic derivatives were developed with great success, docetaxel (**5**) and cabazitaxel (**6**). They were obtained by structural modifications restricted to the variable sections of the original structure and are now available for clinical use (Figure 3).

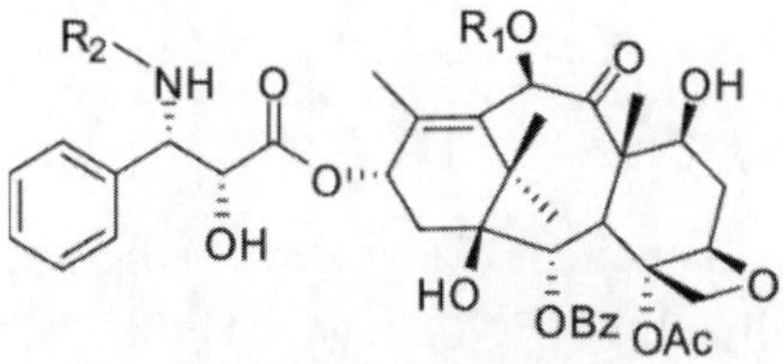

Paclitaxel R_1=Ac, R_2=Bz
Docetaxel R_1=H, R_2=Boc

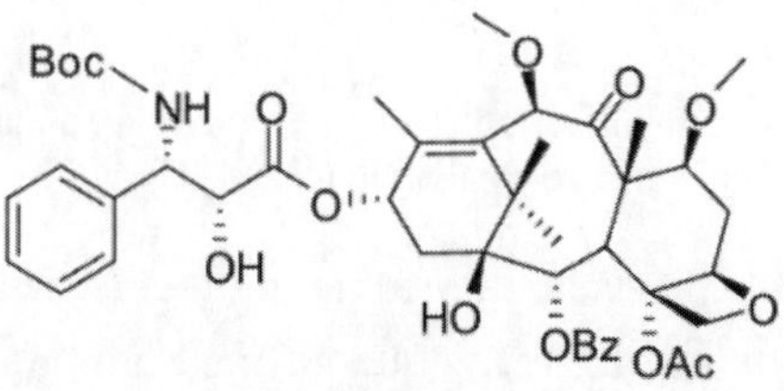

Cabazitaxel

Figure 7. The parts of the paclitaxel structure that could be modified without loss of activity and two of its derivatives, docetaxel and cabazitaxel, available on the market for clinical use.

Although paclitaxel has been applied effectively to treat many cancer diseases, its therapeutic efficacy is starting to be limited due to multidrug resistance (MDR) development [51, 52]. Although the cellular mechanisms involved in the MDR are not fully understood, it appears that the overexpression of ABCB1 (also called P-glycoprotein) and ABCC10 (also named multidrug resistance protein 7) efflux transporters, the α-/β-tubulin mutations and/or alterations in the binding regions are the main cause [51, 52].

The development of new drug delivery systems and new formulations allowed paclitaxel to find its way to the tumor tissue for more direct and safe anticancer activity and to overcome paclitaxel's multidrug resistance, its poor aqueous solubility, clinical neurotoxicity and neutropenia [53–55]. For example, Lipusu®, the first paclitaxel lecithin/cholesterol liposome injectable, has been on the Chinese market since 2006 and is used in the treatment of ovarian, breast, non-SCLC, gastric and head and neck cancers [39]. This liposomal formulation Lipusu® exhibited similar antitumor effects to paclitaxel, but its toxicity is lower than that of paclitaxel under the same dosage [39, 56]. Another example is Abraxane®, an injectable nanoparticle albumin-bound paclitaxel, also named *nab*-paclitaxel developed to improve the solubility of paclitaxel, which was approved in 2005 by FDA and in 2012 by European Medicines Agency (EMA) (EMA/99258/2015, EMEA/H/C/000778) [57]. Higher doses of *nab*-paclitaxel can be administered over a shorter infusion time, and consequently, there is an improvement in neuropathy side effects after the therapy discontinuation [57], although peripheral sensory neuropathy occurred more frequently with *nab*-paclitaxel compared to paclitaxel [55].

The development of paclitaxel-mimics, with a simplified structure, also allowed the discovery of docetaxel, on the market since 1995 under the trade name Taxotere®, a drug that has fewer side effects and improved pharmaceutical properties [58]. It is obtained by semisynthesis from 10-deacetylbaccatin-III and shares with paclitaxel the same mechanism of action and identical ABCB1 affinity, but with different pharmacokinetics and side effects [49]. It is structurally different from paclitaxel only at the C-10 (acetyl group removed) and C-3^0 positions (the *N*-C(O)Ph group is replaced for an *N-tert*-butyl acetate group), (Figure 3) alterations that increase its water solubility and lower its lipophilicity (log $P = 3.20$). It belongs to the first generation of taxanes, used for the treatment of breast, ovarian, prostate and non-SCLCs, and exhibits a longer half-life, more rapid cellular uptake and longer intracellular retention than paclitaxel [59].

Cabazitaxel (Jevtana®) was approved by the FDA in 2010 for the treatment of patients with hormone-refractory metastatic prostate cancer and tumors that are docetaxel- or paclitaxel-resistant [60]. It is also obtained by semisynthesis and is a dimethoxyl derivative of docetaxel, a structural change that increases its lipophilicity (log $P = 3.90$) and consequently its cell penetration through passive influx associated with alteration of the P-gp affinity [61]. This allows the drug to accumulate intracellularly at greater concentrations than docetaxel and explains its improved cytotoxicity and effectiveness in taxane-resistant patients [27, 49].

Paclitaxel is already a blockbuster of the pharmacy industry not only due to the development of new delivery systems in cancer therapy [62] and its application in combination with other anticancer drugs (e.g., ClinicalTrials.gov Identifier: NCT02379416, NCT00584857 and NCT01288261) [63, 64], but also due to its use in clinical trials for other treatments such as psoriasis [65] and botulinum neurotoxin inhibiting [66], just to mention a few examples that ensure this compound's success.

3.1.3. Homoharringtonine

Homoharringtonine (**7**) is an alkaloid with a cephalotaxine nucleus named cephalotaxine 4-methyl-2(*R*)-hydroxy-2-(4-hydroxy-4-methylpentyl)succinate (Figure 4). It was first isolated from *Cephalotaxus harringtonii* (Knight ex J.Forbes) K.Koch and *Cephalotaxus fortunei* Hook. Trees, whose bark extracts were used in Chinese traditional medicine to treat cancer. Homoharringtonine and other cephalotaxine derivatives can also be found in leaves, bark and seeds of other *Cephalotaxus* species [67]. In fact, the cephalotaxine itself is very abundant in *Cephalotaxus* species leaves which can be isolated and transformed by a simple esterification into homoharringtonine, and thus, this procedure constitutes a semisynthetic methodology used for homoharringtonine industrial production [50, 68].

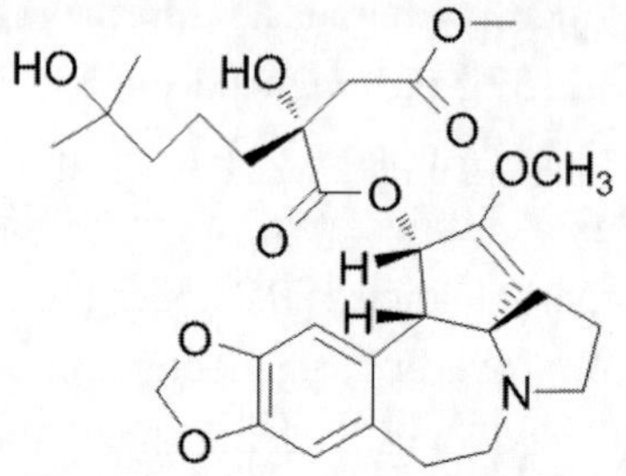

Figure 8. Chemical structure of homoharringtonine also named omacetaxine mepesuccinate (7) with alkaloid nucleus cephalotaxine (red).

The interest in homoharringtonine started when its potent antiproliferative activity against murine P-388 leukemia cells with IC_{50} values of 17 nM was demonstrated [69]. In fact, since the 1970s homoharringtonine or a mixture of cephalotaxine esters has been used in China to treat hematological malignancies [70]. However, only after the development of the above-mentioned semisynthetic procedure did homoharringtonine attract the attention of Western medicine.

Homoharringtonine is a first-in-class protein translation inhibitor, which means that it inhibits the elongation step of protein synthesis. In fact, homoharringtonine binds to the A-site of the large ribosomal subunit, an action that blocks the access of the charged tRNA and consequently the peptide bond formation [71]. Since this drug does not target specific proteins, its success is mainly due to the fact that it can disturb proteins with rapid turnover such as the leukemic cells' upregulated short-lived oncoproteins BCR-ABL1 and antiapoptotic proteins (Mcl-1, Myc) leading to cells apoptosis [71]. Recently, other mechanisms indicated that it could also affect signaling pathways, like the Jak-stat5 pathway, by regulating protein tyrosine kinase phosphorylation [72] and by activating the TGF-β pathway through phosphorylation of smad3 [73].

The identification of several natural cephalotaxine esters structurally similar to homoharringtonine and other derivatives obtained by semisynthesis allowed establishing some structure activity relationships, which were recently reviewed and discussed by Chang et al. [69].

The most important SAR are: (i) the cephalotaxine nucleus is much less active against the P388 cell line than its esters derivatives; (ii) an aliphatic side chain bonded to the hydroxyl group at C-3 seems to be necessary to enhance the activity; (iii) the presence of hydroxyl groups at C-11 or C-3^0 decreases the activity; (iv) a free carboxylic acid at C-4^0 abruptly decreases the activity; however, the methyl group can be replaced by other alkyl groups, even bulky ones, without the loss of the activity and in some cases enhancing it; (v) bulky groups bonded to 8^0-OH are also tolerated; (vi) substituents bonded at 2^0-OH imply a significant loss of activity (Figure 4).

There is a long track record of the clinical efficacy and safety of homoharringtonine use in the treatment of chronic myeloid leukemia. Currently, the focus is on its use in patients that experienced resistance or intolerance to multiple tyrosine kinase inhibitors (sorafenib and imatinib target) [74] and in patients carrying the T315I mutation, a variant that is unresponsive to tyrosine kinase inhibitors [74–76]. In fact, homoharringtonine was approved by the FDA in 2012 (sold under the trade name Synribo®) to be used in the treatment of chronic myeloid leukemia in patients with resistance and/or intolerance to two or more tyrosine kinase inhibitors, and it is the only natural therapeutic agent approved as a commercial drug to treat chronic myeloid leukemia.

The commercial approval of homoharringtonine and continued preclinical and clinical investigations of this compound indicate opportunities for its use in other hematological malignancies. For instance, the produced durable hematologic and cytogenetic responses regardless of mutational status [76, 77] exhibit the ability to effectively kill stem/progenitor cells [77, 78] and have a role in acute myeloid leukemia [79].

The homoharringtonine therapeutic efficiency continues to be evaluated, and its use is expect in the near future in other hematologic malignancies. It is being evaluated in 20 clinical trials, in mono and combined therapy, involving, for example, patients with newly-diagnosed acute myelogenous leukemia (NCT01873495), with relapsed/refractory acute myeloid leukemia carrying FLT3-ITD (NCT03170895), with myelodysplastic syndrome (NCT02159872), and in combined therapy with imatinib mesylate (NCT00114959), with quizartinib (NCT03135054) and with cytarabine and idarubicin (NCT02440568). Moreover, the subcutaneous administration of homoharringtonine does not influence its bioavailability (NCT00675350) [80] and allowed decreasing its cardiac toxicity [77]. Additionally, the FDA in 2014 approved its administration at home by the patient or a caregiver, which is indeed an improvement because patients have the opportunity to self-administer their therapy and due to homoharringtonine's stability [81].

Although homoharringtonine treatment may result in some hematologic toxicity such as myelosuppression, this should not prevent the use of this drug, once the benefits exceed the damage and the latter can be limited mainly by adequate dose adjustment and patient training for symptoms [82]. All these data show a large number of scenarios where homoharringtonine use is applied and suggest many others where it can receive approval in the near future, showing that its long history in cancer therapy is far from over.

3.2. Metabolites in Clinical Trials

In September 2007, a total of 91 plant-derived compounds was in clinical trials [83], whereas at the end of 2013, there were 100 unaltered natural products plus their derivatives involved in clinical trials, with a majority being in oncology [68].

Several semisynthetic derivatives from the plant-derived compounds camptothecin (e.g., gimatecan), combretastatin A (e.g., fosbretabulin tromethamine; combretastatin A1 diphosphate), rohitukine (e.g., alvocidib, riviciclib), triptolide (e.g., minnelide) and daidzein (e.g., phenoxodiol) [50, 68, 83] are in clinical trials, while the lead compounds are not involved in any clinical studies as an anticancer agent, although they exhibit relevant cytotoxic properties. Only the plant-derived lead compounds are presently in clinical trials as anticancer agents, and their derivatives are discussed below.

3.2.1. Ingenol Mebutate

The phytochemical study of *Euphorbia peplus* L. latex sap yielded several macrocyclic diterpenes [84], including ingenol mebutate (**8**, Figure 5) (also known as PEP005, ingenol-3-angelate and 3-ingenyl angelate), which was later on identified as the most active antitumor component [85]. In fact, the *Euphorbia peplus* sap has been shown, in a recent phase I/II clinical study, to be effective against human non-melanoma skin cancer [86]. This ingenene-type diterpene (Figure 5) can also be isolated from other *Euphorbia* species such as *Euphorbia paralias* L., *Euphorbia millii* Des Moul., *Euphorbia palustris* L., *Euphorbia marginata* Pursh and *Euphorbia helioscopia* L., and especially in the lower leafless stems of *Euphorbia myrsinites* L., where it is found in high quantity (547 mg/kg of dry weight) [68, 87]. Ingenol mebutate has been prepared by semisynthesis using ingenol, which is isolated from the seeds of *Euphorbia lathyris* L. (yield ~100 mg/kg). The methodology involves a selective esterification of the hydroxyl group at position 3 with (*Z*)-2-methylbut-2-enoic acid (angelate nucleus) (Figure 5) [88]. Some efforts have been made to accomplish the ingenol total synthesis, but they are not suitable for application in the pharmaceutical industry, so the ingenol mebutate total synthesis remains undone. Ingenol mebutate is a monoester considered, in pharmacological terms, a small molecule.

Its stability is pH dependent and can undergo facile acyl migration involving the hydroxyl groups, mainly the 5- and 20-OH (Figure 5). This characteristic is important from the biological activity point of view, because the free hydroxyl groups and the ester moiety at position 3 are required for the anticancer activity [89].

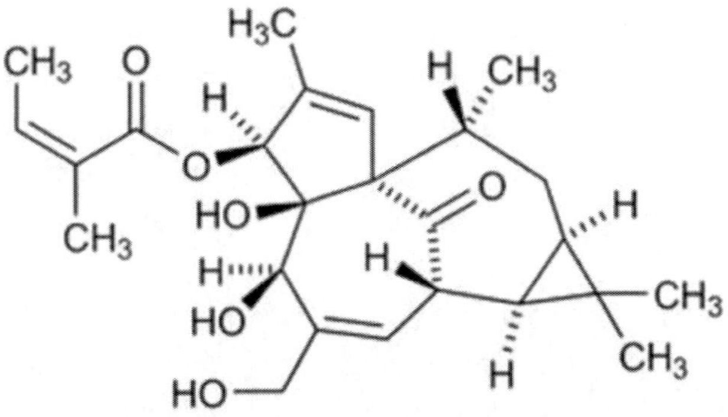

Figure 9. Chemical structure of the diterpene ingenol mebutate.

Ingenol mebutate showed potent antiproliferative effects in a dose- and time-dependent manner against several cell lines [90, 91], especially against colon 205 cells line with IC_{50} = 10 nM, that means more active than staurosporine (IC_{50} = 29 nM) or doxorubicin (IC_{50} = 1.5 μM), known active compounds used as standards [90]. There is evidence that its effectiveness at damaging the tumor vasculature is related to the fact that it can be transported through the epidermis into the deep dermis via a P-glycoprotein [92]. Treatment with this compound, both in vitro (230 μM) and in vivo (42 nmol), rapidly caused swelling of mitochondria probably by loss of mitochondrial membrane potential and cell death by primary necrosis and is, therefore, unlikely to have its activity compromised by the development of apoptosis resistance in tumor cells [86]. There is evidence that this rapid action of ingenol mebutate is due to its dual action combining cytotoxic and immunomodulatory effects in which rapid lesion necrosis and antibody-dependent cellular cytotoxicity mediated by neutrophils occur [93]. The mechanism of action of ingenol mebutate is also partially related to the modulation of protein kinase C (PKC) to which it has a potent binding affinity by activating PKCδ and inhibiting PKCα [91, 94]. In an in vitro assay, low isozyme selectivity was verified with a Ki ranging from 0.105–0.376 nM [95].

The above-mentioned results support the potential of ingenol mebutate for further improvements in cancer therapy; in fact, the cutaneous treatment of non-hyperkeratotic, non-hypertrophic actinic keratosis (a precancerous condition, that if untreated usually leads to a melanoma) with a gel formulation of ingenol mebutate (formerly PEP005 and marketed as Picato®) was approved by both FDA and EMA agencies in 2012 [96, 97]. Unfortunately, adverse reactions associated with this application have been reported, although they are restricted to moderate "local skin responses" and included erythema, flaking/scaling, swelling, crusting, erosion/ulceration and vesiculation/postulation. However, it shows a favorable safety and tolerability profile exhibiting a lack of systemic absorption and photosensitivity [92, 97].

3.2.2. Curcumin

Curcumin (**9**, Figure 6) or diferuloylmethane (bis-α,β-unsaturated β-diketone) is a polyphenolic compound that has been extracted from the rhizome of turmeric (*Curcuma longa* L.), a tropical Southeast Asia plant mainly used as a spice. However, the turmeric powder, which has 2–5% of curcumin, is used in Chinese and Indian traditional medicines [98]. To this ancient remedy have been attributed a wide range of beneficial properties including anti-inflammatory, antioxidant, chemopreventive, chemotherapeutic and chemo-sensitizing activity [98]. Curcumin is an orange-yellow crystalline lipophilic phenolic substance that, in solution, exists in equilibrium with its keto-enol tautomeric forms (Figure 6). It is not very soluble in water and also not very stable, although its degradation increases in basic medium [99].

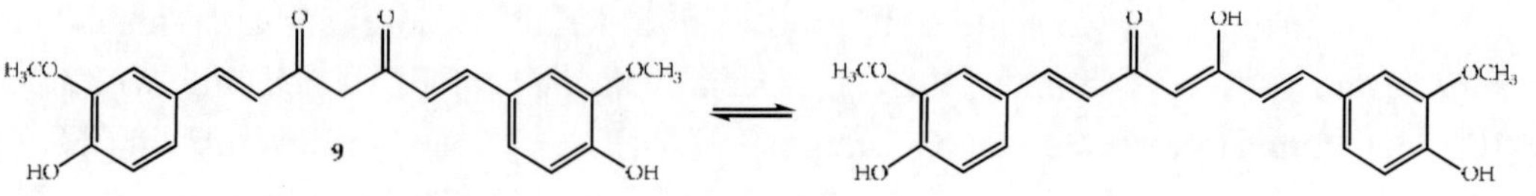

9

Figure 10. Chemical structure of polyphenol curcumin (9).

Research interest in curcumin's anticancer properties has been developed based on the low rate occurrence of gastrointestinal mucosal cancers in Southeast Asian populations and its association with regular turmeric use in their diet [100].

A large volume of experimental data established the therapeutic efficacy of curcumin in in vitro cellular level, as well as in some ex vivo tumor-derived cancer cells/solid tumors like brain tumors, pancreatic, lung, breast, leukemia, prostate, skin cancers and hepatocellular carcinoma, including cytotoxic effects on cancer stem cells and antimetastatic activity [101–103]. This year, its possible application in colorectal, head and neck cancer chemotherapy was also reviewed [104, 105]. Equally important were the assays demonstrating that curcumin was not cytotoxic to normal cells at the dosages required for therapeutic efficacy against the cancer cell lines [106, 107]. The scientific interest and pharmacological potential of curcumin anticancer effects becomes also evident from the number of patents on curcumin-based therapeutics registered in the last five years [108].

Several studies have shown that curcumin can modulate a variety of cancer-related targets or pathways [102, 103, 109, 110], which may be responsible for its effectiveness in combating cancer diseases. Recent studies demonstrate that curcumin's mechanism of action includes: (i) modulation of CYP enzymes by elevation of transcription factor Nrf2 level via the mitogen-activated protein kinase (MAPK) signaling pathway and Akt pathway [111]; (ii) mitotic catastrophe induction due to caspase activation and mitochondrial membrane polarization [14]; (iii) promotion of autophagic cell death, an important death inducer in apoptosis resistant cancer cells by beclin-1-dependent and independent pathways [14, 112]; (iv) arrest of the cell cycle at the check points G1, S-phase and G2/M phase, modulating the cell cycle regulators, including upregulation of cyclin-dependent kinase inhibitors (CDKIs) [113]; (v) promotion of the inhibition of transcription factor NF-κB by preventing nuclear translocation of NF-κB and attenuating the DNA binding ability of NF-κB, contouring the problem of chemoresistance [114]; (vi) promotion of the inhibition of the crucial steps to angiogenesis by downregulation of the PGDF, VEGF and FGF expression and downregulation of MMPs via NF-κB, ERKs, MAPKs, PKC and PI3K inhibition [115]; and (vii) inhibiting tubulin polymerization, that is curcumin binds with DNA [116, 117]. Despite this knowledge about curcumin's multiple mechanisms of action, its biological properties are not fully understood. For example, does curcumin's survival and proliferative effects depend on its concentration, treatment period and cells type? On the other hand, administered doses of curcumin have been studied. Systematic in vivo doses up to 300 mg–3.5 g/kg b.w. (administered for up to 14–90 days) or clinical studies with oral intake of 1.2–12 g daily (for 6 weeks–4 months) did not demonstrate any adverse effects at the populations, animals and patients [118], although these values exceed that normally consumed (granted an acceptable daily intake level of 0.1–3 mg/kg b.w. by the Joint FAO/WHO Expert Committee on Food Additives) and also the typical intake of the Indian population (60–100 mg per day).

Moreover, curcumin has been reported to act as a chemosensitizer for some clinical anticancer drugs (e.g., gemcitabine, paclitaxel and 5-fluorouracil, doxorubicin) and exhibits a synergistic effect in combination with other natural products (e.g., resveratrol, honokiol, epigallocatechin-3-gallate, licochalcone and omega-3), aspects that could be used as an effective strategy to overcome tumor resistance and reduce recurrence [108, 119, 120]. These observations therefore suggest that a superior therapeutic index may be achieved with curcumin when used in combination and could be advantageous in the treatment of some tumors. Anyway, additional studies are still needed to assess the exact mechanism of curcumin's synergic effect.

Nevertheless, the clinical translation of curcumin has been significantly hampered since it is poorly absorbed, improperly metabolized and shows poor systemic bioavailability, which mandates that patients consume up to 8–10 grams of free curcumin orally each day, in order for detectable levels in the circulation [109, 118]. Thus, several strategies have been proposed to counter the bioavailability issue of curcumin involving (i) the use of adjuvants like piperine, which interferes with curcumin metabolism by glucuronidation, (ii) curcumin formulations based on nanotechnology with liposomes, micelles, phospholipid, among others, and (iii) use of curcumin analogues [117, 121–123].

As result of the anticancer potential of curcumin and despite its clinical therapeutic limitations, there are currently 17 open clinical studies involving curcumin, mainly studies of combined curcumin therapy with other substances for the treatment of several types of cancer.

3.2.3. Betulinic Acid

Betulinic acid (3β-hydroxy-lup-20(29)-en-28-oic acid), a lupane-type pentacyclic triterpene (**10**, Figure 7) is biosynthesized from six different isoprene units and was first identified and isolated from *Gratiola officinalis* L. and named "graciolon". It was also isolated from other species, but identified with different names (from the bark of *Platanus acerifolia* (Aiton) Willd. named "platanolic acid" and from *Cornus florida* L. named "cornolic acid"), which led to some confusion. Later on, it was confirmed that all have the same structure, and the compound was named betulinic acid. Nowadays, it is known that this triterpene is extensively spread throughout the plant kingdom (for instance *Betula* spp., *Diospyros* spp., *Syzygium* spp., *Ziziphus* spp., *Paeonia* spp., *Sarracenia flava* L., *Anemone raddeana* Regel and *Lycopodium cernuum* L., among others) and in considerable amounts (up to 2.5%) [124]. However, these sources are not sufficient to meet the growing demand for betulinic acid. Therefore, it can be obtained through a selective oxidation of betulin (lup-20(29)-en-3,28-diol) [125], far more abundant (up to 30%) in birch bark than betulinic acid [126].

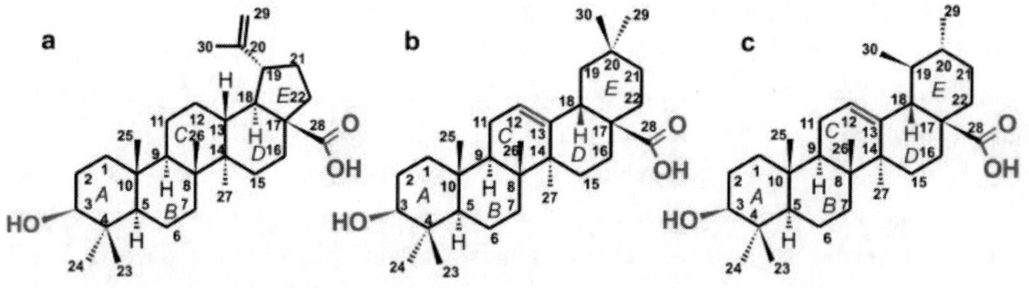

Figure 11. The chemical structure of the pentacyclic triterpene betulinic acid and the main target to structural modifications (in red).

In 1995, the first betulinic acid antitumor activity was reported by a researcher at the University of Illinois. It killed melanoma cells in mice with low IC_{50} values (IC_{50} 0.5–1.5 μg/mL) [127]. Since then, a number of researchers have conducted laboratory tests on betulinic acid to determine its antitumor properties, especially with respect to melanoma cells [128]. More recent studies suggest that betulinic acid possesses a broader spectrum of activity against other cancer cells, and consequently betulinic acid has been selected by the National Cancer Institute for addition into the Rapid Access to Intervention in Development (RAID) program.

Betulinic acid exhibits significant in vitro cytotoxicity in a variety of tumor cell lines and also inhibits the growth of solid tumors in vivo, comparable to some clinically-used drugs and showing a good selectivity index for cancer over normal cells even at doses up to 500 mg/kg b.w. [14, 127, 129, 130]. Its anticancer proprieties have been demonstrated against colorectal lung, colon, breast, prostate, hepatocellular, bladder, head and neck, stomach, pancreatic, ovarian and cervical carcinoma, glioblastoma, chronic myeloid leukemia cells and human melanoma with IC_{50} values mainly between 1 to 13.0 μg/mL [14, 124, 128–132]. Betulinic acid exhibits potent anticancer activity by multiple molecular targets, the best characterized mechanism being the induction of apoptosis by direct regulation of the mitochondrial apoptotic pathway; which can be associated with mitochondrial collapse through direct opening of the permeability transition pore, decreasing mitochondrial outer membrane potential, downregulation of Bcl-2 family members, release of pro-apoptotic factors such as cytochrome c, increase of caspase activities, attenuating both constitutive and inducible STAT3 phosphorylation, nuclear translocation and its DNA binding [124, 130, 133]. However, there is also evidence that, in some cases, apoptosis may be induced by stabilizing p53 and downregulating NF-kB-mediated signaling [124, 134]. The antimetastatic effect of betulinic acid seems to be through the prevention of the epithelial-to-mesenchymal transition in highly aggressive melanoma cells [131], while in breast cancer cells, it be by downregulation of the matrix metalloproteinases expression [133]. Betulinic acid can also induce an antiangiogenic response under hypoxia mediated by the STAT3/HIF-1α/VEGF signaling pathway [124, 130], can block the cell cycle in the G1 phase through inhibition of Cyclin B1 and Hiwi in mRNA and potently induces autophagy as a survival mechanism in response to permeability transition pore opening and mitochondrial damage [14, 133]. Recently, a new cell death pathway was attributed to betulinic acid in which cell death is induced through the inhibition of the stearoyl-CoA-desaturase (SCD-1), an enzyme that is overexpressed in tumor cells [135]. Proteasome inhibition assays suggest the proteasome is the main target for betulinic acid [136]. However, the regulatory effects of betulinic acid on the NF-κB pathway and on Bax or Bak expression are not well clarified [130]. Betulinic acid seems to be a very effective chemosensitizer for anticancer drug treatment in chemoresistant cell lines once it promotes the inhibition of multidrug resistance proteins in vivo and in vitro, as for example in combination with 5-fluorouracil (5-FU) and oxaliplatin [133, 137]. These results clearly demonstrate that in some cases, it is possible to circumvent acquired chemoresistance by combination therapy of anticancer drugs with chemosensitizers as betulinic acid. Moreover, betulinic acid has strong synergy with mithramycin A on the inhibition of migration and invasion of pancreatic cancer cells at nontoxic concentrations by suppressing the Sp1 and uPAR level [138]. Furthermore, a synergistic effect of betulinic acid and tumor necrosis factor-related apoptosis-inducing ligand (TRAIL) combination to inhibit liver cancer progression in vitro and in vivo through targeting the p53 signaling pathway [139] revealed that betulinic acid combined with TRAIL has potential value against liver cancer. Betulinic acid is slightly soluble in water, and therefore, its water solubility is a drawback that should be overcome to improve its absorption and bioavailability. The main targets for structure activity studies were the C-3 hydroxyl, C-20 vinyl and C-28 carboxyl groups (Figure 7). The 3-OH oxidation increased cytotoxic activity, but decreased selectivity; introduction of groups, such as amine or hydroxyl, at the C-28 position increased activity; while modifications at C-20 did not enhance cytotoxicity [14, 124, 140]. It can be conclude that modifications may improve the cytotoxicity and/or the water solubility, but not the selectivity. It seems that the presence of the free hydroxyl group at C-3 and the carboxyl group at C-28 are the most important features. Recently, a clearer and more realistic method, 3D-QSAR by CoMFA and CoMSIA, shows the structure-cytotoxicity relationship of betulinic acid derivatives against human ovarian cancer cell A2780, and the main conclusions were: an electropositive group at the C-2 α-site; an electronegative and hydrogen bond acceptor group at the C-2 β-site; bulky groups at the C-3 β-site; bulky and electronegative groups at the C-3 α-site; bulky, electronegative and hydrogen bond donor or acceptor groups at the C-28 side chain; and would be beneficial to the antitumor potency (Figure 7) [130]. Due to its extraordinary potential as an antitumor agent, betulinic acid was involved in phase I/II clinical trials to evaluate its safety and effectiveness. The study involved topical applications (20% betulinic acid in ointment) to treat dysplastic nevi that can transform into melanoma. Unfortunately, at the end of 2013, the study was suspended due to funding issues (Clinical Trials database).

CONCLUSION

Cancer is becoming a high-profile disease in developed and developing countries, and its treatment is a struggle with some successful cases. Nevertheless, the drugs developed by synthesis and used in chemotherapy have limitations mainly due to their toxic effects on non-targeted tissues and consequently furthering human health problems. Therefore, there is a demand for alternative treatments, and the naturally-derived anticancer agents are regarded as the best choice. As demonstrated herein, with some representative examples, secondary metabolites are themselves suitable anticancer agents leading to the development of new clinical drugs with also new anticancer mechanisms of action. Some have already become cases of success for the pharmaceutical industry. Additionally, they are excellent lead compounds, by which, through structural modifications, alternative formulations and/or using increasingly effective delivery systems, their pharmacological potential is enhanced. Recent new biotechnological solutions, using nanotech approaches, present a new hope for cancer therapy (e.g., plant drug-functionalized nano-diamonds and other nanocarriers based on anticancer drugs). Simultaneously, they provide a further step forward in the successful use of secondary metabolites for cancer therapeutic purposes

[141–144]. In other cases, the success story has not yet reached its high point with its introduction in the market, but the more recent studies presented and discussed in this paper clearly show that this goal is getting closer. On the other hand, demand for plant-derived drugs is putting pressure on high-value medicinal plants and risking their biodiversity, so exploitation of these agents needs to be managed to keep up with demands and be sustainable. Fortunately, there are currently developments using new biotechnological solutions and sustainable alternative methods for the production of high-value plant metabolites.

REFERENCES

[1] Ferlay, J., Soerjomataram, I., Dikshit, R., Eser, S., Mathers, C., Rebelo, M., Parkin, D.M., Forman, D., Bray, F. Cancer incidence and mortality worldwide: Sources, methods and major patterns in GLOBOCAN 2012. *Int. J. Cancer* 2015, *136*, 359–386.

[2] Siegel, R.L., Miller, K.D., Jemal, A. Cancer statistics, 2016. *CA Cancer J. Clin.* 2016, *66*, 7–30.

[3] World Health Organization. *Cancer: Fact Sheets*; WHO: Geneva, Switzerland, 2017. Available online: http://www.who.int/mediacentre/factsheets/fs297/en/

[4] Bray, F. Transitions in human development and the global cancer burden. In *World Cancer Report 2014*; Stewart, B.W., Wild, C.P., Eds.; International Agency for Research on Cancer: Lyon, France, 2014; pp. 54–68. ISBN 978-92-832-0443-5.

[5] Adeloye, D., David, R.A., Aderemi, A.V., Iseolorunkanmi, A., Oyedokun, A., Iweala, E.E., Omoregbe, N., Ayo, C.K. An estimate of the incidence of prostate cancer in Africa: A systematic review and meta-analysis. *PLoS ONE* 2016, *11*, e0153496.

[6] Alves-Silva, J.M., Romane, A., Efferth, T., Salgueiro, L. North African medicinal plants traditionally used in cancer therapy. *Front. Pharmacol.* 2017, *8*, 1–24.

[7] Tariq, A., Sadia, S., Pan, K., Ullah, I., Mussarat, S., Sun, F., Abiodun, O.O., Batbaatar, A., Li, Z., Song, D., et al. A systematic review on ethnomedicines of anticancer plants. *Phytother. Res.* 2017, *31*, 202–264.

[8] Oyebode, O., Kandala, N.-B., Chilton, P.J., Lilford, R.J. Use of traditional medicine in middle-income countries: A WHO-SAGE study. *Health Policy Plan.* 2016, *31*, 984–991.

[9] Diorio, C., Salena, K., Ladas, E.J., Lam, C.G., Afungcwhi, G.M., Njuguna, F., Marjerrison, S. Traditional and complementary medicine used with curative intent in childhood cancer: A systematic review. *Pediatr. Blood Cancer* 2017, *64*, 1–8.

[10] Ma, L., Wang, B., Long, Y., Li, H. Effect of traditional Chinese medicine combined with Western therapy on primary hepatic carcinoma: A systematic review with meta-analysis. *Front. Med.* 2017, *11*, 191–202.

[11] Yan, Z., Lai, Z., Lin, J. Anticancer properties of traditional Chinese medicine. *Comb. Chem. High Throughput Screen.* 2017, *20*, 423–429.

[12] Enioutina, E.Y., Salis, E.R., Job, K.M., Gubarev, M.I., Krepkova, L.V., Sherwin, C.M. Herbal Medicines: Challenges in the modern world. Part 5. Status and current directions of complementary and alternative herbal medicine worldwide. *Expert Rev. Clin. Pharmacol.* 2017, *10*, 327–338.

[13] Mishra, B.B., Tiwari, V.K. Natural products: An evolving role in future drug discovery. *Eur. J. Med. Chem.* 2011, *46*, 4769–4807.

[14] Gali-Muhtasib, H., Hmadi, R., Kareh, M., Tohme, R., Darwiche, N. Cell death mechanisms of plant-derived anticancer drugs: Beyond apoptosis. *Apoptosis* 2015, *20*, 1531–1562.

[15] Khalid, E.B., Ayman, E.E., Rahman, H., Abdelkarim, G., Najda, A. Natural products against cancer angiogenesis. *Tumor Biol.* 2016, *37*, 14513–14536.

[16] Katz, L., Baltz, R.H. Natural product discovery: Past, present and future. *J. Ind. Microbiol. Biotechnol.* 2016, *43*, 155–176.

[17] Kotoku, N., Arai, M., Kobayashi, M. Search for anti-angiogenic substances from natural sources. *Chem. Pharm. Bull.* 2016, *64*, 128–134.

[18] Bernardini, S., Tiezzi, A., Laghezza Masci, V., Ovidi, E. Natural products for human health: An historical overview of the drug discovery approaches. *Nat. Prod. Res.* 2017.

[19] Newman, D.J., Cragg, G.M. Natural products as sources of new drugs from 1981 to 2014. *J. Nat. Prod.* 2016, *79*, 629–661.

[20] Ekor, M. The growing use of herbal medicines: Issues relating to adverse reactions and challenges in monitoring safety. *Front. Pharmacol.* 2014, *4*, 1–10.

[21] Moreira, D.L., Teixeira, S.S., Monteiro, M.H.D., de-Oliveira, A.C.A.X., Paumgartten, F.J.R. Traditional use and safety of herbal medicines. *Rev. Bras. Farmacogn.* 2014, *24*, 248–257.

[22] Nwodo, J.N., Ibezim, A., Simoben, C.V., Ntie-Kang, F. Exploring cancer therapeutics with natural products from African medicinal plants, Part II: Alkaloids, terpenoids and flavonoids. *Anticancer Agents Med. Chem.* 2016, *16*, 108–127.

[23] Habli, Z., Toumieh, G., Fatfat, M., Rahal, O.N., Gali-Muhtasib, H. Emerging cytotoxic alkaloids in the battle against cancer: Overview of molecular mechanisms. *Molecules* 2017, *22*, 250.

[24] Delgoda, R., Murray, J.E. Evolutionary perspectives on the role of plant secondary metabolites. In *Pharmacognosy: Fundamentals, Applications and Strategies*, 1st ed.; Badal, S., Delgoda, R., Eds.; Academic Press: Oxoford, UK, 2017; pp. 93–100. ISBN 9780128020999.

[25] Kabera, J.N., Semana, E., Mussa, A.R., He, X. Plant secondary metabolites: Biosynthesis, classification, function and pharmacological properties. *J. Pharm. Pharmacol.* 2014, *2*, 377–392.

[26] Guo, Z. The modification of natural products for medical use. *Acta Pharm. Sin. B* 2017, *7*, 119–136.

[27] Yao, H., Liu, J., Xu, S., Zhu, Z., Xu, J. The structural modification of natural products for novel drug discovery. *Expert Opin. Drug Discov.* 2017, *12*, 121–140.

[28] Evans, A.E., Farber, S., Brunet, S., Mariano, P.J. Vincristine in the treatment of acute leukaemia in children. *Cancer* 1963, *16*, 1302–1306.

[29] Moore, A., Pinkerton, R. Vincristine: Can its therapeutic index be enhanced? *Pediatr. Blood Cancer* 2009, *53*, 1180–1187.

[30] Almagro, L., Fernández-Pérez, F., Pedreño, M.A. Indole alkaloids from *Catharanthus roseus*: Bioproduction and their effect on human health. *Molecules* 2015, *20*, 2973–3000.

[31] Tang, K., Pan, Q. Strategies for enhancing alkaloids yield in *Catharanthus roseus* via metabolic engineering approaches. In *Catharanthus Roseus: Current Research and Future Prospects*; Naeem, M., Aftab, T., Khan, M., Eds.; Springer International Publishing: Basel, Switzerland, 2017; pp. 1–16.

[32] Mu, F., Yang, L., Wang, W., Luo, M., Fu, Y., Guo, X., Zu, Y. Negative-pressure cavitation extraction of four main vinca alkaloids from *Catharanthus roseus* leaves. *Molecules* 2012, *17*, 8742–8752.

[33] Wang, X., Song, Y., Su, Y., Tian, Q., Li, B., Quan, J., Deng, Y. Are PEGylated liposomes better than conventional liposomes? A special case for vincristine. *Drug Deliv.* 2016, *23*, 1092–1100.

[34] Sertel, S., Fu, Y., Zu, Y., Rebacz, B., Konkimalla, B., Plinkert, P.K., Krämer, A., Gertsch, J., Efferth, T. Molecular docking and pharmacogenomics of Vinca alkaloid and their monomeric precursor, vindoline and catharanthine. *Biochem. Pharmacol.* 2011, *81*, 723–735.

[35] Douer, D. Efficacy and safety of vincristine sulfate liposome injection in the treatment of adult acute lymphocytic leukaemia. *Oncologist* 2016, *21*, 840–847.

[36] Velde, M.E., Kaspers, G.L., Abbink, F.C.H., Wilhelm, A.J., Ket, J.C.F., Berg, M.H. Vincristine-induced peripheral neuropathy in children with cancer: A systematic review. *Crit. Rev. Oncol. Hematol.* 2017, *114*,114–130. Yoshihara, H., Yoshimoto, Y., Hosoya, Y., Hasegawa, D., Kawano, T., Sakoda, A., Okita, H., Manabe, A. Infantile fibrosarcoma treated with postoperative vincristine and dactinomycin. *Pediatr. Int.* 2017, *59*, 371–374.

[37] Weaver, B.A. How Taxol/paclitaxel kills cancer cells. *Mol. Biol. Cell* 2014, *25*, 2677–2681.

[38] Bernabeu, E., Cagel, M., Lagomarsino, E., Moretton, M., Chiappetta, D.A. Paclitaxel: What has been done and the challenges remain ahead. *Int. J. Pharm.* 2017, *526*, 474–495.

[39] Bernabeu, E., Gonzalez, L., Cagel, M., Gergic, E.P., Moretton, M.A., Chiappetta, D.A. Novel Soluplus1®-TPGS mixed micelles for encapsulation of paclitaxel with enhanced in vitro cytotoxicity on breast and ovarian cancer cell lines. *Colloids Surf. B Biointerfaces* 2016, *140*, 403–411.

[40] Howat, S., Park, B., Oh, I.S., Jin, Y.W., Lee, E.K., Loake, G.J. Paclitaxel: Biosynthesis, production and future prospects. *New Biotechnol.* 2014, *31*, 242–245.

[41] Nicolaou, K.C., Yang, Z., Liu, J.J., Ueno, H., Nantermet, P.G., Guy, R.K., Claiborne, C.F., Renaud, J., Couladouros, E.A., Paulvannan, K., et al. Total synthesis of taxol. *Nature* 1994, *367*, 630–634. Fukaya, K., Kodama, K., Tanaka, Y., Yamazaki, H., Sugai, T., Yamaguchi, Y., Watanabe, A., Oishi, T., Sato, T., Chida, N. Synthesis of Paclitaxel. 2. Construction of the ABCD ring and formal synthesis. *Org. Lett.* 2015, *17*, 2574–2577.

[42] Hirai, S., Utsugi, M., Iwamoto, M., Nakada, M. Formal total synthesis of (−)-taxol through Pd-catalyzed eight-membered carbocyclic ring formation. *Chemistry* 2015, *21*, 355–359.

[43] Gallego, A., Malik, S., Yousefzadi, M., Makhzoum, A., Tremouillaux-Guiller, J., Bonfill, M. Taxol from *Corylus avellana*: Paving the way for a new source of this anti-cancer drug. *Plant Cell Tissue Organ Cult.* 2017, *129*, 1–16.

[44] Li, B.-J., Wang, H., Gong, T., Chen, J.-J., Chen, T.-J., Yang, J.-L., Zhu, P. Improving 10-deacetylbaccatin III-10-β-*O*-acetyltransferase catalytic fitness for Taxol production. *Nat. Commun.* 2017, *8*, 1–13.

[45] Baloglu, E., Kingston, D.G.I. A new semisynthesis of paclitaxel from baccatin III. *J. Nat. Prod.* 1999, *62*, 1068–1071.

[46] Mandai, T., Kuroda, A., Okumoto, H., Nakanishi, K., Mikuni, K., Hara, K.J., Hara, K.Z. A semisynthesis of paclitaxel via a 10-deacetylbaccatin III derivative bearing a β-keto ester appendage. *Tetrahedron Lett.* 2000, *41*, 243–246.

[47] Liu, W.C., Gonga, T., Zhu, P. Advances in exploring alternative Taxol sources. *RSC Adv.* 2016, *6*, 48800–48809.

[48] Xiao, Z., Morris-Natschke, S.L., Lee, K.H. Strategies for the optimization of natural leads to anticancer drugs or drug candidates. *Med. Res. Rev.* 2016, *36*, 32–91.

[49] Wang, N.N., Zhao, L.J., Wu, L.N., He, M.F., Qu, J.W., Zhao, Y.B., Zhao, W.Z., Li, J.S., Wang, J.H. Mechanistic analysis of taxol-induced multidrug resistance in an ovarian cancer cell line. *Asian Pac. J. Cancer Prev.* 2013, *14*, 4983–4988.

[50] Barbuti, A.M., Chen, Z.S. Paclitaxel through the ages of anticancer therapy: Exploring its role in chemoresistance and radiation therapy. *Cancers* 2015, *7*, 2360–2371.

[51] Nehate, C., Jain, S., Saneja, A., Khare, V., Alam, N., Dubey, R., Gupta, P.N. Paclitaxel formulations: Challenges and novel delivery options. *Curr. Drug Deliv.* 2014, *11*, 666–686.

[52] Soliman, H.H. *nab*-Paclitaxel as a potential partner with checkpoint inhibitors in solid tumors. *Onco Targets Ther.* 2017, *10*, 101–112.

[53] Zong, Y., Wu, J., Shen, K. Nanoparticle albumin-bound paclitaxel as neoadjuvant chemotherapy of breast cancer: A systematic review and meta-analysis. *Oncotarget* 2017, *8*, 17360–17372.

[54] Xu, X., Wang, L., Xu, H.Q., Huang, X.E., Qian, Y.D., Xiang, J. Clinical comparison between paclitaxel liposome (Lipusu®) and paclitaxel for treatment of patients with metastatic gastric cancer. *Asian Pac. J. Cancer Prev.* 2013, *14*, 2591–2594.

[55] Rivera, E., Cianfrocca, M. Overview of neuropathy associated with taxanes for the treatment of metastatic breast cancer. *Cancer Chemother. Pharmacol.* 2015, *75*, 659–670.

[56] Wen, G., Qu, X.X., Wang, D., Chen, X.X., Tian, X.C., Gao, F., Zhou, X.L. Recent advances in design, synthesis and bioactivity of paclitaxel-mimics. *Fitoterapia* 2016, *110*, 26–37.

[57] Crown, J., O'Leary, M., Ooi, W.S. Docetaxel and paclitaxel in the treatment of breast cancer: A review of clinical experience. *Oncologist* 2004, *9*, 24–32.

[58] Vrignaud, P., Semiond, D., Benning, V., Beys, E., Bouchard, H., Gupta, S. Preclinical profile of cabazitaxel. *Drug Des. Dev. Ther.* 2014, *8*, 1851–1867.

[59] De Morree, E., van Soest, R., Aghai, A., de Ridder, C., de Bruijn, P., Ghobadi Moghaddam-Helmantel, I., Burger, H., Mathijssen, R., Wiemer, E., de Wit, R., et al. Understanding taxanes in prostate cancer, importance of intratumoral drug accumulation. *Prostate* 2016, *76*, 927–936.

[60] Goyal, S., Oak, E., Luo, J., Cashen, A.F., Carson, K., Fehniger, T., DiPersio, J., Bartlett, N.L., Wagner-Johnston, N.D. Minimal activity of nanoparticle albumin-bound (nab) paclitaxel in relapsed or refractory lymphomas: Results of a phase-I study. *Leuk. Lymphoma* 2018, *59*, 357–362.

[61] Ricci, F., Guffanti, F., Damia, G., Broggini, M. Combination of paclitaxel, bevacizumab and MEK162 in second line treatment in platinum-relapsing patient derived ovarian cancer xenografts. *Mol. Cancer* 2017, *16*, 1–13.

[62] Gill, K.K., Kamal, M.M., Kaddoumi, A., Nazzal, S. EGFR targeted delivery of paclitaxel and parthenolide co-loaded in PEG-Phospholipid micelles enhance cytotoxicity and cellular uptake in non-small cell lung cancer cells. *J. Drug Deliv. Sci. Technol.* 2016, *36*, 150–155.

[63] Ehrlich, A., Booher, S., Becerra, Y., Borris, D.L., Figg, W.D., Turner, M.L., Blauvelt, A. Micellar paclitaxel improves severe psoriasis in a prospective phase II pilot study. *J. Am. Acad. Dermatol.* 2004, *50*, 533–540.

[64] Dadgar, S., Ramjan, Z., Floriano, W.B. Paclitaxel is an inhibitor and its boron dipyrromethene derivative is a fluorescent recognition agent for botulinum neurotoxin subtype A. *J. Med. Chem.* 2013, *56*, 2791–2803.

[65] Kantarjian, H.M., O'Brien, S., Cortes, J. Homoharringtonine/omacetaxine mepesuccinate: The long and winding road to food and drug administration approval. *Clin. Lymphoma Myeloma Leuk.* 2013, *13*, 530–533.

[66] Butler, M.S., Robertson, A.A.B., Cooper, M.A. Natural product and natural product derived drugs in clinical trials. *Nat. Prod. Rep.* 2014, *31*, 1612–1661.

[67] Chang, Y., Meng, F.-C., Wang, R., Wang, C.M., Lu, X.-Y., Zhang, Q.-W. Chemistry, bioactivity, and the structure-activity relationship of cephalotaxine-type alkaloids from *Cephalotaxus* sp. In *Studies in Natural Products Chemistry Bioactive Natural Products*, Atta-Ur-Rahman, F.R.S., Ed., Elsevier Science Publishers: Amsterdam, The Netherlands, 2017, Volume 53, pp. 339–373. ISBN 978-0-444-63930-1.

[68] Lü, S., Wang, J. Homoharringtonine and omacetaxine for myeloid hematological malignancies. *J. Hematol. Oncol.* 2014, *7*, 1–10.

[69] Gandhi, V., Plunkett, W., Cortes, J.E. Omacetaxine: A protein translation inhibitor for treatment of chronic myelogenous leucemia. *Clin. Cancer Res.* 2014, *20*, 1735–1740.

[70] Li, X., Yin, X., Wang, H., Huang, J., Yu, M., Ma, Z., Li, C., Zhou, Y., Yan, X., Huang, S., et al. The combination effect of homoharringtonine and ibrutinib on FLT3-ITD mutant acute myeloid leukaemia. *Oncotarget* 2017, *8*, 12764–12774.

[71] Chen, J., Mu, Q., Li, X., Yin, X., Yu, M., Jin, J., Li, C., Zhou, Y., Zhou, J., Shanshan Suo, S., et al. Homoharringtonine targets Smad3 and TGF-β pathway to inhibit the proliferation of acute myeloid leukaemia cells. *Oncotarget* 2017, *8*, 40318–40326.

[72] Pasic, I., Lipton, J.H. Current approach to the treatment of chronic myeloid leukaemia. *Leuk. Res.* 2017, *55*, 65–78.

[73] Chung, C. Omacetaxine for treatment-resistant or treatment-intolerant adult chronic myeloid leukaemia. *Am. J. Health Syst. Pharm.* 2014, *71*, 279–288.

[74] Cortes, J.E., Kantarjian, H.M., Rea, D., Wetzler, M., Lipton, J.H., Akard, L., Khoury, H.J., Michallet, M., Guerci-Bresler, A., Chuah, C., et al. Final analysis of the efficacy and safety of omacetaxine mepesuccinate in patients with chronic- or accelerated-phase chronic myeloid leukaemia: Results with 24 months of follow-up. *Cancer* 2015, *121*, 1637–1644.

[75] Damlaj, M., Lipton, J.H., Assouline, S.E. A safety evaluation of omacetaxine mepesuccinate for the treatment of chronic myeloid leukaemia. *Expert Opin. Drug Saf.* 2016, *15*, 1279–1286.

[76] Allan, E.K., Holyoake, T.L., Craig, A.R., Jørgensen, H.G. Omacetaxine may have a role in chronic myeloid leukaemia eradication through downregulation of Mcl-1 and induction of apoptosis in stem/progenitor cells. *Leukaemia* 2011, *25*, 985–994.

[77] Lam, S.S., Ho, E.S., He, B.L., Wong, W.W., Cher, C.Y., Ng, N.K., Man, C.H., Gill, H., Cheung, A.M., Ip, H.W., et al. Homoharringtonine (omacetaxine mepesuccinate) as an adjunct for FLT3-ITD acute myeloid leukaemia. *Sci. Transl. Med.* 2016, *8*, 1–14.

[78] Heiblig, M., Sobh, M., Nicolini, F.E. Subcutaneous omacetaxine mepesuccinate in patients with chronic myeloid leukaemia in tyrosine kinase inhibitor-resistant patients: Review and perspectives. *Leuk. Res.* 2014, *38*, 1145–1153.

[79] Shen, A.Q., Munteanu, M., Khoury, H.J. Updated product label allows home administration of omacetaxine mepesuccinate. *Oncologist* 2014, *19*, 1.

[80] Akard, L., Kantarjian, H.M., Nicolini, F.E., Wetzler, M., Lipton, J.H., Baccarani, M., Jean Khoury, H., Kurtin, S., Li, E., Munteanu, M., et al. Incidence and management of myelosuppression in patients with chronic- and accelerated-phase chronic myeloid leukaemia treated with omacetaxine mepesuccinate. *Leuk. Lymphoma* 2016, *57*, 654–665.

[81] Saklani, A., Kutty, S.K. Plant-derived compounds in clinical trials. *Drug Discov. Today* 2008, *13*, 161–171.

[82] Rizk, A.M., Hammouda, F.M., El-Missiry, M.M., Radwan, H.M., Evans, F.J. Biologically active diterpene esters from *Euphorbia peplus*. *Phytochemistry* 1985, *24*, 1605–1606.

[83] Ramsay, J.R., Suhrbier, A., Aylward, J.H., Ogbourne, S., Cozzi, S.J., Poulsen, M.G., Baumann, K.C., Welburn, P., Redlich, G.L., Parsons, P.G. The sap from *Euphorbia peplus* is effective against human nonmelanoma skin cancers. *Br. J. Dermatol.* 2011, *164*, 633–636.

[84] Ogbourne, S.M., Parsons, P.G. The value of nature's natural product library for the discovery of new chemical entities: The discovery of ingenol mebutate. *Fitoterapia* 2014, *98*, 36–44.

[85] Béres, T., Dragull, K., Pospíšil, J., Tarkowská, D., Danc˘ák, M., Bíba, O., Tarkowski, P., Doležal, K., Strnad, M. Quantitative analysis of ingenol in *Euphorbia* species via validated isotope dilution ultra-high performance liquid chromatography tandem mass spectrometry. *Phytochem. Anal.* 2018, *29*, 23–29.

[86] Liang, X., Grue-Sørensen, G., Petersen, A.K., Högberg, T. Semisynthesis of ingenol 3-angelate (PEP005): Efficient stereoconservative angeloylation of alcohols. *Synlett* 2012, *23*, 2647–2652.

[87] Liang, X., Grue-Sørensen, G., Månsson, K., Vedsø, P., Soor, A., Stahlhut, M., Bertelsen, M., Engell, K.M., Högberg, T. Syntheses, biological evaluation and SAR of ingenol mebutate analogues for treatment of actinic keratosis and non-melanoma skin cancer. *Bioorg. Med. Chem. Lett.* 2013, *23*, 5624–5629.

[88] Serova, M., Ghoul, A., Benhadji, K.A., Faivre, S., Le Tourneau, C., Cvitkovic, E., Lokiec, F., Lord, J., Ogbourne, S.M., Calvo, F., et al. Effects of protein kinase C modulation by PEP005, a novel ingenol angelate, on mitogen-activated protein

kinase and phosphatidylinositol 3-kinase signaling in cancer cells. *Mol. Cancer Ther.* 2008, *7*, 915–922.

[89] Benhadji, K.A., Serova, M., Ghoul, A., Cvitkovic, E., Le Tourneau, C., Ogbourne, S.M., Lokiec, F., Calvo, F., Hammel, P., Faivre, S., et al. Antiproliferative activity of PEP005, a novel ingenol angelate that modulatesPKC functions, alone and in combination with cytotoxic agents in human colon cancer cells. *Br. J. Cancer* 2008, *99*, 1808–1815.

[90] Collier, N.J., Ali, F.R., Lear, J.T. Ingenol mebutate: A novel treatment for actinic keratosis. *Clin. Pract.* 2014, *11*, 295–306.

[91] Rosen, R.H., Gupta, A.K., Tyring, S.K. *Dual mechanism of action of ingenol mebutate gel for topical treatment of actinic keratoses: Rapid lesion necrosis followed by lesion-specific immune response.*

[92] *Am. Acad. Dermatol.* 2012, *66*, 486–493.

[93] Matias, D., Bessa, C., Simões, M.F., Reis, C.P., Saraiva, L., Rijo, P. Natural products as lead protein kinase c modulators for cancer therapy. In *Studies in Natural Products Chemistry Bioactive Natural Products*, Atta-Ur-Rahman, F.R.S., Ed., Elsevier Science Publishers: Amsterdam, The Netherlands, 2017, Volume 53, pp. 45–79. ISBN 978-0-444-63930-1.

[94] Kedei, N., Lundberg, D.J., Toth, A., Welburn, P., Garfield, S.H., Blumberg, P.M. Characterization of the interaction of ingenol 3-angelate with protein kinase C. *Cancer Res.* 2004, *64*, 3243–3255. [CrossRef] [PubMed]

[95] Doan, H.Q., Gulati, N., Levis, W.R. Ingenol mebutate: Potential for further development of cancer immunotherapy. *J. Drugs Dermatol.* 2012, *11*, 1156–1157.

[96] Tzogani, K., Nagercoil, N., Hemmings, R.J., Samir, B., Gardette, J., Demolis, P., Salmonson, T., Pignatti, F. The European Medicines Agency approval of ingenol mebutate (Picato) for the cutaneous treatment of non-hyperkeratotic, non-hypertrophic actinic keratosis in adults: Summary of the scientific assessment of the Committee for Medicinal Products for Human Use (CHMP). *Eur. J. Dermatol.* 2014, *24*, 457–463.

[97] Kocaadam, B., S¸anlier, N. Curcumin, an active component of turmeric (*Curcuma longa*), and its effects on health. *Crit. Rev. Food Sci. Nutr.* 2017, *57*, 2889–2895.

[98] Wang, Y.J., Pan, M.H., Cheng, A.L., Lin, L.I., Ho, Y.S., Hsieh, C.Y., Lin, J.K. Stability of curcumin in buffer solutions and characterization of its degradation products. *J. Pharm. Biomed. Anal.* 1997, *15*, 1867–1876.

[99] Sinha, R., Anderson, D.E., McDonald, S.S., Greenwald, P. Cancer risk and diet in India. *J. Postgrad. Med.* 2003, *49*, 222–228.

[100] Perrone, D., Ardito, F., Giannatempo, G., Dioguardi, M., Troiano, G., Lo Russo, L., De Lillo, A., Laino, L., Lo Muzio, L. Biological and therapeutic activities and anticancer properties of curcumin. *Exp. Ther. Med.* 2015, *10*, 1615–1623.

[101] Pavan, A.R., Silva, G.D., Jornada, D.H., Chiba, D.E., Fernandes, G.F., Man Chin, C., Dos Santos, J.L. Unraveling the anticancer effect of curcumin and resveratrol. *Nutrients* 2016, *8*, 628.

[102] Imran, M., Saeed, F., Nadeem, M., Arshad, U.M., Ullah, A., Suleria, H.A. Cucurmin, anticancer and antitumor perspectives—A comprehensive review. *Crit. Rev. Food Sci. Nutr.* 2016, *22*, 1–23.

[103] Redondo-Blanco, S., Fernández, J., Gutiérrez-del-Río, I., Villar, C.J., Lombó, F. New insights toward colorectal cancer chemotherapy using natural bioactive compounds. *Front. Pharmacol.* 2017, *8*, 1–22.

[104] Borges, G.Á., Rêgo, D.F., Assad, D.X., Coletta, R.D., De Luca Canto, G., Guerra, E.N. In vivo and in vitro effects of curcumin on head and neck carcinoma: A systematic review. *J. Oral Pathol. Med.* 2017, *46*, 3–20.

[105] Sordillo, P.P., Helson, L. Curcumin and cancer stem cells: Curcumin has asymmetrical effects on cancer and normal stem cells. *Anticancer Res.* 2015, *35*, 599–614.

[106] Yu, H.J., Ma, L., Jiang, J., Sun, S.Q. Protective effect of curcumin on neural myelin sheaths by attenuating interactions between the endoplasmic reticulum and mitochondria after compressed spinal cord. *J. Spine* 2016, *5*, 1–6.

[107] Di Martino, R.M.C., Luppi, B., Bisi, A., Gobbi, S., Rampa, A., Abruzzo, A., Bellutia, F. Recent progress on curcumin-based therapeutics: A patent review (2012–2016). Part I: Curcumin. *Expert Opin. Ther. Pat.* 2017, *27*, 579–590.

[108] Kumar, G., Mittal, S., Sak, K., Tuli, H.S. Molecular mechanisms underlying chemopreventive potential of curcumin: Current challenges and future perspectives. *Life Sci.* 2016, *148*, 313–328.

[109] Kunnumakkara, A.B., Bordoloi, D., Harsha, C., Banik, K., Gupta, S.C., Aggarwal, B.B. Curcumin mediates anticancer effects by modulating multiple cell signaling pathways. *Clin. Sci.* 2017, *131*, 1781–1799.

[110] Schwertheim, S., Wein, F., Lennartz, K., Worm, K., Schmid, K.W., Sheu-Grabellus, S.Y. Curcumin induces.

[111] G2/M arrest, apoptosis, NF-κB inhibition, and expression of differentiation genes in thyroid carcinoma cells.

[112] *Cancer Res. Clin. Oncol.* 2017, *143*, 1143–1154.

[113] Yang, C., Ma, X., Wang, Z., Zeng, X., Hu, Z., Ye, Z., Shen, G. Curcumin induces apoptosis and protective autophagy in castration-resistant prostate cancer cells through iron chelation. *Drug Des. Dev. Ther.* 2017, *11*, 431–439.

[114] Dasiram, J.D., Ganesan, R., Kannan, J., Kotteeswaran, V., Sivalingam, N. Curcumin inhibits growth potential by G1 cell cycle arrest and induces apoptosis in p53-mutated COLO 320DM human colon adenocarcinoma cells. *Biomed. Pharmacother.* 2017, *86*, 373–380.

[115] Uwagawa, T., Yanaga, K. Effect of NF-κB inhibition on chemoresistance in biliary–pancreatic cancer. *Surg. Today* 2015, *45*, 1481–1488.

[116] Fu, Z., Chen, X., Guan, S., Yan, Y., Lin, H., Hua, Z.C. Curcumin inhibits angiogenesis and improves defective hematopoiesis induced by tumor-derived VEGF in tumor model through modulating VEGF-VEGFR2 signaling pathway. *Oncotarget* 2015, *6*, 19469–19482.

[117] Haris, P., Mary, V., Aparna, P., Dileep, K.V., Sudarsanakumar, C. A comprehensive approach to ascertain the binding mode of curcumin with DNA. *Spectrochim. Acta A Mol. Biomol. Spectrosc.* 2017, *175*, 155–163.

[118] Ramya, P.V., Angapelly, S., Guntuku, L., Singh Digwal, C., Nagendra Babu, B., Naidu, V.G., Kamal, A. Synthesis and biological evaluation of curcumin inspired indole analogues as tubulin polymerization inhibitors. *Eur. J. Med. Chem.* 2017, *127*, 100–114.

[119] Gupta, S.C., Patchva, S., Aggarwal, B.B. Therapeutic roles of curcumin: Lessons learned from clinical trials. *AAPS J.* 2013, *15*, 195–218.

[120] Klippstein, R., Bansal, S.S., Al-Jamal, K.T. Doxorubicin enhances curcumin's cytotoxicity in human prostate cancer cells in vitro by enhancing its cellular uptake. *Int. J. Pharm.* 2016, *514*, 169–175. [CrossRef] [PubMed]

[121] Pimentel-Gutiérrez, H.J., Bobadilla-Morales, L., Barba-Barba, C.C., Ortega-De-La-Torre, C., Sánchez-Zubieta, F.A., Corona-Rivera, J.R., González-Quezada, B.A., Armendáriz-Borunda, J.S., Silva-Cruz, R., Corona-Rivera, A. Curcumin potentiates the effect of chemotherapy against acute lymphoblastic leukaemia cells via downregulation of NF-κB. *Oncol. Lett.* 2016, *12*, 4117–4124.

[122] Rahimi, H.R., Nedaeinia, R., Shamloo, A.S., Nikdoust, S., Oskuee, R.K. Novel delivery system for natural products: Nano-curcumin formulations. *Avicenna J. Phytomed.* 2016, *6*, 383–398.

[123] Liu, W., Zhai, Y., Heng, X., Che, F.Y., Chen, W., Sun, D., Zhai, G. Oral bioavailability of curcumin: Problems and advancements. *J. Drug Target* 2016, *24*, 694–702.

[124] Puneeth, H.R., Ananda, H., Kumar, K.S.S., Rangappa, K.S., Sharada, A.C. Synthesis and antiproliferative studies of curcumin pyrazole derivatives. *Med. Chem. Res.* 2016, *25*, 1842–1851.

[125] Ali-Seyed, M., Jantan, I., Vijayaraghavan, K., Bukhari, S.N. Betulinic acid: Recent advances in chemical modifications, effective delivery, and molecular mechanisms of a promising anticancer therapy. *Chem. Biol. Drug Des.* 2016, *87*, 517–536.

[126] Pichette, A., Liu, H., Roy, C., Tanguay, S., Simard, F., Lavoie, S. Selective oxidation of betulin for the preparation of betulinic acid, an antitumoral compound. *Synth. Commun.* 2004, *34*, 3925–3937.

[127] Holonec, L., Ranga, F., Crainic, D., Truţta, A., Socaciu, C. Evaluation of betulin and betulinic acid content in birch bark from different forestry areas of western carpathians. *Not. Bot. Horti Agrobot.* 2012, *40*, 99–105.

[128] Pisha, E., Chai, H., Lee, I.S., Chagwedera, T.E., Farnsworth, N.R., Cordell, G.A., Beecher, C.W., Fong, H.H., Kinghorn, A.D., Brown, D.H. Discovery of betulinic acid a selective inhibitor of human-melanoma that functions by induction of apoptosis. *Nat. Med.* 1995, *10*, 1046–1051.

[129] Singh, S., Sharma, B., Kanwar, S.S., Kumar, A. Lead phytochemicals for anticancer drug development. *Front. Plant Sci.* 2016, *7*, 1–13.

[130] Lee, S.Y., Kim, H.H., Park, S.U. Recent studies on betulinic acid and its biological and pharmacological activity. *EXCLI J.* 2015, *14*, 199–203.

[131] Zhang, D.M., Xu, H.G., Wang, L., Li, Y.J., Sun, P.H., Wu, X.M., Wang, G.J., Chen, W.M., Ye, W.C. Betulinic acid and its derivatives as potential antitumor agents. *Med. Res. Rev.* 2015, *35*, 1127–1155.

[132] Gheorgheosu, D., Duicu, O., Dehelean, C., Soica, C., Muntean, D. Betulinic acid as a potent and complex antitumor phytochemical: A minireview. *Anticancer Agents Med. Chem.* 2014, *14*, 936–945.

[133] Ali, M.T.M., Zahari, H., Aliasak, A., Lim, S.M., Ramasamy, K., Macabeoacabeo, A.P.G. Synthesis, characterization and cytotoxic activity of betulinic acid and *sec*-betulinic acid derivatives against human colorectal carcinoma. *Orient. J. Chem.* 2017, *33*, 242–248.

[134] Luo, R., Fang, D., Chu, P., Wu, H., Zhang, Z., Tang, Z. Multiple molecular targets in breast cancer therapy by betulinic acid. *Biomed. Pharmacother.* 2016, *84*, 1321–1330.

[135] Shankar, E., Zhang, A., Franco, D., Gupta, S. Betulinic acid-mediated apoptosis in human prostate cancer cells involves p53 and nuclear factor-kappa b (NF-κB) pathways. *Molecules* 2017, *22*, 264.

[136] Potze, L., Di Franco, S., Grandela, C., Pras-Raves, M.L., Picavet, D.I., van Veen, H.A., van Lenthe, H., Mullauer, F.B., van der Wel, N.N., Luyf, A., et al. Betulinic acid induces a novel cell death pathway that depends on cardiolipin modification. *Oncogene* 2016, *35*, 427–437.

[137] Waechter, F., Silva, G.S., Willig, J., de Oliveira, C.B., Vieira, B.D., Trivella, D.B., Zimmer, A.R., Buffon, A., Pilger, D.A., Gnoatto, S. Design, synthesis, and biological evaluation of betulinic acid derivatives as new antitumor agents for leukaemia. *Anticancer Agents Med. Chem.* 2017.

[138] Jung, G.R., Kim, K.J., Choi, C.H., Lee, T.B., Han, S.I., Han, H.K., Lim, S.C. Effect of betulinic acid on anticancer drug-resistant colon cancer cells. *Basic Clin. Pharmacol. Toxicol.* 2007, *101*, 277–285.

[139] Gao, Y., Jia, Z.L., Kong, X.Y., Li, Q., Chang, D.Z., Wei, D.Y., Le, X.D., Huang, S.D., Huang, S.Y., Wang, L.W., Xie, K.P. Combining betulinic acid and

mithramycin a effectively suppresses pancreatic cancer by inhibiting proliferation, invasion, and angiogenesis. *Cancer Res.* 2011, *71*, 5182–5193.

[140] Xu, Y., Li, J., Li, Q.J., Feng, Y.L., Pan, F. Betulinic acid promotes TRAIL function on liver cancer progression inhibition through p53/Caspase-3 signaling activation. *Biomed. Pharmacother.* 2017, *88*, 349–358.

[141] Yogeeswari, P., Sriram, D. Betulinic acid and its derivatives: A review on their biological properties. *Curr. Med. Chem.* 2005, *12*, 657–666.

[142] Gismondi, A., Reina, G., Orlanducci, S., Mizzoni, F., Gay, S., Terranova, M.L., Canini, A. Nanodiamonds coupled with plant bioactive metabolites: A nanotech approach for cancer therapy. *Biomaterials* 2015, *38*, 22–35.

[143] Gismondi, A., Nanni, V., Reina, G., Orlanducci, S., Terranova, M.L., Canini, A. Nanodiamonds coupled with 5,7-dimethoxycoumarin, a plant bioactive metabolite, interfere with the mitotic process in B16F10 cells altering the actin organization. *Int. J. Nanomed.* 2016, *11*, 557–574.

[144] Gupta, C., Prakash, D., Gupta, S. Cancer treatment with nano-diamonds. *Front. Biosci. (Sch. Ed.)* 2017, *9*, 62–70.

[145] Raj, R., Mongia, P., Sahu, S.K., Ram, A. Nanocarriers based anticancer drugs: Current scenario and future perceptions. *Curr. Drug Targets* 2016, *17*, 206–228.

Chapter 7

TRADITIONAL SYSTEM OF MEDICINE AND NUTRITIONAL SUPPLEMENTATION: USE VS REGULATION

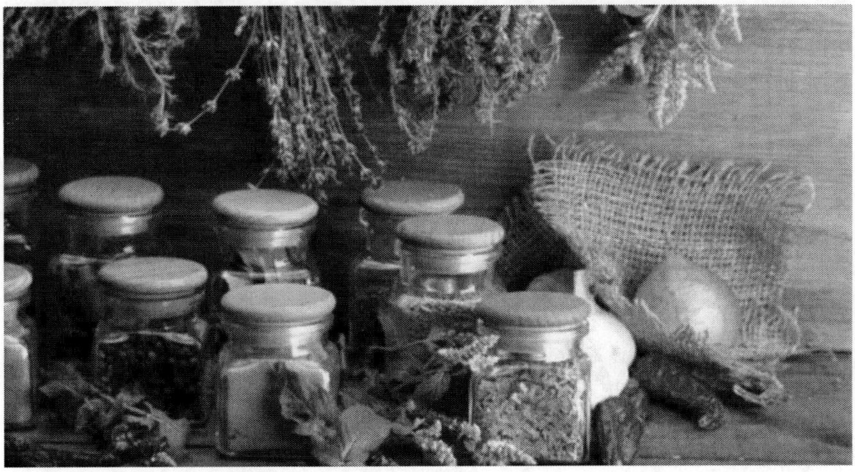

ABSTRACT

Food is the major source for serving the nutritional needs, but with growing modernization some traditional ways are being given up. Affluence of working population with changing lifestyles and reducing affordability of sick care, in terms of time and money involved, are some of the forces that are presently driving people towards thinking about their wellness. There has been increased global interest in traditional medicine. Efforts to monitor and regulate traditional herbal medicine are underway. Ayurveda, the traditional Indian medicine, remains the most ancient yet living traditions. Although India has been successful in promoting its therapies with more research and science-based approach, it still needs more extensive research and evidence base. Increased side effects, lack of curative treatment for several chronic diseases, high cost of new drugs, microbial resistance and emerging, diseases are some reasons for renewed public interest in complementary and alternative medicines. Numerous nutraceutical combinations have entered the international market through exploration of ethnopharmacological claims made by different traditional practices. This review gives an overview of the Ayurvedic system of medicine and its role in translational medicine in order to overcome malnutrition and related disorders. Many of the scientific and regulatory challenges that exist in research on the safety, quality and efficacy of dietary supplements are common to all countries as the marketplace for them becomes increasingly global. This article summarizes some of the challenges in supplement science and provides a case study of research at the Office of Dietary Supplements at the National Institutes of Health, USA, along with some resources it has developed that are available to all scientists. It includes examples of some of the regulatory challenges faced and some resources for those who wish to learn more about them.

Keywords: dietary supplements, food supplements, supplement science, scientific challenges, regulatory challenges, natural health product, complementary medicine, traditional medicines, National Institutes of Health, Office of Dietary Supplements

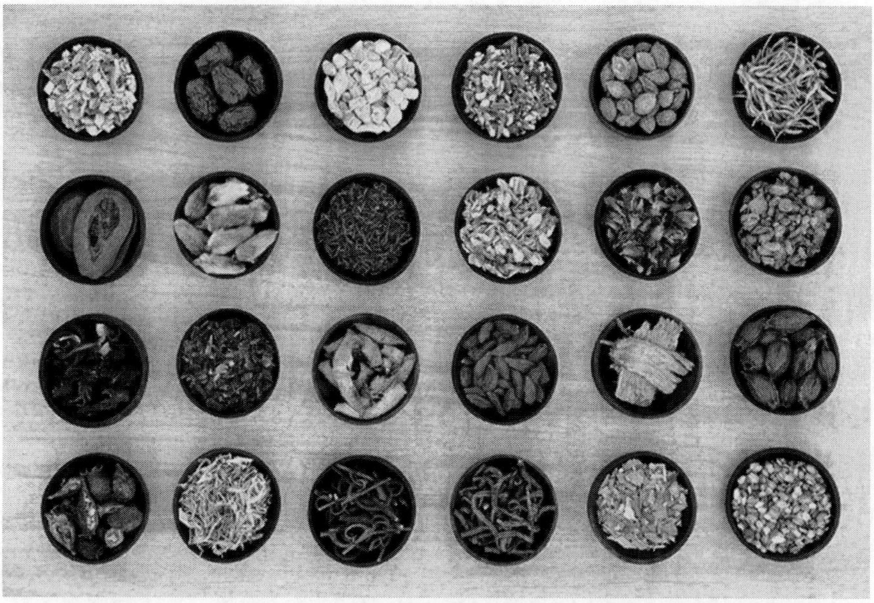

Figure 1. Dietary supplements. Herbal supplements are regulated by the FDA, but not as drugs or as foods. They fall under a category called dietary supplements. Manufacturers don't have to seek FDA approval before selling dietary supplements. Companies can claim that products address a nutrient deficiency, support health or are linked to body functions — if they have supporting research and they include a disclaimer that the FDA hasn't evaluated the claim. The FDA is responsible for monitoring dietary supplements that are on the market. If the FDA finds a product to be unsafe, it can take action against the manufacturer or distributor or both, and may issue a warning or require that the product be removed from the market. These regulations provide assurance that: Herbal supplements meet certain quality standards; The FDA can intervene to remove dangerous products from the market. (Source: Herbal supplements: What to know before you buy. MAYO CLINIC Nov. 08, 2017.)

1. Introduction

India is known for its traditional medicinal systems— Ayurveda, Siddha, and Unani. Medical systems are found mentioned even in the ancient Vedas and other scriptures. The Ayurvedic concept appeared and developed between 2500 and 500 BC in India. The fundamental challenge in any discussion about the regulation of dietary supplements is that there is no global consensus on how the category of products known variously as dietary supplements, natural health products (NHPs), complementary medicines or food supplements in different countries is defined. For example, a product considered to be a dietary supplement and regulated as a food in the USA, in another jurisdiction may be considered a food supplement or a therapeutic good (complementary medicine) or a therapeutic good (prescription medicine) or potentially even a controlled substance. The situation is even more complicated when countries like China or India that have an existing regulatory framework for traditional medicine or phytomedicine that includes crude botanicals are considered. To add further to the confusion, many regulatory frameworks are changing. Another challenge is that while all regulatory scientists want to protect consumers from harm, ensure that consumers have the ability to make informed choices about the products they use, and do the right thing, the scientific challenges and regulatory systems that have arisen to deal with them vary greatly from country to country. Even in countries with similar cultures, legal systems, and levels of economic development, regulations applying to dietary supplements vary considerably. Some of these differences are explored below, using examples from Australia, Canada and the USA, all English-speaking countries with largely similar cultures and legal systems to illustrate this point. The discussion of other countries with similar legal systems such as the United Kingdom, New Zealand and South Africa or other nations in the Americas, Europe, Africa and Asia, often with different cultures, legal systems, and levels of economic development is left for others with greater expertise and experience. A final challenge is that "dietary supplement" health products are often very emotive and polarizing topics, evoking a diverse range of opinions and viewpoints. While some observers may contend that these products should be considered in a similar fashion to conventional drugs and foods, others believe that a more tailored approach is necessary since there is often a traditional or historical evidence base and products often contain multiple ingredients. Increasingly, this situation has become even more complex because of the lucrative nature of the global dietary supplement sector, increased involvement of a growing industry sector producing them, and the introduction of many new and innovative products onto the market. A detailed discussion of the politics of the subject is outside the scope of this paper. However, it must be recognized that politics may play both a positive and negative role in shaping both regulatory frameworks and research agendas. Irrespective of the reader's point of view, this context is important in any discussion of dietary supplement products.

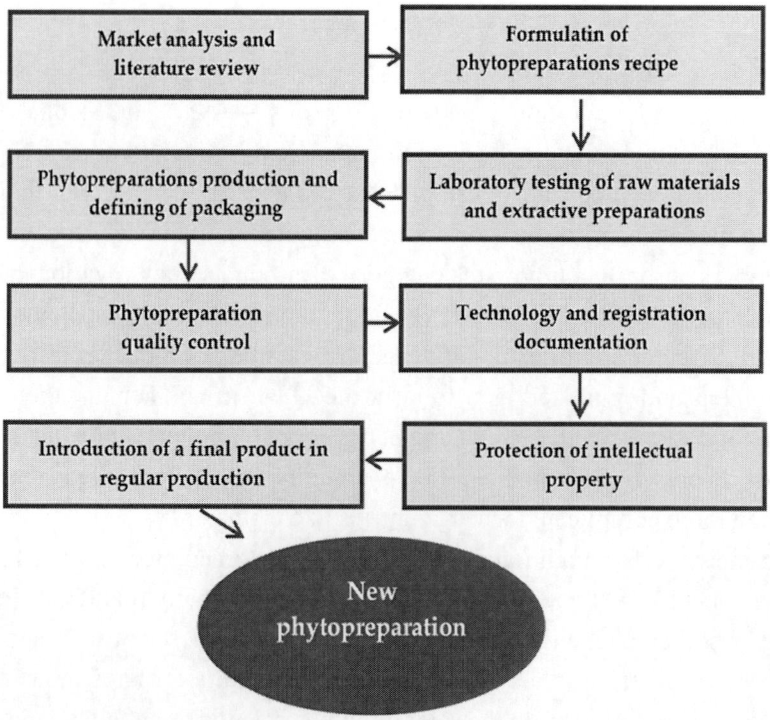

Figure 2. Planning and development of new herbal preparation. Analysis of active substances in the selected plant raw materials and quality control prescribed by Pharmacopoeia or another relevant document are performed. Then, the quality control of semifinal product is conducted. In the case of capsules, the analysis of the active substance in dry extract is performed, and also the analysis of other parameters that define its quality, and that is defined by Pharmacopoeia monographs or summarized in an internal specification or a certificate. Afterwards, the preparation formulation is conducted (formulation of teas or herbal drops, herbal creams, capsules, etc.). In addition to the main plant raw materials, secondary raw materials are selected, which will synergistically facilitate the functioning of the dominant plant drugs, and auxiliary pharmaceutical raw materials are selected. Auxiliary raw materials are used as the basis for semi-solid galenic forms (creams, ointments, and gels), and capsule fillers (Djordjevic SM. From Medicinal Plant Raw Material to Herbal Remedies. In: IntechOpen Limited DOI: 10.5772/66618).

1.1. Importance of Research on Dietary Supplements

Internationally, herbal products are regulated under different classifications, some of which are: complimentary medicines; natural health products; prescription medicines; over the counter medicines; supplements; traditional herbal medicines, etc. Until relatively recently, there was limited scientific research on dietary supplements and so little was known about them [1]. However, the prevalence of supplement use has increased dramatically over the past 20 years [2], and they have become a matter of consumer interest [3, 4]. At the same time, the application of state-of-the art scientific methods to explore issues involving dietary supplements has advanced rapidly. The other invited articles in

Exhibit 1. International regulatory overview of herbal supplements

India	Herbal drugs are regulated under the Drug and Cosmetic Act (D and C) 1940 and Rules 1945 in India, where regulatory provisions for Ayurveda, Unani, Siddha medicine are clearly laid down.
Malaysia	Herbal products in Malaysia fall under the category of regulated products. Any marketer intending to place the herbal products in the market require to register the product first. The applicant is required to be registered with the Malaysia Registrar of Business or Suruhanjaya Syarikat Malaysia under two classifications
Philippines	The Bureau of Food and Drugs (BFAD), who are the regulators in the country, mandate registration of the traditionally used herbal products before manufacture, import or market. The extent of control of BFAD includes the brand names of the traditional herbal products as well, and their prior clearance is required, before filing for product registration.
Nigeria	Nigeria, the trade of herbal products is regulated by National Agency for Food and Drug Administration and Control (NAFDAC) who has classified these products as "Herbal Medicines and Related Products." Premarketing registration of herbal medicines and related products is mandatory in Nigeria. No advertisement can be made as a cure for any disease conditions listed in "Schedule 1" to the Food and Drug Act 1990.
Australia	Complementary medicines which do not require medical supervision are permitted and have to be entered on the Australian Register for Therapeutic Goods (ARTG) before marketing. The low-risk medicines require to be listed while the medicines for comparatively higher risk therapeutic conditions require registration on the ARTG. Only evidence-based claims which are entered on the ARTG are allowed.
United States	As per FDA, the drug must be marketed under an approved New Drug Application (NDA). FDA regulates the dietary supplements under the Dietary Supplement Health and Education Act of 1994. The claims need to comply with the regulatory guidelines issued by the FDA. The manufacturing of dietary supplements should be done as per the current GMP for dietary supplements.
Canada	Complete data on product composition, standardization, stability, microbial and chemical contaminant testing methods and tolerance limits, safety and efficacy along with ingredient characterization, quantification by assay or by input needs to be submitted to Natural Health Product Directorate (NHPD). The authority mandates that NHPs must comply with the contaminant limits and must be manufactured as per the GMP norms.
European Union	The European Medicine Agency have laid down two ways of registration of herbal medicinal products: (1) A full marketing authorization by submission of a dossier, which provides the information on quality, safety and efficacy of the medicinal products including the physicochemical, biological or microbial tests and pharmacological, toxicological and clinical trials data; under directive 2001/83/EC. (2) For traditional herbal medicinal products, which do not require medical supervision, and where evidence of long traditional of use of medicinal products exists, and adequate scientific literature to demonstrate a well-established medicinal use cannot be provided, a simplified procedure under directive 2004/24/EC exists.

Source: Sharma S. Current status of herbal product: Regulatory overview. J Pharm Bioallied Sci. 2015;7(4):293-6.

this special issue illustrate progress in our understanding of supplement science as it applies to several nutrients, including vitamin D, iron, omega-3 fatty acids, and iodine. Progress on botanicals and other non-nutrient ingredients (e.g., glucosamine, methyl-sulfonyl-methane (MSM), coenzyme Q10) has been more challenging [5]. There is no global consensus in terminology for the category of products known variously as dietary supplements, NHPs, and food supplements in different countries and while we recognize this limitation, for the purpose of this article the term dietary supplement will be used to refer to such products as nutritional supplements, herbal medicines and traditional medicines. This article summarizes some of the scientific challenges in supplement research and some resources that may be useful in studying them. Most of the scientific challenges in supplement science are ubiquitous and global, so it is vital for scientists to collaborate across nations to help meet them without duplicating effort. A case study is provided by the work of the NIH Office of Dietary Supplements (ODS) which has been pursuing this goal since 2000. Some freely available resources and tools that ODS has developed for advancing health-related scientific knowledge on supplements are presented. The supplement marketplace is increasingly international, making collaboration between regulators essential since national decisions have international implications. Since products are consumed world-wide, calls for global quality standards are emerging. The remainder of the article focuses on regulatory challenges involving dietary supplements, and perspectives on how the regulatory systems in a number of different countries deal with them. Key resources for learning more about these approaches are provided.

1.2. Areas of Scientific Consensus about Supplement Science

Although there is broad consensus on the need for advances in science to make progress, opinions vary on the best paths to take and on priority areas for consideration.

1.2.1. Quality

The supply of ingredients used in supplements has outpaced the availability of methods and trained personnel to analyze them [6]. For example, in 1994, when the Dietary Supplement Health and Education Act (DSHEA) first became law in the USA, about 600 U.S. manufacturers of supplements were producing an estimated 4000 products. By 2000, more than 29,000 supplement products were on the US market but few documented analytical methods or reference materials (RM) were available for these products. This growth in the market has also been evident internationally. For example, there are anecdotal reports that over 100,000 product license applications have been approved in Canada since the Natural Health Products Regulations came into force in 2005. The need for improving quality continues today, since now there are estimated to be more than 85,000 supplement products in the US marketplace and concerns about ingredient misidentification, safety concerns, and quality assurance/control problems continue to be important for the industry and the public [7, 8]. The first step in characterizing supplement products is generally identifying the ingredients [9]. Plant identification is a particular challenge. Even when easily identified whole plants or plant parts are used, unless the chain of custody is tight, and the exact manufacturing process is known and well characterized, the quality of extracts and blends such as those found in many botanical products is difficult to ascertain. Reliable analytical methods to characterize the bioactive components in supplements are helpful, but even for the nutrients in supplements, specific analytical chemistry methods must be often developed [10]. The bio-actives in supplements differ from those in foods in their matrices in that the forms, combinations, and doses in which they are consumed, and the circumstances under which they are used are likely to differ. Analytical techniques for other bio-actives in supplements are further complicated because the active compound(s) are often unknown, and even when they are known, validated analytical methods may not exist for determining their content. Reference materials are often unavailable to compare results between different laboratories for research purposes and to monitor data and supplement quality.

1.2.2. Safety

Manufacturers are prohibited from marketing supplement products that are unsafe or contain unsafe ingredients. This includes assuring that safe upper levels of intake for nutrients or maximum dosages for other constituents are not exceeded and ensuring that toxic contaminants are absent. Improved accuracy and precision of the nutrient measurements, bioactive marker compounds for other ingredients, natural toxins, toxic elements and/or pesticides in dietary supplement ingredients and finished products will be helpful to regulatory agencies.

1.2.3. Efficacy

Demonstration of efficacy typically depends on a number of research approaches ranging from basic in-vitro research on the mechanisms of action to animal and human studies. For example, in the past, large and expensive clinical trials using poorly characterized herbal supplement products for which the mechanisms of action were not understood were performed, leading to results that were inconclusive and irreproducible [11–13]. These experiences led publishers and funders to demand better product characterization and funders to demand more mechanistic evidence of bioactivity. Once mechanistic plausibility is established, animal and small phase 1 and phase 2 trials should precede the launch of large phase 3 studies of efficacy. More and better clinical studies of the safety and efficacy of dietary supplements on “hard” health outcomes are also sorely needed. Health outcomes such as changes in validated surrogate markers for performance, functions, morbidity, and mortality from diseases or conditions are required rather than changes in biochemical measures in blood with unvalidated surrogate markers. The question of the use of evidence from traditional forms of health and healing such as Traditional Chinese Medicine (TCM) makes the question of efficacy often more complex. This is briefly explored in the regulatory section below.

1.2.4. Translation of the Science

Widespread consensus exists on the need to translate the scientific evidence on supplements into appropriate recommendations, regulations, and policies that ensure the public health. Population-based prevalence estimates of supplement use are needed to estimate total exposures to nutrients or other bioactives that can be related to health outcomes [14]. Monitoring is especially important when supplementation is used as a public health strategy to fill nutrient gaps in deficient populations. It is also needed in other countries such as the USA where use of certain supplements is high, and where substantial proportions of total intakes of nutrients such as vitamin D and calcium come from supplements, especially among older adults [15].

Exhibit 2. Parameters of quality control for herbal preparations

Herbal drugs	1. Definition: the name of the herbal drugs and content of active substances 2. Characters: appearance, taste, odor, solubility 3. Identification: macroscopic and microscopic examination, TLC 4. Tests: water, loss on drying, total ash, foreign matter, insoluble matter, extractable matter, swelling index, microbiological purity, bitterness value, broken drug 5. Assay: essential oils, tannins, declared active substances (GC, LC, UV-VIS)
Herbal drug preparations	Dry extract *(Extractum siccum)* 1. Definition: standardized dry extract prepared from..., content of active substances 2. Production: method of extraction and solvents 3. Characters: appearance 4. Identification: TLC 5. Tests: loss on drying, total ash, microbiological purity 6. Assay: declared active substances (LC) Liquid extract (*Extractum fluidum*) 1. Definition: liquid extract produced from …, and content of active substances 2. Production: method of extraction and solvents 3. Characters: appearance, taste, odor 4. Identification: TLC 5. Tests: ethanol, methanol and 2-propanol, loss on drying, microbiological purity 6. Assay: declared active substances (LC, UV-VIS) Tincture (*Tinctura*) 1. Definition: tincture produced from…, and content of active substances 2. Production: method of extraction and solvents 3. Characters: appearance, taste, odor 4. Identification: TLC 5. Tests: ethanol, methanol and 2-propanol, dry residue, microbiological purity 6. Assay: declared active substances (LC, UV-VIS) Essential oil (*Aetheroleum*) 1. Definition: essential oil obtained by …, and content of dominant components 2. Production: method of extraction and solvents 3. Characters: appearance, odor, solubility 4. Identification: TLC and chromatographic profile (GC and GC-MS) 5. Tests: relative density, refractive index, optical rotation, chromatographic profile

Source: European Pharmacopoeia 8.

Exhibit 3. Parameters of quality control of phyto-preparation

Phyto-Preparations	Parameters of Quality Control
Mono-component tea and tea mixture	1. Identification 2. Appearance 3. Verification of components, declared mass ratio of components 4. Verification of package weight 5. microbiological purity
Liquid herbal preparations (liquid extracts, tinctures, and mixtures of extracts or tinctures), herbal drops, solutions, syrups	1. Identification 2. Appearance 3. Loss on drying 4. Content of ethanol 5. Relative density 6. Refractive index 7. Verification of package weight 8. Qualitative and quantitative analysis 9. microbiological safety and/or complete health safety control
Semi-solid forms (herbal gels, cream, and unguent)	1. Identification 2. Appearance 3. Verification of package weight 4. pH value 5. microbiological safety and/or complete health safety control
Solid-dosage forms (capsules, tablets, etc.)	1. Identification 2. Appearance 3. Declared mass of single-dose preparations 4. Disintegration 5. Qualitative and quantitative analysis of the declared active components 6. microbiological safety and/or complete health safety control

Source: European Pharmacopoeia 8.

2. Challenges and Resources: Regulatory Perspectives

As with other categories of regulated goods such as foods and drugs, the development of regulations is a balancing act where many different factors need to be taken into account. Notable among these are ensuring that products are of high quality and safe, that any claims made are truthful and not misleading, and that there is reasonable and appropriate access to the marketplace. All regulatory scientists want to both protect consumers from harm and support them in making informed choices about the products they include—or as importantly do not include—in their healthcare options. Appropriate regulatory oversight of this category is very challenging, and requires that scientists and regulators work together, as the former director general of the World Health Organization, Margaret Chan, MD urged [16]. This section provides a concise overview of how these regulations have been developed, and common themes as well as challenges faced in a global market.

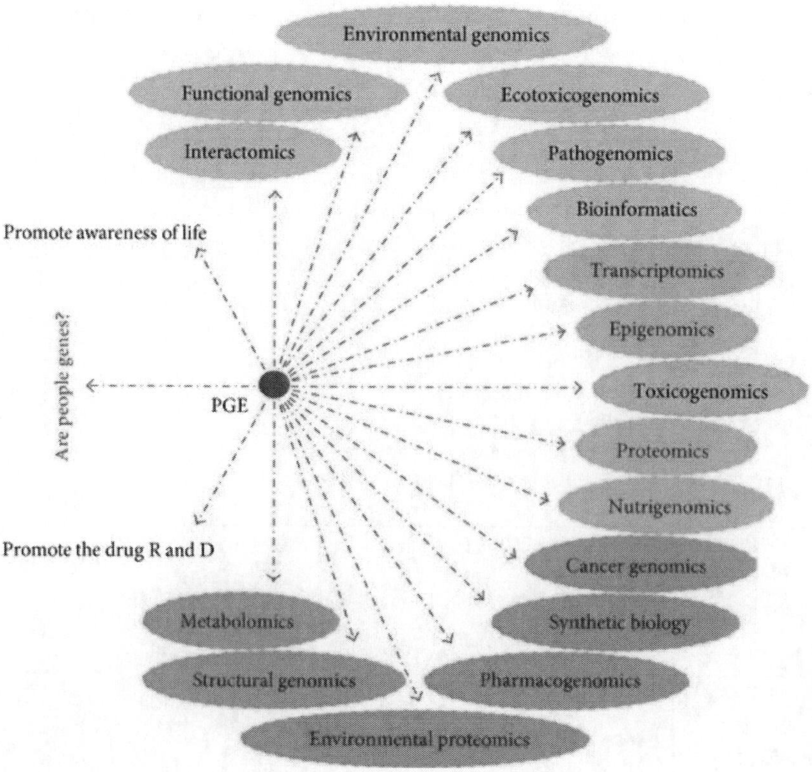

Figure 3. "Postgenomic" era (PGE) and the associated new disciplines of study. Firstly, in this "postgenomic" era, the screening of herbal ingredients should be accelerated. Due to the development of related disciplines in the "postgenomic" era, the pace of drug discovery from herbal medicine is likely to be hastened and become more efficient than ever, with a resultant higher success rate. Unlike synthetic drugs, drugs derived from herbal medicine are developed by isolating and identifying the active chemical entities in the crude herbal extract, rather than by going through processes of drug design and synthesis. Although many aids and tools for advanced drug design are now available and the in vivo properties of a drug can also be predicted using quantum mechanics and statistical mechanics, the complexity of biological systems often defies some of the basic assumptions of rational drug design. As such, it is impossible to estimate all drug-related parameters in an accurate manner during the "pregenomic" era. It is estimated that a single herbal preparation may contain more than 100 active compounds, and their bioactivities and/or drug-like properties are difficult to be accurately identified and evaluated by conventional pharmacological methods or drug screening approaches. (Source: Pan SY, Zhou SF, Gao SH, et al. New Perspectives on How to Discover Drugs from Herbal Medicines: CAM's Outstanding Contribution to Modern Therapeutics. Evid Based Complement Alternat Med. 2013;2013:627375.)

2.1. Definition of "Dietary Supplements"

Although the definition of dietary supplement within a specific jurisdiction such as the USA is quite precise [17, 18], a fundamental challenge to any discussion on regulation is that there is no global consensus on either what falls within this category or even what the category is called. Intuitively many equate a dietary supplement in the USA with a NHP in Canada or a traditional herbal medicine in the European Union or a complementary medicine in Australia, but this is not the case. For example, while melatonin is regulated in the USA as a dietary supplement and in Canada as a NHP, in Australia it is considered as a prescription medicine [19–21]. Dehydroepiandrosterone (DHEA) is readily available as a dietary supplement in the US, while in many other jurisdictions it is regulated as a controlled substance and is subject to significant regulatory oversight [22].

This situation is even more complicated when one considers that in addition to dietary supplements such as vitamins and minerals, many of these products come from traditional systems of health and healing such as TCM in China and Ayurvedic/Unani/Siddha medicine in India. For this reason, we must differentiate between the manner in which nations regulate the practice of medicine and the manner in which they regulate marketed products used in medical practice or as foods. In the U.S., the practice of medicine is regulated by the states, while marketed food and drug products in interstate commerce are regulated by the Federal government. Approaches and regulatory frameworks in many parts of the world, notably in Asia, reflect this fact with terminology and categories developed accordingly [23].

Table 1. Useful global resources on dietary supplement regulatory issues and definitions

Name	URL	Comments
USA		
FDA Food and Drug Administration Dietary Supplements	www.fda.gov/food/dietarysupplements/	Details on regulations, policies and guidelines dealing with dietary supplements
Australia		
Therapeutic Goods Administration (TGA)	www.tga.gov.au/complementary-medicines	Details of existing complementary medicine regulations, policies and guidelines
Food Standards Australia and New Zealand	www.foodstandards.gov.au/Pages/ default.aspx	Details on food standards, policies and guidelines.
Canada		
Health Canada	www.canada.ca/en/health-canada/services/drugshealth-products/ natural-non-prescription.html	Details on the existing NHP regulations, policies and guidelines as well as work underway with regards to a comprehensive approach to self care products
	www.canada.ca/en/health-canada/services/foodnutrition/legislation-guidelines/guidancedocuments/category-specific-guidance-temporarymarketing-authorization-supplemented-food.html	Information on supplemented food category.
EU European Union		
EU Parliament and Council	ec.europa.eu/health/human-use/herbalmedicines_en	Details on the traditional herbal medicine directive re: member states.
European Food Safety Authority (EFSA)	www.efsa.europa.eu	Provides details and links to regulation of foods and food supplements.

Table 1. (Continued)

Name	URL	Comments
China		
China Food and Drugs Administration (CFDA)	eng.sfda.gov.cn/WS03/CL0755/	Information on health food regulations including 'blue hat' process. (Note: English translation was not available).
China—Special Administrative Region of Hong Kong		
Health Ministry—Chinese Medicine Division	www.cmd.gov.hk/html/eng/important_info/ regulation.html	Information on policies and regulation related to Chinese proprietary medicines.
Japan	www.mhlw.go.jp/english/topics/foodsafety/fhc/02.html	
Singapore		
Health Sciences Authority	www.hsa.gov.sg/content/hsa/en.html	Information on policies, regulation and guidelines related to health products and Chinese proprietary medicines. As a member state, resource to access work on regulatory harmonization of products within Association of South East Asian Nations (ASEAN).
New Zealand		
Medsafe	www.medsafe.govt.nz/regulatory/DietarySupplements/Regulation.asp	Provides information related to regulation, policies and guidelines dealing with dietary supplements.
India		
Food Safety and Standards Authority of India (FSSAI)	fssai.gov.in/home	Government direction, standards and regulation of health supplements and nutraceuticals. New regulations published in November 2016 take effect in January 2018. Health supplements are intended to supplement the diet of healthy individuals over 5 year, and levels of nutrients should not exceed RDA amounts.
Ministry of Ayurveda, Yoga, Unani, Siddha and Homeopathy (AYUSH)	ayush.gov.in	Policies, guidelines and regulations dealing with Indian traditional medicines.
WHO	who.int/medicines/areas/traditional/en/	Provides links to on-going work by the WHO including the Traditional Medicine Strategy 2014-2023, the International Regulation on the Cooperation of Herbal Medicines and various technical guidelines.
World Self Medication Industry	www.wsmi.org	Industry association website providing details on international approaches to over-the-counter medicines including dietary supplements.
International Alliance of Dietary/Food Supplement Associations (IADSA)	www.iadsa.org	Industry association website providing details on international approaches to dietary supplements.

Exhibit 4. An overview of the regulatory options for regulating practitioners of traditional/complementary medicine

Area of Regulation	Regulatory Options
Education and	Type of qualification: university education, specific training for practitioners of traditional/complementary medicine and for conventional health care practitioners
Training	Educational setting: schools, colleges or universities Specify standards in terms of length of training vs content of core curriculum Shared biomedical curriculum vs alternative curriculum Private/professional associations accredit courses vs independent accreditation (by registering body or government) Training component of conventional medical training aimed at familiarization vs integration
Licensing and	Individual registration vs associations of practitioners register (and all members automatically registered)
Registration	Automatic registration with accredited qualification vs licensing exam vs both Recognition of prior non-accredited training or experience vs licensing exam Lifetime membership vs re-licensing (associated with continuing medical education) Joint or dual licensing of practitioners of traditional/complementary medicine and conventional medical practitioners practicing traditional/complementary medicine vs no additional licensing requirements for conventional medical practitioners
Practice	Generic laws that also cover the practice of traditional/complementary medicine vs specific traditional/complementary medicine legislation De-criminalization of practice vs professionalization of practice Mono-therapeutic (that is, individual traditional/complementary medicine practitioner regulators) vs multi-therapeutic (that is, umbrella regulator for all such practitioners) vs integrated (that is, single regulator for traditional/ complementary and conventional medicine practitioners) National vs regional/local standards of practice Setting specific standards (for example, hospital vs primary care; public hospital vs private practice) Delegate standard setting to professionals vs specify in legislation Statement of minimum standards vs statement of limits of practice Protection or title vs protection of practice

* Regulating Complementary Medical Practitioners An International Review. Web Kingfund.co.uk.

To assist in development of its Traditional Medicine Strategy 2014–2023, the World Health Organization refers to this category as Traditional and Complementary Medicines (T & CM) [16]. Although this classification does have significant limitations, it recognizes the fact that definitions for this category vary significantly globally. Descriptions of specific national/regional definitions and categories can be found through the list of resources in Table 1.

While it would be easy just to consider that the substance itself is the defining factor in determining whether or not a product is a dietary supplement, this is not the case. Two other important factors considered are the claim that the product is making and how the product is supplied or recommended (intended use). In many jurisdictions such as the USA, Canada and Australia, dietary supplements are considered suitable for self-selection without the need for the intervention of a practitioner or prescription. Here the claims that can be made are limited to minor conditions and to the support of health and wellness depending on the jurisdiction [24, 25]. In other jurisdictions, notably those where a traditional form of health and healing is recognized, traditional and complementary medicine products are often prescribed, and in some cases supply is limited only to trained practitioners.

2.2. Regulatory Models

As with the definition of the products themselves, there is no consistent global approach to regulation, with many different frameworks developed that largely reflecting national and regional priorities and needs. That being said, there are a number of common themes and approaches that have been taken internationally.

2.2.1. Where Does the Category Fall within Existing Legislation?

With a few exceptions, notably where traditional forms of health and healing exist, most countries do not regulate dietary supplements as a stand-alone category. Rather, they include them as a subset of existing legislation [17, 18]. That is, they "hang from the hook" that is set in existing legislation. In the past, this was largely a question of whether these products should be considered a subset of drugs or foods; increasingly though, a third option is to capture them under existing regulations for biologics. It is important to note that overarching legislation is often one of the most important factors impacting the type of claim that can be made and what level of scrutiny and oversight will exist. For example, countries that regulate these products as a subset of drugs or therapeutic goods such as Australia, Canada and the European Union (EU) for traditional herbal medicines allow far more specific clinical claims to be made than in a jurisdiction such as the USA, where dietary supplements are captured in regulations under the existing food legislation, with their advertising regulated by trade regulations [20, 25, 26].

2.2.2. Should They Be Regulated as a Group?

As noted above in many jurisdictions dietary supplements are simply captured under the existing food or drug regulations and legislation with no specific consideration for these products, in some cases specific regulations have developed to reflect the category. In these cases, two different regulatory models have typically been adopted that reflect their domestic use, national priorities and public health needs. In many jurisdictions, the first model applies. Dietary supplements are simply captured under the existing food or drug regulations and legislation. In that model, a wide range of products (typically herbal medicines, traditional medicines and dietary or nutritional supplements) reside under an umbrella term such as dietary supplements in the USA, complementary medicines in Australia or NHP in Canada [20, 24, 25]. In the second model, specific regulations are developed to deal with these products. In this case, specific categories are developed with very structured regulatory frameworks for specific types of T&CMs. This is particularly the case in countries with a strong traditional form of health and healing such as Chinese proprietary medicines in China (TCM), Ayurvedic medicines in India and Kampo medicines in Japan [23].

Irrespective of the approach taken, it is rare that one set of regulations will encompass all products commonly considered to be dietary supplement-like. Typical examples of this are guidelines and legislation related to advertising that apply irrespective of whether or not a product is considered to be a dietary supplement.

2.2.3. Common Elements of Regulatory Frameworks

As with other forms of regulations, independent and irrespective of the approach taken, frameworks that deal with dietary supplements may contain a number of common elements, in this case often specifically developed to reflect the challenges and nature of the products. These common elements include: process for approval of a product to be sold; provisions related to manufacture and Good Manufacturing Practices (GMPs); reporting of adverse events; controls on labeling related to indications, contraindications and warnings; and, where claims are permitted, the type and quality of supporting evidence required. Again, the number and nature of these elements applied are determined by the specific regulations in place.

2.2.4. Risk-Based Approach

Operationally, the regulation of dietary supplements faces a number of issues and challenges not shared with conventional drugs or even food products. Notable amongst these are the sheer number of individual dietary supplements on the domestic markets, often numbering in the tens of thousands, and the fact that the sector contains many different types of products often posing very different risks that are grouped together often by the fact that they do not fit under any other regulatory regime. In particular, considerable challenges are posed especially by herbal and traditional medicine products that contain crude botanicals and a complex milieu of potentially active moieties, unlike conventional allopathic pharmaceuticals.

While a completely pre-market approach, where all products and manufacturing sites are 'approved' before the dietary supplement is marketed would be the optimal situation, given the challenges mentioned above, this is often impractical. This has led to the development of regulatory frameworks that increasingly blend elements looking at products and sites both before they come to market as well as once they are available to consumers, or post-market. This regulatory oversight is sometimes referred to as a "life-cycle" approach. Examples of post-market regulatory approaches (i.e., once the dietary supplement is on the market) include target audits where dietary supplements already on the market are analyzed for quality or manufacturers are requested to submit evidence they may hold that supports a specific claim. The determining factor on which approach is applied is largely determined by risk posed to the consumer. Since most dietary supplements when appropriately manufactured are considered to be inherently low risk, increasingly regulatory frameworks are increasingly focused more on post-market review than pre-market licensure. Even in countries that are in many ways socially, economically and legally similar, different approaches to the definition and regulation of dietary supplement health products are evident although they contain some common elements. Illustrative examples of this are evident in the different regulatory frameworks in place in the United States, Australia and Canada.

In the United States, dietary supplements are regulated under the Dietary Supplements Health Education Act of 1994 (DSHEA) as a subset of foods and limited to those taken orally. This approach is primarily post-market in nature. However, it does contain pre-market elements. For example, manufacturers must hold evidence to support their claims and they cannot make specific disease treatment claims but only claims related to nutritional support (which includes physiological structure and function) [20]. All products must carry a disclaimer on the label stating that claims have not been reviewed by the US Food and Drug Administration (FDA). Provisions also include a post-market site audit process for manufacturing sites for Good Manufacturing Practice compliance and mandatory reporting of serious adverse effects by manufacturers. Companies must notify the Food and Drug Administration before marketing products with new dietary ingredients (NDI) [27]. There is at present no indication that DSHEA will be substantially changed or modified by Congress, in recent years the regulatory authority has given more attention to the notification and classification of NDIs as well as the importance of Good Manufacturing Practices (GMP) [20].

In Australia, although a small number of these products are captured by a food standard, most are regulated as therapeutic goods under the Australian Therapeutic Goods Act. Products are referred to as complementary medicines and are legally defined as being a listed therapeutic good or a registered therapeutic good. The legislation itself does not define these terms, but a comprehensive set of guidelines describes how they are considered. Most complementary medicines are listed medicines and are managed through an online portal called the Electronic Listing Facility (ELF). Permitted claims are limited to minor, self-limited considerations and those traditional forms of health and healing such as traditional Chinese medicine. Evidence for efficacy is assured through a random and targeted post-market audit system and new listable substances are evaluated pre-market. As with all registered therapeutic goods, registered complementary medicines are evaluated pre-market for safety, quality and efficacy. Manufacturers of either finished listed or registered complementary medicines must undergo an on-site audit to ensure GMP [28].

In 2014, complementary medicines were included within a comprehensive review of regulations for all therapeutic goods and medical devices to be conducted by an external expert panel [29]. The Commonwealth government accepted the majority of the recommendations from the panel and preliminary draft legislation was made public in September 2017. Although one of the recommendations was to keep complementary medicines as a distinct category, some significant changes are proposed, allowing mid-level claims through a new third regulatory route between the listed and registered therapeutic goods process as well as changes to how advertising is approved and compliance management [25, 30].

In Canada, the majority of these dietary supplement products are referred to as natural health products (NHPs) and are considered a subset of drugs under a specific set of regulations—the Natural Health Products Regulations. Products must undergo a premarket assessment for safety, quality and efficacy. This is done in part through an online submission process with permissible claims supported by Health Canada monographs. Producers of NHPs who wish to make novel claims not supported through the monograph process must submit a full dossier of evidence for review. The products can make therapeutic claims, but their use is limited to self-care situations. While manufacturers are required to have a valid site license following approved GMP guidelines, no pre-market site audit is needed; the process being primarily paper based [24]. To address the growing number of NHPs sold in a food-like format, Health Canada has created a new category of food currently defined through regulatory policy called "supplemented foods". The category does allow for some health claims, but they are limited reflecting the nature of the products [31].

Unlike Australia, Canada is proposing to take different approach and rather than keeping NHPs as a distinct category, will include them in a self-care health product category together with non-prescription medicines and cosmetics. The intent of this initiative is to support informed consumer choice through a more consistent regulatory approach to these product categories that is based on risk. Key questions being explored deal with topics including evidence needed to support claims, provisions ensuring safety and quality and introduction of cost recovery framework [32]. The overviews above are brief and concise with more detailed information on these country specific approaches to be found through the list of resources in Table 1.

2.2.5. Competing Types of Evidence

While it is clear that high quality scientific evidence is always required to support the quality of a dietary supplement, from a regulatory perspective the same may not always be true with regard the type and nature of the evidence required to support a product claim. Given the nature of the dietary supplement sector and the fact that it often encompasses traditional medicines with a long history of use, the question faced by regulators is how to balance the need for robust scientific evidence with a respect for diverse forms of health and healing.

Globally, no consistent approach has been taken in answering this question. In some jurisdictions such as Canada and Australia, the approach has been to link the form of evidence, whether it be traditional or evidence based from scientific research, to the level and type of claim that can be made. In these cases, typically products based on traditional evidence making traditional health care claims are 'approved' according to pre-cleared and approved sources of information such as monographs or labeling standards. For products making higher level, clinical claims, in a way similar to that for conventional pharmaceuticals, companies must supply a full dossier with appropriate supporting evidence such as that from randomized controlled trials (RCTs) [24, 28]. In many countries such as the United States with no pre-market approval framework system, claims that can be made are more limited [17, 18]. In countries with long-established traditional forms of medicines such as in China, India, and Japan, specific regulatory frameworks have been developed for these types of products with the type of claim that can be made and the evidence required to reflect this approach [23].

As the dietary supplement sector matures and develops and the market for raw ingredients becomes more global, establishing a balance between evidence generated by scientific research and that coming from traditional forms of health and healing is becoming increasingly demanding. This will be discussed later.

2.3. Evolving Regulatory Landscape—Challenging Issues

International regulatory frameworks are still considered by many to be a new and novel sector, although many of them are now more than two decades old. They were developed to reflect a time when the sector and nature of the market, not to mention the needs and demands of the consumer, were very different. This has meant that some decisions made in the past around policies and regulatory decisions may need to be revisited. These include the need to evaluate evidence of the "grandfathering" of dietary supplements already on the market when new regulations were implemented, the need to ensure that approaches are sustainable through cost-recovery mechanisms and the more global nature of the market place. Table 1 provides links to some of the regulatory frameworks of different countries that provide insights into the ways issues are dealt with in them. Some of the key issues that commonly arise are detailed in the next session.

2.3.1. Evaluating Evidence for Product Claims

As the market for dietary supplements has increased, so has the amount and diversity of scientific evidence and research to support, or not support, their use. This market is made more complex when there are conflicting evidence bases and conflicting ways for evaluating them. For example, how, or should, traditional evidence be evaluated within the framework of traditional healing theories or those of allopathic evidence based medicine; what should be done when evidence from traditional forms of health and healing are not supported by more conventional evaluation mechanisms such as randomized clinical trials;

and how can consumers, often wanting to explore both conventional and traditional medicine, be supported in making informed choices about including, or not including, these products in their health care options.

The original concept of Evidence Based Medicine is based on three basic premises—individual clinical expertise, the best external evidence and patients' values and expectations [33]. The challenge faced by the regulator is to ensure that these are in play and to support consumers in making informed choices that are often made in a self-care setting.

2.3.2. Questions at the Regulatory Interface

It has never been easy to distinguish between a dietary supplement and other categories such as conventional foods, drugs and biologics. As all these sectors have evolved, this question of product classification has become even more complex. Two of the main questions at the regulatory interface are: what are the boundaries are between dietary supplements and conventional foods and between dietary supplements and over-the-counter drugs? As the popularity of dietary supplements available in a food-like format such as a pre-prepared drink or bar has increased, the line between what a consumer would understand to be a food as compared to a dietary supplement has become increasingly blurred. In essence, how does the regulator provide for appropriate regulatory oversight? This has been particularly challenging for those jurisdictions that consider these products as a sub-set of drugs with regulation and often legislation governing them that is very different from that for foods. In these cases, the regulatory frameworks are more specific to such dosage forms as capsules, tablets and tinctures. The challenge is one primarily of balance in providing a regulatory approach that is appropriate and not unnecessarily restrictive with the need to ensure that consumers are aware that these food-like dietary supplements that they are considering are not typical foods. This lack of clarity is also challenging for the private sector in determining what regulatory framework applies to a product, either food or drug, that they wish to develop and bring to market. In Canada, this concern required the government to create a new category called "supplemented foods" distinct from NHPs where products in a food like format are considered as a subset of foods and not as natural health products [31]. In other jurisdictions such as Australia, authority has been given to the respective regulators to deem something to be either a therapeutic good or a food based a specific set of criteria [34].

The challenge at the over-the-counter (OTC)/dietary supplement interface is even more pronounced. A number of herbal medicines with a long history of use within the conventional health care model, such as senna and cascara, are regulated in most countries as OTC drugs rather than dietary supplements. As described above, Health Canada is proposing to address this issue in part by considering both NHPs and OTC drugs within a single regulatory approach for self-care products [32].

2.3.3. Working on the Global Stage

Although science and research may be global, regulations are still made primarily to reflect domestic needs and pressures. This poses a challenge regarding dietary supplements and dietary supplement ingredients that are now often sourced and/or manufactured outside of the country where they are sold. In spite of calls for regulatory harmonization, examples of true harmonization are limited to regions such as countries in the Association of South East Asian Nations (ASEAN) with the lack of a coherent and consistent regulatory approach prohibiting this globally [35]. Even if regulatory harmonization is not possible, regulatory cooperation is often a viable option, taking into account inputs from stakeholder groups such as industry and not just governments. For example, to support cooperation between regulators, in 2005 in Ottawa, the World Health Organization supported the creation of the International Cooperation on Herbal Medicine (IRCH). IRCH now has over twenty members and provides a forum and mechanism for regulators to share information on safety issues and common challenges they all face [36]. Increasingly governments are working together as well as with other stakeholders such as industry and consumers to address common problems and in some cases to provide regulatory decisions in one jurisdiction that can be used as a basis for action in another.

2.3.4. Strengthening Product Quality

As the dietary supplement market has become more global and lucrative, so have the importance of ensuring product quality and the challenges in doing so. There are increasing numbers of cases of adverse reactions and some fatalities due to contaminants or adulterants in the product rather than in the dietary supplement ingredients themselves. In some cases this has been due to intentional fraud by producers of these poor quality products who have developed sophisticated methods for overcoming existing regulations and oversight. This situation is explored in greater depth elsewhere in this paper.

2.4. Need for Continued Science in Support of Regulation

Irrespective of whether the goal is to support production of high quality products or to develop, apply or modify methods for evaluation of evidence in support of claims, the need for robust and relevant science and research on dietary supplements has never been more necessary. As regulatory frameworks evolve, many of the questions posed above will need to be addressed, balancing the need for robust science with a respect for traditional forms of health and healing.

3. Challenges: Scientific Perspectives

3.1. Issues Involving Human Requirements

Scientists often disagree about definitions of human requirements for bioactives and the implications for supplements. They differ on whether some non-nutrient bioactives are required for certain population subgroups and also on the health effects associated with the use of non-nutrient bioactives. It has been known for over 100 years that inborn errors of nutrient metabolism exist that can be remediated by supplying the lacking nutrient that has become conditionally essential. However, it is not clear that such a model based on single gene defects is useful for the amelioration of multigenic complex diseases. It is unclear that there are large numbers of individuals with common diseases and conditions such as type 2 diabetes or depression whose unique genetic characteristics cause them to have special nutritional requirements requiring supplements or medical foods [37].

Discoveries of genetic polymorphisms and the advent of inexpensive genetic tests that are widely available to consumers have nutritional implications. They have led to the rise of personalized or "precision nutrition" [38] and to the proliferation of boutique "personalized" eating plans and "precision" dietary supplements supposedly tailored to an individual's genetic profile. The extent to which such supplements are efficacious in reducing chronic degenerative disease remains to be determined.

3.2. Supplement Quality, Safety and Efficacy

Challenges remain on the appropriate means for assuring supplement quality, safety and efficacy.

3.2.1. Quality

Regulators, health professionals and manufacturers often disagree on how much quality testing is necessary for supplements. This is echoed by the World Health Organization's Strategy on Traditional Medicines 2014–2023 [39] where quality is seen as a cornerstone of the sector. Botanical extracts and blends present particular challenges for detecting misidentification and contamination. The presence of adulterants and contaminants of both a biological and chemical nature in supplements is also challenging. Certain categories of supplements, such as athletic performance, sexual performance, and weight loss products, are particularly prone to the deliberate "spiking" with unlabeled extraneous or synthetic substances to confuse analytical techniques and even occasionally the addition of active synthetic drugs. Purity is a special problem for individuals with inborn errors of metabolism for specific nutrients such as vitamin B-6 or choline who require reliable, high quality sources of the nutrient. In countries that do not require that added nutrients be pharmaceutical grade or provide nutrients free to such patients, afflicted individuals must buy products that vary greatly in their quality on the open market.

The scientific challenges involved in all of the problems cited above depend in part on the adequacy and application of analytical methods. Analytical methods and reference standards are lacking for many of the thousands of different bioactive ingredients in dietary supplements. There is still disagreement about whether only a single officially endorsed method of analysis is acceptable. Any analytical method that is appropriately calibrated to a recognized reference standard should suffice but the onus is on the user of the method to demonstrate that affirmative requirements are met and that the method is suitable for its intended use and yields results that are accurate and precise. Methods that are suitable for foods may not be so for dietary supplements. Opinions also differ on whether government or the private sector is responsible for developing reference standards and analytical methods, and, if the private sector develops them, how they can be both kept independent and objective and made publicly available to avoid duplication of effort while preserving the marketing advantage of the developer. Tension also exists between researchers who desire ever more precise analytical methods for ingredients in dietary supplements and manufacturers who are concerned about the expertise and monetary costs required to apply some of the methods. A balance needs to be struck between the two.

3.2.2. Safety

Apart from concerns related to product quality, the safety of dietary supplements depends largely on dose. High doses of some nutrients are more likely to pose problems than others, although there is disagreement about the levels at which problems arise. For example, some dialysis patients who are receiving very large doses of calcium and the active form of vitamin D on a chronic basis may exceed the Tolerable Upper Level (UL) and incur adverse effects on health, including calcification of the soft tissues [40]. Very high doses of vitamin D may also cause adverse effects in people with normal kidney function [41]. There is little evidence that usual doses and forms of these nutrients give rise to health problems [42]. The possibilities of excessive intakes of nutrients from dietary supplements are greater in countries with programs to fortify their food supplies than in others, and therefore they must also be evaluated [43–46].

Dose-response data for establishing safe levels of intakes of non-nutrient bioactives in supplements is frequently lacking [47, 48]. Some dietary supplements containing non-target herbs added intentionally (like germander as an adulterant for skullcap), or others such as black cohosh, kava extract, green tea and others have been associated with liver injures of various types even after taking into account concomitant use with acetaminophen and alcohol and consumption while fasting [49]. Extracts that are used in bodybuilding and weight loss have also been linked to liver injury. This has led to studies of the composition of different supplements [50, 51]. Causes of liver toxicity from supplements appear to be due to insufficient regulatory authority, inaccurate product labeling, adulterants and inconsistent sourcing of ingredients [52]. There is controversy about whether evidence of causality is sufficient for regulators to take action against supplements that seem to pose a hepatotoxic risk [53]. Some possible actions include requirements for warning labels with usage instructions as is done for drugs, or/and removal of products from the market. Adulterated or fraudulent tainted products sold as dietary supplements are already illegal and subject to recall [54].

Interactions of some ingredients in supplements with other dietary supplements, nutrients, prescription or over-the-counter drugs are well documented. Of particular concern are adverse reactions occurring with commonly used medications, such as anti-hypertensive and cardiovascular preparations [55]. In addition, much interest focuses around concomitant use of herbal medicines such as St. John's Wort which has been shown to alter drug metabolism of a number of drugs notably those used in the treatment of HIV/AIDS, warfarin, insulin, aspirin and digoxin [56].

3.2.3. Efficacy

Among the most hotly debated issues in supplement research is the type and amount of evidence needed to demonstrate the efficacy of dietary supplements. Many of the issues involving efficacy include those common in testing of all medications such as study designs, significance testing, appropriate outcomes, effect sizes, acceptable biomarkers of effect, and the differences between statistical and clinical significance. In order to be efficacious, dietary supplements must be bioavailable, and yet in some countries regulations do not require testing of supplements for disintegration and dissolution and some products on the market fail such tests. This is a matter of concern both to researchers and regulators since such results have a negative impact on studies of dietary supplement efficacy. In-vitro methods are available for testing disintegration and dissolution of drugs, and these are adaptable for use with dietary supplement products. Regulators in some countries insist on changes in health outcomes or in validated surrogate biochemical markers of effect on the causal pathway to a health or performance outcome. Others accept changes in intermediary biochemical markers that may or may not be surrogates of health outcomes. These considerations have come to the fore because supplements on the market in some countries apparently have little or no demonstrated efficacy. For example, one recent review of 63 randomized, placebo-controlled clinical trials of dietary supplements in Western adults found that in 45 of them no benefits were found, 10 showed a trend toward harm and 2 showed a trend toward benefit, while 4 reported actual harm, and 2 both harms and benefits; only vitamin D and omega 3 fatty acids had strong enough benefits and lack of harm to suggest possible efficacy [3]. This is an area of controversy that is highly polarized with questions being raised that depend on the type of dietary supplement being used, notably herbal medicines, the quality of the studies included in the review, and additional factors such as product quality of the supplement being evaluated that need to be taken into account [57].

3.2.4. Standards of Efficacy for Traditional Natural Products

The traditional use of Chinese medicines, Ayurvedic medicines and other remedies is embedded in larger healing systems and cultural or metaphysical beliefs that are part of users' larger and more holistic world views. Should usual standards for efficacy should apply to them when they are used in the traditional manner? Clearly such uses are quite different than the use of a single product or ingredient at much higher traditional doses and without such a cultural context.

3.3. Policy

Although policy issues arise with all types of dietary supplements, the examples below will focus on nutrient-containing dietary supplements since these are particularly germane to discussions of nutritional status.

3.3.1. Nutrient Supplements Are Only One of Many Strategies for Improving Nutrient Intakes

There are many strategies for filling nutrient gaps in dietary intakes. They include nutrition education on appropriate food choices, fortification and enrichment that add nutrients to staple foods, genetic engineering that increases the nutrient content of a commodity itself either by genetic engineering/biotechnology, biofortification involving conventional breeding, and the use of nutrient containing dietary supplements. Dietary supplements provide concentrated sources of bioactives that are low or lacking in some individuals' ordinary dietary intakes. The supplements can be used selectively by those whose diets have gaps in them. However, supplements have disadvantages. Their use depends upon individual motivations. Because they provide concentrated sources of bioactives at relatively high levels, they may increase the risks that some individuals will ingest excessive quantities and suffer health risks. Moreover, since dietary supplements can contain ingredients that lack a history of safe use, their long-term health effects may be unknown. The advantages and disadvantages of dietary supplements as a strategy to improve dietary intakes therefore must be carefully considered.

3.3.2. Supplementation as a Strategy to Achieve Nutritional Adequacy

The cost-effectiveness of using supplements to fill gaps in nutrient intakes as opposed to other means such as fortification or nutrition education varies from one nutrient to another and by country, and so each situation is unique and must be evaluated independently. There are also questions about what the supplement should be, if supplementation is chosen. In countries where nutrient containing dietary supplements are common, the use of multivitamin-multi-mineral (MVM) supplements is often associated with a greater proportion of the population reaching the estimated average requirement (EAR) for nutrients [58]. However, for some of these nutrients, intakes are already adequate, so that the increased intakes may do little good, and in some cases supplements may increase the risk of exceeding the upper safe level (UL) of intakes.

3.3.3. Monitoring of Supplement Use

Monitoring of supplement use is particularly important in countries where premarket approval is not required to detect potential adverse reactions. Dietary indicators are known to be imprecise and estimates of usual intake are lacking for many nutrients [59]. Biochemical indicators of deficiency are often not well linked with adverse health outcomes, underscoring the need for more attention to be paid to the development of agreed on measures of deficiency and excess [60]. Recent work on key nutrient biomarkers is now available, facilitating the monitoring of high risk groups, such as pregnant women for folate status [61, 62].

3.3.4. Authoritative Recommendations for Dietary Supplements

Health and nutrition experts differ on whether it is appropriate to include recommendations for nutrient containing dietary supplements in national health promotion and disease prevention recommendations. Many countries opt to recommend that adequate nutrient intake for the general public be achieved solely from foods, and reserve recommendations of specific nutrient supplements for specific subgroups in the population. Others recommend only food alone with no recommendations for special populations.

3.3.5. Inclusion of Dietary Supplements in Food Programs to Reduce Malnutrition

There is pressure by industry to include MVM or other dietary supplements in food programs. However, there is little evidence that the target groups are deficient in the ingredients in the supplements, nor has it been demonstrated that provision of a supplement leads to better health outcomes.

3.3.6. Stimulating Innovation

The development of new and more highly bioavailable forms of the nutrients, timed release, dosage forms, novel bioactive constituents and the appropriate application of new technologies such as nanotechnology are all important, but some pose new scientific and regulatory challenges.

4. Case Study: Office of Dietary Supplements (ODS), National Institutes of Health (NIH), USA

This case study highlights some examples of dietary supplement research supported by or conducted at the ODS, and provides some research tools it has developed that may be useful resources for scientists both there and abroad.

4.1. Background

Since its establishment in 1995 as part of the implementation of the Dietary Supplement and Health Education Act [17, 18] of 1994, the ODS is the lead federal agency devoted to the scientific exploration of dietary supplements. Its mission is to support, conduct and coordinate scientific research and provide intellectual leadership to strengthen the knowledge and understanding of dietary supplements in order to enhance the US population's health and quality of life. ODS's four goals are to: expand the scientific knowledge base on dietary supplements by stimulating and supporting a full range of biomedical research and by developing and contributing to collaborative initiatives, workshops, meetings and conferences; enhance the dietary supplement research workforce through training and career development; foster development and dissemination of research resources and tools to enhance the quality of dietary supplement research; and translate dietary supplement research findings into useful information for consumers, health professionals, researchers, and policymakers. Several of its major initiatives that have expanded the scientific knowledge base on dietary supplements are described elsewhere in this special issue of NUTRIENTS. They include studies to clarify the implications for public health of omega-3 fatty acids [63], iodine [64], vitamin D [65], and iron [66].

4.2. Research Resources and Tools

This section provides the details on freely available research resources developed by ODS that are available for scientists to use to enhance the quality of dietary supplement research and meet public health priorities, with a focus on those that may be useful to scientists in other countries.

4.3. Analytical Methods for Dietary Supplements

The rigorous assessment of dietary supplement ingredients requires accurate, precise and reliable analytical methods and matching reference materials. The ODS Analytical Methods and Reference Materials program accelerates the creation and dissemination of validated methods and reference materials. It provides resources for characterization and verification of supplement product content that enhance the reliability and reproducibility of research using these products and supports product quality [67]. The genesis of the program was the paucity of publicly available methods for the analysis of supplement ingredients [68, 69]. In 2000, the US dietary supplement community tended to use proprietary or compendial methods for quality control operations, and scientists and laboratories often kept their proprietary methods to themselves. Negative publicity about discrepancies between label claims and the results of product testing performed by third parties led to some unsuccessful efforts on the part of the industry to pay a laboratory to develop and validate methods through the Association of Official Analytical Chemists International (AOACI). The program was not successful for several reasons, including lack of expert technical guidance and conflicting sponsor priorities. However, this early effort led to a collaboration between trade associations, ODS, the AOACI, the United States Pharmacopoeia (USP), NSF International, and others in an attempt to establish standard methods for dietary supplement analysis. The ODS became involved because explicit wording in DSHEA required the Government to use "publicly available" analytical methods for enforcement actions involving dietary supplements. In response to the need for such publicly available methods and to support efforts to validate methods used in biomedical research on dietary supplement ingredients, ODS established the Analytical Methods and Reference Materials (AMRM) program in 2002. ODS has been involved in sponsoring the creation of AOAC Official Methods of Analysis for dietary supplements and in the development and dissemination of numerous analytical methods and reference materials for 15 ingredients in dietary supplements in the USA, 32 botanical identification and documentation projects, and 45 studies determining contamination and adulterants. It has also helped to develop guidance on the validation of identity methods for botanical ingredients [70] and the conduct of single-laboratory validation studies for dietary supplements, Appendix K, AOAC Official Methods of Analysis, and provided guidance to evaluation of the literature on botanical supplements [71, 72]. The portion of the ODS website includes a searchable database of analytical methods; these can be accessed at: https://ods.od.nih.gov/Research/AMRMProgramWebsite.aspx. ODS also supports the Dietary Supplement Laboratory Quality Assurance Program in which participants measure concentrations of active and/or marker compounds and nutritional and toxic elements in practice and test materials. Exercises have included water and fat-soluble vitamins, nutritional and toxic elements, fatty acids, contaminants (e.g., aflatoxins, polyaromatic hydrocarbons (PAH's)) and botanical markers (e.g., phytosterols and flavonoids).

4.4. Reference Materials

ODS supports the development of certified reference materials for dietary supplement ingredients with assigned values for concentrations of active and/or marker compounds, pesticides, and toxic metals to assist in the verification of product label claims and in quality control during the manufacturing process. A reference material is a material that is sufficiently homogeneous and stable with respect to one or more specified properties, which have been established to be fit for its intended use in a measurement process. A certified reference material (CRM) is a reference material characterized by a metrologically valid procedure for one or more specified properties, accompanied by a certificate that provides the value of the specified property, its associated uncertainty, and a statement of metrological traceability. Certified reference materials can be used for laboratory proficiency studies, methods development, method verification, and method validation studies. Calibration standards are the single chemical entities necessary for construction of calibration curves for quantitative analysis and for confirming analyte identity. Several processes are used to produce calibration standards. ODS provided funding to the U.S. Department of Commerce's National Institute of Standards and Technology (NIST) for the development and distribution of calibration standard solutions and matrix standard reference materials (SRM®; a NIST-trademarked type of CRM). The materials fall into one of the following categories: (1) pure chemical entities or their mixtures, including many nutrients and other ingredients in dietary supplements for use in establishing analyte identity and for calibrating instruments; (2) natural matrix materials that represent the supply chain of a particular dietary supplement, e.g., biomass (ginkgo leaves and powder), processed botanical ingredient (ginkgo extract), finished product; (3) natural matrix materials that cover a range of analytes including nutritional compounds, botanical marker compounds, and compounds with known health concerns (heavy metals, pesticides, plant toxins); and (4) Clinical materials that can be used to assist clinical laboratories assess nutrient status or exposure, such as the measure of measure of vitamin D status commonly used around the world, serum 25-hydroxyvitamin D [73–75]. ODS is now expanding efforts to develop biomarkers of nutrient exposure and status in blood and other biological specimens in relation to chronic disease risk in individuals and populations. ODS has worked with NIST to produce and make available reference materials for calibration of various laboratory methods. Supplementary Table S1 shows NIST Standard Reference Materials (SRM®) now available. Supplementary Table S2 shows dietary supplement and nutritional assessment SRMs that are currently in progress.

4.5. Dietary Supplement Databases

Two databases have been developed by ODS that are described elsewhere in detail [76–80]. The goal of the Dietary Supplement Label Database (DSLD) is to include labels for virtually all dietary supplements sold in the USA. This provides all the information on the product label including composition, claims, and manufacturer contact information. It now contains over 72,000 dietary supplement labels, with new labels added at the rate of 1000 per month. Used together with food composition databases it is possible to estimate total daily intakes of nutrients and other bioactive ingredients from both foods and dietary supplements. A mobile version of DSLD is now available for use on smartphones to enhance consumer access to it [78, 80]. It is primarily aimed at researchers and so contains information about products that are currently on the market, as well as those that have been removed from the market. The Dietary Supplement Ingredient Database (DSID) provides analytically derived information on the amount of labeled ingredients of a representative sample of commonly used categories of supplement products sold in the USA, including adult, child and prenatal MVM supplements and omega-3 fatty acids. DSID is now being expanded to examine botanicals and other ingredients in supplements that are of public health interest, such as green tea products. Calculators included with the DSID permit a consumer to examine how closely the labeled contents of a nutrient in a product compare to chemical analyses of all products in the category [79].

4.6. Nutrition Research Methods and Review Methodology

Systematic reviews of dietary supplements require special techniques. ODS has sponsored a series of technical reports on the application of review methodology to the field of nutrition and dietary supplements [81–86]. Staff have also collaborated in performing systematic reviews with other groups [87, 88].

4.7. Population-Based Monitoring of Dietary Supplement Use

In collaboration with the National Health and Nutrition Examination Survey (NHANES) of the National Center for Health Statistics, ODS investigates patterns of dietary supplement use using national and other large cohorts, and assesses supplements' effects on total nutrient intakes. Several studies have focused on adults [89], children [90, 91], and others in the population and their supplement use. Other studies have focused on the contributions to total intakes of nutrients made by dietary supplements. Investigators at ODS have been active in funding monitoring efforts on the links between intakes of folic acid and health [92]. They have devoted particular attention to blood levels of folic acid and dietary intake patterns that are associated with very low and very high intakes of the nutrient [93–95]. The survey methods used are well documented and they may be useful for those in other countries planning similar population-based surveys to consult [96].

The motivations for use of dietary supplements are also documented; they often differ from those specified in regulations. NHANES contains several items that are consumer tested and available for use in other surveys on motivations. Knowledge of motivations can improve understanding of how people use these products and may provide clues for encouraging appropriate supplement use.

4.8. Translation of Supplement Science for Health Professionals and the Public

ODS has produced and periodically updates a library of more than two dozen fact sheets on the ingredients in supplements such as vitamin D, magnesium, and special products such as MVM supplements and products marketed for weight loss. There is a detailed version for professionals that is complete with detailed references, as well as easy-to-read versions for consumers in both English and Spanish. ODS also works with the National Library of Medicine (NLM) to produce and update a Dietary Supplement Subset of NLM's PubMed. The National Center for Complementary and Integrative Health (NCCIH) at NIH produces a series of fact sheets on many botanicals and other non-nutrient bioactives in supplements that are also useful. They can be accessed at https: //www.nccih.nih.gov. ODS also hosts an intensive, free 3-day course on issues in dietary supplement research annually for researchers. Further information about these and other projects is accessible at: https://www.ods.od.nih.gov.

4.9. Other Resources

In order to foster the development of appropriate study methods for dietary supplement research, ODS sponsors workshops on the latest knowledge and emerging approaches to the study of dietary supplements. It also supports the development of cutting–edge approaches to elucidate the mechanisms of action of complex botanical dietary supplements. It co-funds the Centers for Advancing Research on Natural Products (CARBON) with the NCCIM, including its program to develop high content high throughput methods to rapidly generate hypotheses on active compounds and the cellular targets. These and other resources are announced as they become available on the ODS website.

4.10. Fostering Use of Systematic Evidence Reviews in Policy Making and Clinical Practice

ODS has strengthened the scientific framework for developing dietary recommendations by encouraging the incorporation of systematic reviews into the development of the DRI. It has sponsored 18 systematic reviews on topics related to dietary supplements. These include ephedra, B vitamins, MVM supplements, omega-3 fatty acids, soy, probiotics, and vitamin D. The ephedra systematic review was helpful to the US government in banning ephedra products from the US market. The systematic reviews of omega-3 fatty acids funded over a decade ago and more recent updates on their associations with cardiovascular disease and infant health outcomes have been useful for planning intervention programs as well as for regulatory purposes. Current AHRQ reviews are available on the AHRQ website (https://www.ahrq.gov).

5. Medicinal Plants Used in Alternative/ Traditional Medicines

India is the largest producer of medicinal plants. There are currently about 250,000 registered medical practitioners of the Ayurvedic system, as compared to about 700,000 of the modern medicine. In India, around 20,000 medicinal plants have been recorded; however, traditional practitioners use only 7,000–7,500 plants for curing different diseases. The proportion of use of plants in the different Indian systems of medicine is Ayurveda 2000, Siddha 1300, Unani 1000, Homeopathy 800, Tibetan 500, Modern 200, and folk 4500. In India, around 25,000 effective plant-based formulations are used in traditional and folk medicine. More than 1.5 million practitioners are using the traditional medicinal system for health care in India. It is estimated that more than 7800 manufacturing units are involved in the production of natural health products and traditional plant-based formulations in India, which requires more than 2000 tons of medicinal plant raw material annually. More than 1500 herbals are sold as dietary supplements or ethnic traditional medicines [97, 98].

More than 80 percent of people in developing countries cannot afford the most basic medical procedures, drugs, and vaccines. Among wealthier populations in both developed and developing countries, complementary and alternative practices are popular although proof of their safety and effectiveness is modest. Evidence-based research in Ayurveda is receiving larger acceptance in India and abroad [98-101]. The National Center for Complementary and Alternative Medicine has been inaugurated as the United States Federal Government's lead agency for scientific research in this arena of medicine. Its mission is to explore complementary and alternative healing practices in the context of rigorous science, support sophisticated research, train researchers, disseminate information to the public on the modalities that work, and explain the scientific rationale underlying discoveries. The center is committed to explore and fund all such therapies for which there is sufficient preliminary data, compelling public health need and ethical justifications [102, 103].

Table 2. Impact of modern food concept in required nutrition [97-103]

Nutrients	Intake by Traditional Ways	Intake by Modern Ways	Effect on Nutrient Intake
Water soluble vitamins (vitamins B and C) and minerals	Vegetables used for cooking were/are fresh	Freezing and packaging of the cut vegetables	Loss of ascorbic acid, water soluble vitamins, and minerals
Proteins, minerals, and vitamin B complex	Manual processing of cereals, without polishing	Milling and polishing of cereals	Reduces protein, minerals, and vitamin B complex
Calcium, iron, thiamine, and niacin	Fresh grinding at home	Heavy milling and poor storage conditions	Loss of calcium, iron, thiamin, and niacin
Iron	Cooking in iron pot	Food generally cooked in cookware like nonstick and Teflon-coated utensils	The benefit of organic iron from the conventional iron pot is not obtained by using modern cookware
Copper	Storing of water and cooking use of copper vessels	Stainless steel utensils and plastic wares	Copper required in minor amount which is not gained from modern utensils used today. Deficiency is known to cause chronic diarrhea, malabsorption problems, and reduce immunity. Use of plastic containers is also harmful

Table 3. Some common medicinal plants having nutraceutical potential and their primary use in traditional medicine [97-104]

Plant Name	Common Name	Uses
Asparagus racemosus Willd	Shatavari	A potent Ayurvedic rejuvenative. It supplies many female hormones and mostly recommended for those women who have hysterectomies. It also helps to maintain urinary tract and strengthens the immune system and also purifies the blood.
Commiphora mukul Engl.	Guggul	A major ingredient in joint and immunocare and regarded as a remedy in Ayurvedic medicine; it increase white blood cell count to possess strong 264arieg-modulating properties. It also protects against the common cold as well as used in various other conditions like lower cholesterol and triglycerides, while maintaining the HDL to LDL ratio.
Cyperus scariosus Br.	Nagarmusta	Useful in supporting healthy genitourinary system and have hepatoprotective properties.
Garcinia cambogia Dr	Garcinia	Fruits contain biologically active compounds (¯) hydroxycitric acid, which is known to inhibit the synthesis of lipids and fatty acids. HCA inhibits the enzyme ATP-citrate lyase that leads to reduce production of acetyl CoA, which is a key substance in fat and carbohydrate metabolism. Therefore, formation of LDL and triglycerides is very low. It also suppresses appetite by promoting synthesis of glycogen. That way the brain gets signals of fullness and satisfaction sooner. Garcinia contains significant amounts of vitamin C and used as a heart tonic.
Glycyrrhiza glabra L.	Yashtimadhu, Licorice	It is a versatile medicine in India and China, for gastrointestinal health. It is a mild laxative, soothes and tones the mucous membranes, and relieves muscle spasms. It is

Plant Name	Common Name	Uses
		an antioxidant, cancer protecting, botanical boosting, and certain immune functions such as interferon production. Its mode of action is as an antimutagen, preventing damage to genetic material that can eventually result in cancer.
Gymnema sylvestre R. Br.	Gurmarar	Its Sanskrit name means literally "sugar destroyer," has a glycolytic action, and reduces the strength of a glucose solution. It has been used in Ayurveda to regulate sugar metabolism for several centuries. It increases insulin production, regeneration of pancreas cells, and the site of insulin production. Another property is abolishing the taste of sugar, so that Gurmarar has been effective to suppress and neutralize the craving for sweets.
Melia azadirachta L.	Nimba, Neem	It has strong health alleviating activity, used as a tonic and astringent that promotes healing. The extract has antispasmodic action. Its usage in Ayurvedic medicine for thousands of years has proved its detoxifying properties. It has shown most beneficial effects for the circulatory, digestive, respiratory, and urinary systems.
Momordica charantia L.	Karela, Bitter melon	Karela has been widely used in Ayurvedic medicine. It contains Gurmarin, a polypeptide considered to be similar to bovine insulin, and has a strong sugar regulating effect by suppressing the neural responses to sweet taste stimuli.
Moringa pterygosperma Gaertn	Shigru, Horseradish tree	Shigru contains physiologically active principles that is effective in a broad range of health needs. It contains "Pterygospermin," an antibiotic-like substance.
Mucuna pruriens Baker	Kiwanch, Kapikachchhu, Cow-itch plant	It is a good natural source of *L. dopa*. In the Ayurvedic system it is reported as an effective tonic for nervous system. Studies have demonstrated its usefulness maintaining optimum performance of the nervous system.
Nardostachys jatamansi DC.	Jatamansi, Musk root	Jatamansi is a relaxing plant, effectiveness for mental health. It is used in various Ayurvedic formulations as a potent ingredient. It has been shown effective in maintaining a restful sleep and with many menopausal symptoms.
Piper longum L.	Pippali, Indian Long Pepper	Pippali is a powerful stimulant for both the digestive and the respiratory systems and has a rejuvenating effect on lungs. It plays an important role in release of metabolic heat energy. This effect is the result of increased thyroid hormone level in the body. Pippali a typical Ayurvedic complementary component whose benefit is to increase the bioavailability and enhance absorption of the other active ingredients.
Piper nigrum L.	Maricha, Black pepper	The black pepper is one of the most important spices which is widely used to amplify the body's ability to absorb nutrients contained in the food and aid the digestive process.
Bergenia ligulata Wall	Pasanavheda	It has the unique property like diuretic action with optimum urinary tract health. This important drug supports bladder by acting on the crystalloid-colloid balance and keeping calcium salts in solution.
Terminalia chebula Retz.	Haritaki	Haritaki is a safe and effective purgative, expectorant, and tonic. It is an important ingredient of the classical Ayurvedic formulation "Triphala" which has a combination of three fruits. Tiphalpha is an important Ayurvedic medicine, which promotes health through successive steps of purification and detoxification. It is known to have strong antimutagenic activity, because of its very rich content vitamin C.
Tinospora cordifolia Miers	Guduchi	Guduchi is a rich source of natural vitamin C and effective in inhibiting the growth of bacteria and in building up the immune resistance and has immune-boosting ability. Use of this plant increases white blood cells the killing ability of macrophages, the immune cells responsible for fighting invaders.
Withania somnifera (L.) Dunal	Ashwagandha	In Ayurvedic medicines Ashwagandha holds a place similar to Ginseng in traditional Chinese medicinal therapies. It is also called the "Indian Ginseng". It has been used for thousands of years as a popular remedy in Ayurvedic systems for many conditions. It is one of the best health tonics and restorative agents that have been used to treat general debility.
Zingiber officinale Rosc	Sunthi, Ginger	Ginger is considered an adjuvant in many Ayurvedic formulas in which it enhances absorption and prevents gastrointestinal side effects. It is a very common spice which is used in Ayurvedic medicine to improve digestion and to prevent nausea. These properties help bowel movements and relax the muscles which control the digestive system.

Table 4. Some important herbal formulations frequently used in traditional Ayurvedic system in India [105]

Disease	Formulation's Ingredients/Ratio	Dose/Method of Use
Anemia	*Asparagus racemosus* (roots) 20% *Withania somnifera* (roots) 20% *Phyllanthus emblica* (fruits) 15% *P. amarus* (leaves) 10% *Tephrosia purpurea* (leaves) 10% *Plumbago zeylanica* (roots) 5% *Glycyrrhiza glabra* (roots) 15% *Piper longum* (fruits) 5%	4 gm of powder is given to the patient, twice daily with water
Asthma/bronchitis	*Solanum xanthocarpum* (whole plant) 25% *Piper longum* (fruits) 10% *Adhatoda vasica* (leaves) 25% *Zingiber officinale* (roots) 10% *Curcuma zedoaria* (roots) 10% *Ocimum sanctum* (leaves) 10% *Phyllanthus emblica* (fruits) 10%	4 gm (one teaspoonful) of mixed powder given to the patient, twice a day (morning and at bedtime) with water
Arthritis	*Piper longum* (fruits) 10% *xanthocarpum* (whole plant) 15% *Withania somnifera* (roots) 10% *Terminalia chebula* (fruits) 10% *bellerica* (fruits) 10% *Curcuma zedoaria* (roots) 15% *Phyllanthus emblica* (fruits) 15% *Ricinus communis* (roots) 15%	4 gm of mixed powder should be given to the patient, twice daily (morning and evening, one hour before meals) with ginger juice for rheumatic problems
Blood circulation	*Zingiber officinale* (roots) 20% *Piper longum* (roots) 10% *Withania somnifera* (roots) 10% *Phyllanthus emblica* (fruits) 10% *Curcuma longa* (roots) 10% *Terminalia bellerica* (fruits) 10% *T. chebula* (fruits) 10% *Ocimum sanctum* (leaves) 10% *Tephrosia purpurea* (leaves) 10%	4 gm of mixed powder is given to the patient, twice daily with water
Cancer	*Azadirachta indica* (bark) 20% *Bauhinia 266ariegate* (bark) 15% *Crataeva nurvala* (bark) 15% *Terminalia chebula* (fruits) 15% *T. bellerica* (fruits) 10% *Holarrhena antidysenterica* (bark) 10% *Tinospora cordifolia* (stems) 15%	4 gm of mixed powder should be given to the patient, twice a day (morning and night) with lukewarm honey for cancer cure
Chronic constipation	*Holarrhena antidysenterica* (bark) 10% *Plumbago ovata* (husk) 20% *Terminalia bellerica* (fruits) 10% *T. chebula* (fruits) 15% *Phyllanthus emblica* (fruits) 15% *Cassia angustifolia* (leaves) 20% *Glycyrrhiza glabra* (roots) 10%	4 gm of mixed powder is given to the patient, at night before going to bed, with water
Chronic fever	*Tinospora cordifolia* (stems) 15% *Ocimum sanctum* (leaves) 15% *Adhatoda vasica* (leaves) 15% *Azadirachta indica* (leaves) 15% *Holarrhena antidysenterica* (bark) 10% *Piper longum* (fruits) 10% *Zingiber officinale* (roots) 10%	4 gm of mixed powder is given to the patient, twice daily before meals with water

Disease	Formulation's Ingredients/Ratio	Dose/Method of Use
	Terminalia bellerica (fruits) 10%	
Cough	*Phyllanthus emblica* (fruits) 25% *Adhatoda vasica* (leaves) 20% *Ocimum sanctum* (leaves) 10% *Piper longum* (fruits) 10% *Zingiber officinale* (roots) 10% *Glycyrrhiza glabra* (roots) 15% *Solanum xanthocarpum* (whole plant) 10%	3 gm of mixed powder should be given to the patient twice daily (morning and at night before going to bed) with lukewarm mixed with honey to cure cold
Cysts	*Terminalia chebula* (fruits) 20% *Azadirachta indica* (bark) 20% *Holarrhena antidysenterica* (bark) 10% *Terminalia bellerica* (fruits) 10% *Withania somnifera* (roots) 20% *Tinospora cordifolia* (stems) 20%	4 gm of mixed (one teaspoonful) powder is given to the patient, twice a day (morning and evening) with water
Cysts	*Terminalia chebula* (fruits) 20% *Azadirachta indica* (bark) 20% *Holarrhena antidysenterica* (bark) 10% *Terminalia bellerica* (fruits) 10% *Withania somnifera* (roots) 20% *Tinospora cordifolia* (stems) 20%	4 gm of mixed (one teaspoonful) powder is given to the patient, twice a day (morning and evening) with water
Dental diseases	*Azadirachta indica* (leaves) 15% *A. arabia* (bark) 15% *Areca catechu* (bark) 15% *Achyranthes aspera* (leaves) 10% *Ficus benghalensis* (bark) 15% *Quercus infectoria* (fruits) 15% *Symplocos 267ariegat* (bark) 15%	The powder is applied to the gums and teeth, two times a day. Additionally a gargle of the decoction (3 gm of powder mixed in 150 mL of water)
Diarrhoea	*Holarrhena antidysenterica* (bark) 25% *Aegle marmelos* (fruits) 25% *Zingiber officinale* (roots) 10% *Terminalia chebula* (fruits) 10% *Cyperus rotundus* (roots) 10% *Syzygium cumini* (seeds) 10% *Phyllanthus emblica* (fruits) 10%	3 gm of mixed powder is given to the patient, three times a day, with curd for dysentery and diarrhoea
Dislocation of bones	*Asparagus racemosus* (roots) 15% *Withania somnifera* (roots) 15% *Azadirachta 267ariega* (bark) 20% *Terminalia arjuna* (bark) 20% *T. chebula* (fruits) 10% *T. bellerica* (fruits) 10% *Phyllanthus emblica* (fruits) 10%	3 gm of mixed powder is given to the patient, twice a day with water for dislocation of bones and fractures
Diabetes	*Gymnema sylvestre* (leaves) 30% *Tinospora cordifolia* (stems) 15% *Azadirachta indica* (leaves) 10% *Phyllanthus emblica* (fruits) 20% *Curcuma longa* (roots) 10% *Aegle marmelos* (leaves) 15%	4 gm of mixed powder should be given to the patient, twice a day with water
Fistula	*Glycyrrhiza glabra* (roots) 20% *Terminalia chebula* (fruits) 20% *T. bellerica* (fruits) 15% *Tinospora cordifolia* (stems) 15% *Azadirachta indica* (leaves) 15% *Withania somnifera* (roots) 15%	3 gm of mixed powder should be given to the patient, twice daily with water to treat fistula

Table 4. (Continued)

Disease	Formulation's Ingredients/Ratio	Dose/Method of Use
Female sterility	*Asparagus racemosus* (roots) 20% *Withania somnifera* (roots) 20% *Glycyrrhiza glabra* (roots) 20% *Phyllanthus emblica* (fruits) 10% *Ficus glomerata* (bark) 10% *F. religiosa* (bark) 10%	3 gm of mixed powder is given to the patient twice daily, half an hour before meals with milk
General health tonic	*Withania somnifera* (roots) 20% *Asparagus racemosus* (roots) 10% *Glycyrrhiza glabra* (roots) 10% *Tribulus terrestris* (fruits) 10% *Phyllanthus emblica* (fruits) 15% *Terminalia arjuna* (bark) 15% *Centella asiatica* (leaves) 10%	4 gm of powder is given to the patient, twice daily (morning and evening) with milk
Gastritis	*Zingiber officinale* (roots) 10% *Piper longum* (fruits) 10% *Mentha piperita* (leaves) 10% *Terminalia chebula* (fruits) 15% *T. bellerica* (fruits) 15% *Phyllanthus emblica* (fruits) 15% *Plumbago zeylanica* (roots) 10% *Tinospora cordifolia* (stems) 15%	4 gm of (one teaspoonful) mixed powder is given to the patient twice daily, half an hour before meals with water
Hair problems	*Eclipta alba* (leaves) 15% *Centella asiatica* (leaves) 15% *Terminalia chebula* (fruits) 10% *T. bellerica* (fruits) 10% *Phyllanthus emblica* (fruits) 15% *Glycyrrhiza glabra* (roots) 15% *Tinospora cordifolia* (stems) 10% *Tribulus terrestris* (fruits) 10%	4 gm of mixed powder is given to the patient, twice a daily with honey
High blood pressure	*Terminalia arjuna* (bark) 35% *T. chebula* (fruits) 15% *Asparagus racemosus* (roots) 15% *Zingiber officinale* (roots) 10% *Withania somnifera* (roots) 25%	4 gm of powder is given to the patient, twice a day (morning and night) with honey
Heart tonic	*Withania somnifera* (roots) 10% *Terminalia arjuna* (bark) 30% *T. bellerica* (fruits) 10% *T. chebula* (fruits) 10% *Cyperus rotundus* (roots) 10% *Phyllanthus emblica* (fruits) 10% *Ocimum sanctum* (leaves) 10%	3 gm of mixed powder is given to the patient, twice a day with water
Intestinal worms	*Holarrhena antidysenterica* (bark) 10% *Mentha piperita* (leaves) 10% *Tinospora cordifolia* (stems) 20% *Butea monosperma* (seeds) 20% *Azadirachta indica* (leaves) 10% *Phyllanthus emblica* (fruits) 20% *Tribulus terrestris* (fruits) 10%	3 gm of mixed powder is given to the patient, twice daily (morning and night) with water
Epilepsy	*Centella asiatica* (leaves) 30% *Withania somnifera* (roots) 20% *Tribulus terrestris* (fruits) 15% *Piper longum* (roots) 10%	3 gm mixed powder is given to the patient, twice daily (morning and evening) with fruit juice to treat Hysteria

Disease	Formulation's Ingredients/Ratio	Dose/Method of Use
	Achyranthes aspera (leaves) 15% *Plumbago zeylanica* (roots) 10%	
Leucorrhoea	*Symplocos 269ariegat* (bark) 35% *Asparagus racemosus* (roots) 15% *Adhatoda vasica* (leaves) 10% *Aegle marmelos* (fruits) 10% *Phyllanthus emblica* (fruits) 10% *Azadirachta indica* (bark) 10%	3 gm of mixed powder is given to the patient, twice daily with water
Leucoderma	*Psoralea corylifolia* (seeds) 20% *Terminalia chebula* (fruits) 10% *Phyllanthus emblica* (fruits) 20% *Azadirachta indica* (bark) 20% *Areca catechu* (bark) 10% *Tinospora cordifolia* (stems) 10% *Eclipta alba* (leaves) 10%	3 gm of mixed powder should be given to the patient, twice a day before meals with water
Liver tonic	*Holarrhena antidysenterica* (bark) 10% *Eclipta alba* (leaves) 20% *Tephrosia purpurea* (leaves) 20% *Tinospora cordifolia* (stems) 10% *Azadirachta indica* (bark) 10% *Phyllanthus amarus* (whole plant) 20% *Plumbago zeylanica* (roots) 10%	4 gm of mixed powder is given to the patient twice daily, half an hour before meals with water
Lack of appetite	*Zingiber officinale* (roots) 10% *Piper longum* (fruits) 10% *Phyllanthus emblica* (fruits) 30% *Terminalia chebula* (fruits) 15% *Tinospora cordifolia* (stems) 15% *Cassia angustifolia* (leaves) 10% *Mentha piperita* (leaves) 10%	4 gm of mixed powder is given to the patient, two times a day after meals with water for indigestion
Male sterility	*Withania somnifera* (roots) 15% *Mucuna pruriens* (seeds) 25% *Tribulus terrestris* (fruits) 20% *Glycyrrhiza glabra* (roots) 10% *Terminalia arjuna* (bark) 10% *Phyllanthus emblica* (fruits) 10% *Zingiber officinale* (roots) 5% *Piper longum* (fruits) 5%	4 gm of mixed powder is given to the patient, twice a day with honey
Migraine	*Curcuma longa* (roots) 15% *Glycyrrhiza glabra* (roots) 15% *Azadirachta indica* (bark) 15% *Tinospora cordifolia* (stems) 15% *Terminalia chebula* (fruits) 10% *Ocimum sanctum* (leaves) 15% *Eclipta alba* (leaves) 15%	4 gm of mixed powder is given to the patient, twice a day with honey
Obesity	*Terminalia chebula* (fruits) 15% *Terminalia bellerica* (fruits) 15% *Phyllanthus emblica* (fruits) 10% *Crataeva nurvala* (bark) 25% *Tribulus terrestris* (fruits) 25% *Zingiber officinale* (roots) 10%	4 gm of powder is given to the patient, twice a day with warm water

Table 4. (Continued)

Disease	formulation's Ingredients/Ratio	Dose/Method of Use
Paralysis	*Curcuma zedoaria* (roots) 20% *Withania somnifera* (roots) 20% *Tribulus terrestris* (fruits) 20% *Zingiber officinale* (roots) 20% *Piper longum* (fruits) 5% *Crataeva nurvala* (leaves) 10% *Plumbago zeylanica* (roots) 5%	3 gm of mixed powder is given to the patient, three times a day with honey
Prostate enlargement	*Tinospora cordifolia* (stems) 15% *Tribulus terrestris* (fruits) 15% *Phyllanthus emblica* (fruits) 15% *Zingiber officinale* (roots) 10% *Butea monosperma* (seeds) 10% *Adhatoda vasica* (leaves) 5% *Terminalia chebula* (fruits) 10% *T. bellerica* (fruits) 10% *Glycyrrhiza glabra* (roots) 10%	4 gm of mixed powder is given to the patient twice a day, morning and evening before meals with water
Piles	*Eclipta alba* (leaves) 35% *Terminalia chebula* (fruits) 15% *Terminalia bellerica* (fruits) 10% *Phyllanthus emblica* (fruits) 10% *Adhatoda vasica* (leaves) 10% *Plumbago zeylanica* (roots) 5% *Piper longum* (fruits) 5% *Aegle marmelos* (fruits) 10%	4 gm of mixed powder is given to the patient, twice daily (morning and at bedtime) with water
Sleeplessness	*Withania somnifera* (roots) 20% *Centella asiatica* (leaves) 30% *Piper longum* (roots) 20% *Glycyrrhiza glabra* (roots) 10% *Terminalia bellerica* (fruits) 10%	3 gm mixed powder is given to the patient, at night before going to bed, with milk
Skin diseases	*Cyperus rotundus* (roots) 10% *Tinospora cordifolia* (stems) 20% *Azadirachta indica* (bark) 20% *Terminalia chebula* (fruits) 10% *T. bellerica* (fruits) 10% *Curcuma longa* (roots) 10% *Phyllanthus emblica* (fruits) 10% *Centella asiatica* (leaves) 10%	3 gm of powder is given to the patient, twice a day before meals with water to cure allergy problems
Sexual debility	*Withania somnifera* (roots) 10% *Mucuna pruriens* (seeds) 20% *Asparagus racemosus* (roots) 10% *Sida cordifolia* (seeds) 10% *Tribulus terrestris* (fruits) 20% *Glycyrrhiza glabra* (roots) 10%	About 4 gm of mixed powder should be given to the patient, twice daily (morning and at night before going to bed) with milk
Throat diseases	*Glycyrrhiza glabra* (roots) 30% *Terminalia chebula* (fruits) 10% *T. bellerica* (fruits) 10% *Solanum xanthocarpum* (whole plant) 20% *Piper longum* (fruits) 10% *Sida cordifolia* (roots) 10% *Phyllanthus emblica* (fruits) 10%	4 gm of mixed powder is given to the patient twice daily, morning and at bedtime with honey
Thyroid problems	*Crataeva nurvala* (bark) 20% *Bauhinia 270ariegate* (bark) 20% *Sida cordifolia* (leaves) 15%	3 gm of mixed powder is given to the patient, twice daily with lukewarm water

Disease	formulation's Ingredients/Ratio	Dose/Method of Use
	Terminalia chebula (fruits) 10% *T. bellerica* (fruits) 10% *Glycyrrhiza glabra* (roots) 15% *Zingiber officinale* (roots) 10%	
Urinary tract	*Tribulus terrestris* (fruits) 25% *Zingiber officinale* (roots) 10% *Solanum xanthocarpum* (whole plant) 10% *Crataeva nurvala* (bark) 25% *Tinospora cordifolia* (stems) 10% *Asparagus racemosus* (roots) 10% *Tephrosia purpurea* (leaves) 10%	4 gm of mixed powder is given to the patient, twice a day with water

The nomenclature for nutraceuticals is based on the segments it constitutes. In Canada, this term is natural health products; in USA, it is called dietary supplements, and in Japan it is called foods for special health use. There are distinct definitions and regulations for dietary supplements and functional foods in USA, Canada, and Europe. In Japan, dietary supplements and functional foods are governed under the same set of regulations. USA and Canada actually list the constituents that a product must have to be called a nutraceutical, whereas Europe and Japan just provide general guidelines on the properties that a product should have to be called a nutraceutical. Traditional and herbal medicines are included in the definition of dietary or nutritional supplements in Canada. Japan does not mention traditional herbal medicines under functional foods for special health use.

6. Future Needs

Attitudes toward safety, efficacy, and values about what is important in food and life will be important in determining future needs involving supplement science in the countries we have discussed and perhaps elsewhere in the world. Safety is critical, and requires better chains of custody and product characterization that exists at present for these products, particularly those involving global markets. Efficacy, that is that the health promotion claims for the product are true and not misleading is also critical. Demonstrating efficacy requires clinical studies with well defined products and rigorous experimental designs, and the studies must be replicable. To that end, many publishers now require that submitted manuscripts comply with established guidelines for the reporting of clinical trial results (e.g., CONSORT guidelines), while funders require demonstration of product integrity by applicants [106, 107]. Finally, there are issues of personal choice and values, sometimes involving the efficacy of supplements as complementary and alternative therapies that are part of a larger philosophical or religious world views and systems. These must be accommodated without abandoning safety.

Both basic and more applied challenges will continue well into the future. Much remains to be learned about the effects of bioactive constituents such as flavonoids in foods and dietary supplements on health outcomes, as many recent papers in Nutrients and elsewhere indicate [108-110]. More and better biomarkers need to be developed and their associations with health outcomes clarified [111]. Supplements intended to enhance sports performance [112] botanicals used for disease treatment [113] and those ingredients thought to slow aging [114] all require identification of valid biomarkers of efficacy as well as of exposure. The role of supplements and the gut microbiome also must be explored for its associations with common diseases and conditions [115]. The associations between supplement ingredients and health outcomes in chronic degenerative disease must be clarified [47, 1014, 116–118]. High risk groups need more attention. Certain subgroups within the population such as athletes consume very high amounts of some supplements and it is important to monitor them to prevent adverse outcomes and study the effects, if any, on athletic performance [119]. Others use supplements in the hope that they will improve cognitive performance [112]. Those who practice polypharmacy with prescription, non-prescription drugs and dietary supplements represent another high-risk group, and interventions to limit the potential for adverse events are needed [120, 121]. Collaborations among scientists in many countries are needed to drive supplement science forward. Irrespective of the type of health product, high quality science is fundamental to the success of any regulatory framework. Assessments of the safety, quality and efficacy of nutrients and other bioactives are needed to provide the scientific information that regulators need. As mentioned earlier, the nature and diversity of the sector means that regulators face a number of very specific challenges for these low risk products. These include evaluating traditional evidence, dealing with products that contain multiple bioactives and addressing the growing challenges of ensuring product quality. It is critical that scientists and regulators work together and learn from each other in both identifying issues and developing ways in which they can be addressed. Although regulatory challenges must be met at the national level, there must be due regard paid to the fact that national regulatory decisions about supplements have global implications [121-123].

CONCLUSION

If the situation prevailing in this sector is analyzed taking into consideration different aspects- it becomes clear that there is a perceptible trend towards increased usage of drugs used in Indian Traditional Systems especially those which are based on herbal products not only in India but in different parts of the world. However, one of the basic problems that still remained to be solved is related to proving efficacy of the products used in these systems on the basis of controlled clinical trial and complementary pharmacological studies. It is difficult to ensure consistency in the results and components in the products. This is traced mainly to lack of standardization of the inputs used and the process adopted for preparation of the formulations. Government of India has taken these aspects in to consideration and has initiated many projects for standardization of single and compound formulations along with standardization of operating procedures for important formulations. Though standardization is very difficult it is not an un-attainable goal. Science is vital in regulatory settings, and there is no reason that science and regulation should be incompatible. The challenges in supplement science and its regulation provide new opportunities for scientists and regulators to work together both nationally and internationally, to learn from each other, and to cooperate and when appropriate harmonize approaches to improve the public health.

References

[1] White, A. Growth-inhibition produced in rats by the oral administration of sodium benzoate: Effects of various dietary supplements. *Yale J. Biol. Med.* 1941, *13*, 759–768.

[2] Kantor, E.D., Rehm, C.D., Du, M., White, E., Giovannucci, E.L. Trends in dietary supplement use among US adults from 1999–2012. *JAMA Intern. Med.* 2016, *316*, 1464–1474.

[3] Marik, P.E., Flemmer, M. Do dietary supplements have beneficial health effects in industrialized nations: What is the evidence? *JPEN J. Parenter. Enter. Nutr.* 2012, *36*, 159–168.

[4] Manson, J.E., Brannon, P.M., Rosen, C.J., Taylor, C.L. Vitamin D deficiency—is there really a pandemic? *N. Engl. J. Med.* 2016, *375*, 1817–1820.

[5] Balentine, D.A., Dwyer, J.T., Erdman, J.W., Jr., Ferruzzi, M.G., Gaine, P.C., Harnly, J.M., Kwik-Uribe, C.L. Recommendations on reporting requirements for flavonoids in research. *Am. J. Clin. Nutr.* 2015, *101*, 1113–1125.

[6] Betz, J.M., (NIH Office of Dietary Supplements, Bethesda, MD, USA). *Personal communication,* 2017.

[7] Mudge, E.M., Betz, J.M., Brown, P.N. The importance of method selection in determining product integrity for nutrition research. *Adv. Nutr.* 2016, *7*, 390–398.

[8] Orhan, I.E., Senol, F.S., Skalicka-Wozniak, K., Georgiev, M., Sener, B. Adulteration and safety issues in nutraceuticals and dietary supplements: Innocent or risky? In *Nutraceuticals, Nanotechnology in the Agri-Food Industry*; Grumezescu, A.M., Ed., Academic Press: Amsterdam, The Netherlands, 2016; Volume 4, pp. 153–182.

[9] AOAC International. AOAC International guidelines for validation of botanical identification methods. *J. AOAC Int.* 2012, *95*, 268–272.

[10] Dwyer, J.T., Holden, J., Andrews, K., Roseland, J., Zhao, C., Schweitzer, A., Perry, C.R., Harnly, J., Wolf, W.R., Picciano, M.F., et al. Measuring vitamins and minerals in dietary supplements for nutrition studies in the USA. *Anal. Bioanal. Chem.* 2007, *389*, 37–46.

[11] Swanson, C.A. Suggested guidelines for articles about botanical dietary supplements. *Am. J. Clin. Nutr.* 2002, *75*, 8–10.

[12] Wolsko, P.M., Solondz, D.K., Phillips, R.S., Schachter, S.C., Eisenberg, D.M. Lack of herbal supplement characterization in published randomized controlled trials. *Am. J. Med.* 2005, *118*, 1087–1093.

[13] Gagnier, J.J., DeMelo, J., Boon, H., Rochon, P., Bombardier, C. Quality of reporting of randomized controlled trials of herbal medicine interventions. *Am. J. Med.* 2006, *119*, 800.e1–800.e11.

[14] Dwyer, J., Costello, R.B., Merkel, J. Assessment of dietary supplements. In *Nutrition in the Prevention and Treatment of Disease*, 4th ed., Coulston, A.M., Boushey, C.J., Rerruzai, M.G., Delahaty, L.M., Eds., Academic Press: London, UK, 2017; pp. 49–70.

[15] Ahluwalia, N., Dwyer, J., Terry, A., Moshfegh, A., Johnson, C. Update on NHANES dietary data: Focus on collection, release, analytical considerations, and uses to inform public policy. *Adv. Nutr.* 2016, *7*, 121–134.

[16] Chan, M. Forward. In *WHO Traditional Medicine Strategy: 2014–2023*; WHO: Hong Kong, China, 2013; pp. 7–8. 17. Dickinson, A. History and overview of DSHEA. *Fitoterapia* 2011, *82*, 5–10. [CrossRef] [PubMed]

[17] Taylor, C.L. Regulatory frameworks for functional foods and dietary supplements. *Nutr. Rev.* 2004, *62*, 55–59.

[18] Australian Government Department of Health Therapeutic Goods Administration. *The Poisons Standard* (the SUSMP). Available online: https://www.tga.gov.au/publication/poisons-standard-susmp (accessed on 17 September 2017).

[19] U.S. Food and Drug Administration. *Dietary Supplements.* Available online: https://www.fda.gov/food/ dietarysupplements/

[20] *Health Canada. Monograph: Melatonin—Oral.* Available online: http://webprod.hc-sc.gc.ca/nhpidbdipsn/monoReq.do?id=136 (accessed on 17 September 2017).

[21] Ventola, C.L. Current issues regarding complementary and alternative medicine (CAM) in the United States: Part 2: Regulatory and safety concerns and proposed governmental policy changes with respect to dietary supplements. *P T* 2010, *35*, 514–522.

[22] World Health Organization. *National Policy on Traditional Medicine and Regulation of Herbal Medicines—Report of a WHO Global Survey.* Available online: http://apps.who.int/medicinedocs/en/d/Js7916e/ (accessed on 6 November 2017).

[23] Health Canada Natural and Non-prescription Health Products Directorate (NNHPD) *About Natural Health Product Regulation in Canada.* Available online: https://www.canada.ca/en/health-canada/services/drugs-health-products/natural-non-prescription/regulation.html.

[24] Australian Government Department of Health Therapeutic Goods Administration. *Exposure Drafts: Therapeutic Goods Amendment (2017 Measures No. 1) Bill 2017 and Therapeutic Goods (Charges) Amendment Bill* 2017. Available online: https://www.tga.gov.au/consultation/consultation-exposure-drafts-2017.

[25] European Commission Directorate-General for Health and Food Safety. *Herbal Medicinal Products.* Available online: https://ec.europa.eu/health/human-use/herbal-medicines_en.

[26] U.S. Food and Drug Administration. *New Dietary Ingredients (NDI) Notification Process.* Available online: https://www.fda.gov/food/dietarysupplements/new dietaryingredientsnotificationprocess/default.htm.

[27] Australian Government Department of Health Therapeutic Goods Administration. *Australian Regulatory Guidelines for Complementary Medicines (ARGCM).* Available online: https://www.tga.gov.au/publication/australian-regulatory-guidelines-complementary-medicines-argcm.

[28] Australian Government Department of Health Therapeutic Goods Administration. *Medicines and Medical Devices Regulation Review.* Available online: https://www.tga.gov.au/mmdr

[29] Australian Government Department of Health Therapeutic Goods Administration. *Australian Government Response to the Review of Medicines and Medical Devices Regulation.* Available online: https://www.tga.gov.au/australian-government-response-review-medicines-and-medical-devices-regulation.

[30] Government of Canada. *Category Specific Guidance for Temporary Marketing Authorization: Supplemented Food.* Available online: https://www.canada.ca/en/health-canada/services/food-nutrition/legislationguidelines/uidance-documents/category-specific-guidance-temporary-marketing-authorization supplemented-food.html.

[31] Government of Canada Health Canada. *Consulting Canadians on the Regulation of Self-Care Products in Canada.* Available online: https://www.canada.ca/en/health-canada/programs/consultation-regulation-selfcare-products/consulting-canadians-regulation-self-care-products-canada.html.

[32] Physiopedia. *Evidence Based Practice (EBP).* Available online: https://www.physio-pedia.com/Evidence_ Based_Practice_(EBP).

[33] Australian Government Department of Health Therapeutic Goods Administration. *Complementary Medicine Interface Issues.* Available online: https://www.tga.gov.au/complementary-medicine-interfaceissues.

[34] Singapore Government Health Science Authority. *ASEAN Harmonization of Traditional Medicines and Health Supplements.* Available online: http://www.hsa.gov.sg/content/hsa/en/Health_Products_Regulation/Complementary_Health_Products/Overview/ASEAN_Harmonization_of_Traditional_Medicines_and_Health_Supplements.html.

[35] World Health Organization. *International Regulatory Cooperation for Herbal Medicines* (IRCH). Available online: http://www.who.int/medicines/areas/traditional/irch/en/

[36] Gorman, U., Mathers, J.C., Grimaldi, K.A., Ahlgren, J., Nordstrom, K. Do we know enough? A scientific and ethical analysis of the basis for genetic-based personalized nutrition. *Genes Nutr.* 2013, *8*, 373–381.

[37] De Toro-Martin, J., Arsenault, B.J., Despres, J.P., Vohl, M.C. Precision nutrition: A review of personalized nutritional approaches for the prevention and management of metabolic syndrome. *Nutrients* 2017, *9*, 913.

[38] World Health Organization. *WHO Traditional Medicine Strategy: 2014–2023.* Available online: http://www.who.int/medicines/publications/traditional/trm_strategy14_23/en/

[39] Drueke, T.B., Massy, Z.A. Role of vitamin D in vascular calcification: Bad guy or good guy? *Nephrol. Dial. Transplant.* 2012, *27*, 1704–1707.

[40] Rooney, M.R., Harnack, L., Michos, E.D., Ogilvie, R.P., Sempos, C.T., Lutsey, P.L. Trends in use of high-dose vitamin D supplements exceeding 1000 or 4000 international units daily, 1999–2014. *JAMA Intern. Med.* 2017, *317*, 2448–2450.

[41] Prentice, R.L., Pettinger, M.B., Jackson, R.D., Wactawski-Wende, J., Lacroix, A.Z., Anderson, G.L., Chlebowski, R.T., Manson, J.E., Van Horn, L., Vitolins, M.Z., et al. Health risks and benefits from calcium and vitamin D supplementation: Women's Health Initiative clinical trial and cohort study. *Osteoporos. Int.* 2013, *24*, 567–580.

[42] Fulgoni, V.L., 3rd; Keast, D.R., Bailey, R.L., Dwyer, J. Foods, fortificants, and supplements: Where do Americans get their nutrients? *J. Nutr.* 2011, *141*, 1847–1854.

[43] Boyles, A.L., Yetley, E.A., Thayer, K.A., Coates, P.M. Safe use of high intakes of folic acid: Research challenges and paths forward. *Nutr. Rev.* 2016, *74*, 469–474.

[44] Dwyer, J.T., Wiemer, K.L., Dary, O., Keen, C.L., King, J.C., Miller, K.B., Philbert, M.A., Tarasuk, V., Taylor, C.L., Gaine, P.C., et al. Fortification and health: Challenges and opportunities. *Adv. Nutr.* 2015, *6*, 124–131.

[45] Dwyer, J.T., Woteki, C., Bailey, R., Britten, P., Carriquiry, A., Gaine, P.C., Miller, D., Moshfegh, A., Murphy, M.M., Smith Edge, M. Fortification: New findings and implications. *Nutr. Rev.* 2014, *72*, 127–141.

[46] Yetley, E.A., MacFarlane, A.J., Greene-Finestone, L.S., Garza, C., Ard, J.D., Atkinson, S.A., Bier, D.M., Carriquiry, A.L., Harlan, W.R., Hattis, D., et al. Options for basing Dietary Reference Intakes (DRIs) on chronic disease endpoints: Report from a joint US-/Canadian-sponsored working group. *Am. J. Clin. Nutr.* 2017, *105*, 249s–285s.

[47] Gaine, P.C., Balentine, D.A., Erdman, J.W., Jr., Dwyer, J.T., Ellwood, K.C., Hu, F.B., Russell, R.M. Are dietary bioactives ready for recommended intakes? *Adv. Nutr.* 2013, *4*, 539–541.

[48] Brown, A.C. Liver toxicity related to herbs and dietary supplements: Online table of case reports. Part 2 of 5 series. *Food Chem. Toxicol.* 2017, *107*, 472–501.

[49] Saldanha, L., Dwyer, J., Andrews, K., Betz, J., Harnly, J., Pehrsson, P., Rimmer, C., Savarala, S. Feasibility of including green tea products for an analytically verified dietary supplement database. *J. Food Sci.* 2015, *80*, H883–H888.

[50] Sander, L.C., Bedner, M., Tims, M.C., Yen, J.H., Duewer, D.L., Porter, B., Christopher, S.J., Day, R.D., Long, S.E., Molloy, J.L., et al. Development and certification of green tea-containing standard reference materials. *Anal. Bioanal. Chem.* 2012, *402*, 473–487.

[51] De Boer, Y.S., Sherker, A.H. Herbal and dietary supplement-induced liver injury. *Clin. Liver Dis.* 2017, *21*, 135–149.

[52] Avigan, M.I., Mozersky, R.P., Seeff, L.B. Scientific and regulatory perspectives in herbal and dietary supplement associated hepatotoxicity in the United States. *Int. J. Mol. Sci.* 2016, *17*, 331.

[53] Brown, A.C. An overview of herb and dietary supplement efficacy, safety and government regulations in the United States with suggested improvements. Part 1 of 5 series. *Food Chem. Toxicol.* 2017, *107*, 449–471.

[54] Gardiner, P., Phillips, R., Shaughnessy, A.F. Herbal and dietary supplement-drug interactions in patients with chronic illnesses. *Am. Fam. Physician* 2008, *77*, 73–78.

[55] Tsai, H.H., Lin, H.W., Simon Pickard, A., Tsai, H.Y., Mahady, G.B. Evaluation of documented drug interactions and contraindications associated with herbs and dietary supplements: A systematic literature review. *Int. J. Clin. Pract.* 2012, *66*, 1056–1078.

[56] Gagnier, J.J., Boon, H., Rochon, P., Moher, D., Barnes, J., Bombardier, C., Group, C. Reporting randomized, controlled trials of herbal interventions: An elaborated CONSORT statement. *Ann. Intern. Med.* 2006, *144*, 364–367.

[57] Blumberg, J.B., Frei, B.B., Fulgoni, V.L., Weaver, C.M., Zeisel, S.H. Impact of frequency of multi-vitamin/multi-mineral supplement intake on nutritional adequacy and nutrient deficiencies in U.S. adults. *Nutrients* 2017, *9*, 849.

[58] Raghavan, R., Ashour, F.S., Bailey, R. A review of cutoffs for nutritional biomarkers. *Adv. Nutr.* 2016, *7*, 112–120.

[59] Centers for Disease Control and Prevention National Center for Environmental Health Division of Laboratory Sciences. *Second National Report on Biochemical Indicators of Diet and Nutrition in the U.S. Population*; Centers for Disease Control and Prevention: Atlanta, GA, USA, 2012.

[60] Bailey, L.B., Stover, P.J., McNulty, H., Fenech, M.F., Gregory, J.F., 3rd; Mills, J.L., Pfeiffer, C.M., Fazili, Z., Zhang, M., Ueland, P.M., et al. Biomarkers of nutrition for development-folate review. *J. Nutr.* 2015, *145*, 1636s–1680s.

[61] Branum, A.M., Bailey, R., Singer, B.J. Dietary supplement use and folate status during pregnancy in the United States. *J. Nutr.* 2013, *143*, 486–492.

[62] Balk, E.M., Lichtenstein, A.H. Omega-3 fatty acids and cardiovascular disease: Summary of the 2016 Agency of Healthcare Research and Quality evidence review. *Nutrients* 2017, *9*, 865.

[63] Ershow, A.G., Skaeff, S., Merkel, J., Pehrsson, P. Development of databases on iodine in foods and dietary supplements. *Nutrients* 2018, in press.

[64] Taylor, C.L., Sempos, C.T., Davis, C.D., Brannon, P.M. Vitamin D: Moving forward to address emerging science. *Nutrients* 2017, *9*, 1308.

[65] Brannon, P.M., Taylor, C.L. Iron supplementation during pregnancy and infancy: Uncertainties and implications for research and policy. *Nutrients* 2017, *9*, 1327.

[66] Kuszak, A.J., Hopp, D.C., Williamson, J.S., Betz, J.M., Sorkin, B.C. Approaches by the U.S. National Institutes of Health to support rigorous scientific research on dietary supplements and natural products. *Drug Test. Anal.* 2016, *8*, 413–417.

[67] Betz, J.M., Fisher, K.D., Saldanha, L.G., Coates, P.M. The NIH analytical methods and reference materials program for dietary supplements. *Anal. Bioanal. Chem.* 2007, *389*, 19–25.

[68] Betz, J.M., Brown, P.N., Roman, M.C. Accuracy, precision, and reliability of chemical measurements in natural products research. *Fitoterapia* 2011, *82*, 44–52.

[69] LaBudde, R.A., Harnly, J.M. Probability of identification: A statistical model for the validation of qualitative botanical identification methods. *J. AOAC Int.* 2012, *95*, 273–285.

[70] Betz, J.M., Hardy, M.L. Evaluating the botanic dietary supplement literature. In *The HERBAL Guide: Dietary Supplement Resources for the Clinician*; Bonakdar, R.A., Ed., Lippincott Williams and Wilkins: Philadelphia, PA, USA, 2010; pp. 175–184.

[71] Betz, J.M., Hardy, M.L. Evaluating the botanical dietary supplement literature: How healthcare providers can better understand the scientific and clinical literature on herbs and phytomedicines. *HerbalGram* 2014, *101*, 58–67.

[72] Brooks, S.P.J., Sempos, C.T. The importance of 25-hydroxyvitamin D assay standardization and the Vitamin D Standardization Program. *J. AOAC Int.* 2017, *100*, 1223–1224.

[73] Phinney, K.W., Tai, S.S., Bedner, M., Camara, J.E., Chia, R.R.C., Sander, L.C., Sharpless, K.E., Wise, S.A., Yen, J.H., Schleicher, R.L., et al. Development of an improved standard reference material for vitamin D metabolites in human serum. *Anal. Chem.* 2017, *89*, 4907–4913.

[74] Phinney, K.W., Bedner, M., Tai, S.S., Vamathevan, V.V., Sander, L.C., Sharpless, K.E., Wise, S.A., Yen, J.H., Schleicher, R.L., Chaudhary-Webb, M., et al. Development and certification of a standard reference material for vitamin D metabolites in human serum. *Anal. Chem.* 2012, *84*, 956–962.

[75] Dwyer, J.T., Picciano, M.F., Betz, J.M., Fisher, K.D., Saldanha, L.G., Yetley, E.A., Coates, P.M., Milner, J.A., Whitted, J., Burt, V., et al. Progress in developing

analytical and label-based dietary supplement databases at the NIH Office of Dietary Supplements. *J. Food Compost. Anal.* 2008, *21*, S83–S93.

[76] Dwyer, J.T., Saldanha, L.G., Bailen, R.A., Bailey, R.L., Costello, R.B., Betz, J.M., Chang, F.F., Goshorn, J., Andrews, K.W., Pehrsson, P.R., et al. A free new dietary supplement label database for registered dietitian nutritionists. *J. Acad. Nutr. Diet.* 2014, *114*, 1512–1517.

[77] Dwyer, J.T., (NIH Office of Dietary Supplements, Bethesda, MD, USA). *Personal communication*, 2017.

[78] Andrews, K.W., (USDA-ARS Beltsville Human Nutrition Research Center, Beltsville, MD, USA). *Personal communication,* 2017.

[79] Saldanha, L.G., (NIH Office of Dietary Supplements, Bethesda, MD, USA). *Personal communication,* 2017.

[80] Lichtenstein, A.H., Yetley, E.A., Lau, J. *Application of Systematic Review Methodology to the Field of Nutrition: Nutritional Research Series*; Agency for Healthcare Research and Quality: Rockville, MD, USA, 2009; Volume 1.

[81] Helfand, M., Balshem, H. AHRQ series paper 2: Principles for developing guidance: AHRQ and the effective health-care program. *J. Clin. Epidemiol.* 2010, *63*, 484–490.

[82] Trikalinos, T.A., Lee, J., Moorthy, D., Yu, W.W., Lau, J., Lichtenstein, A.H., Chung, M. *Effects of Eicosapentanoic Acid and Docosahexanoic Acid on Mortality across Diverse Settings: Systematic Review and Meta-Analysis of Randomized Trials and Prospective Cohorts: Nutritional Research Series*; Agency for Healthcare Research and Quality: Rockville, MD, USA, 2012; Volume 4.

[83] Trikalinos, T.A., Moorthy, D., Chung, M., Yu, W.W., Lee, J.H., Lichtenstein, A.H., Lau, J. *Comparison of Translational Patterns in Two Nutrient-Disease Associations*; Agency for Healthcare Research and Quality: Rockville, MD, USA, 2011.

[84] Moorthy, D., Chung, M., Lee, J., Yu, W.W., Lau, J., Trikalinos, T.A. *Concordance between the Findings of Epidemiological Studies and Randomized Trials in Nutrition: An Empirical Evaluation and Citation Analysis*; Agency for Healthcare Research and Quality: Rockville, MD, USA, 2013.

[85] Brannon, P.M., Taylor, C.L., Coates, P.M. Use and applications of systematic reviews in public health nutrition. *Annu. Rev. Nutr.* 2014, *34*, 401–419.

[86] Ko, R., Low Dog, T., Gorecki, D.K., Cantilena, L.R., Costello, R.B., Evans, W.J., Hardy, M.L., Jordan, S.A., Maughan, R.J., Rankin, J.W., et al. Evidence-based evaluation of potential benefits and safety of beta-alanine supplementation for military personnel. *Nutr. Rev.* 2014, *72*, 217–225.

[87] Brooks, J.R., Oketch-Rabah, H., Low Dog, T., Gorecki, D.K., Barrett, M.L., Cantilena, L., Chung, M., Costello, R.B., Dwyer, J., Hardy, M.L., et al. Safety and performance benefits of arginine supplements for military personnel: A systematic review. *Nutr. Rev.* 2016, *74*, 708–721.

[88] Bailey, R.L., Gahche, J.J., Miller, P.E., Thomas, P.R., Dwyer, J.T. Why US adults use dietary supplements. *JAMA Intern. Med.* 2013, *173*, 355–361.

[89] Bailey, R.L., Gahche, J.J., Thomas, P.R., Dwyer, J.T. Why US children use dietary supplements. *Pediatr. Res.* 2013, *74*, 737–741.

[90] Berner, L.A., Keast, D.R., Bailey, R.L., Dwyer, J.T. Fortified foods are major contributors to nutrient intakes in diets of US children and adolescents. *J. Acad. Nutr. Diet.* 2014, *114*, 1009–1022.e8.

[91] Taylor, C.L., Bailey, R.L., Carriquiry, A.L. Use of folate-based and other fortification scenarios illustrates different shifts for tails of the distribution of serum 25-hydroxyvitamin D concentrations. *J. Nutr.* 2015, *145*, 1623–1629.

[92] Pfeiffer, C.M., Hughes, J.P., Lacher, D.A., Bailey, R.L., Berry, R.J., Zhang, M., Yetley, E.A., Rader, J.I., Sempos, C.T., Johnson, C.L. Estimation of trends in serum and RBC folate in the U.S. population from pre- to postfortification using assay-adjusted data from the NHANES 1988–2010. *J. Nutr.* 2012, *142*, 886–893.

[93] Pfeiffer, C.M., Sternberg, M.R., Hamner, H.C., Crider, K.S., Lacher, D.A., Rogers, L.M., Bailey, R.L., Yetley, E.A. Applying inappropriate cutoffs leads to misinterpretation of folate status in the US population. *Am. J. Clin. Nutr.* 2016, *104*, 1607–1615.

[94] Pfeiffer, C.M., Lacher, D.A., Schleicher, R.L., Johnson, C.L., Yetley, E.A. Challenges and lessons learned in generating and interpreting NHANES nutritional biomarker data. *Adv. Nutr.* 2017, *8*, 290–307.

[95] Gahche, J.J., (NIH Office of Dietary Supplements, Bethesda, MD, USA*). Personal communication,* 2017.

[96] M. M. Pandey, S. Rastogi, and A. K. S. Rawat, "Indian herbal drug for general healthcare: an overview," *The Internet Journal of Alternative Medicine,* vol. 6, no. 1, p. 3, 2008.

[97] B. Patwardhan, D. Warude, P. Pushpangadan, and N. Bhatt, "Ayurveda and traditional Chinese medicine: a comparative overview," *Evidence-Based Complementary and Alternative Medicine*, vol. 2, no. 4, pp. 465–473, 2005.

[98] R. A. Mashelkar, "Second world Ayurveda congress (theme: Ayurveda for the future)—inaugural address: part III," *Evidence-Based Complementary and Alternative Medicine*, vol. 5, no. 4, pp. 367–369, 2008.

[99] E. L. Cooper, "Ayurveda is embraced by eCAM," *Evidence-Based Complementary and Alternative Medicine,* vol. 5, no. 1, pp. 1–2, 2008.

[100] E. L. Cooper, "Ayurveda and eCAM: a closer connection," *Evidence-Based Complementary and Alternative Medicine*, vol. 5, no. 2, pp. 121–122, 2008.

[101] K. Joshi, Y. Ghodke, and B. Patwardhan, "Traditional medicine to modern pharmacogenomics: Ayurveda Prakriti type and CYP2C19 gene polymorphism associated with the metabolic variability," *Evidence-Based Complementary and Alternative Medicine*, vol. 2011, Article ID 249528, 5 pages, 2011.

[102] E. L. Cooper, "CAM, eCAM, bioprospecting: the 21st century pyramid," *Evidence-Based Complementary and Alternative Medicine,* vol. 2, no. 2, pp. 125–127, 2005.

[103] H. Gavaghan, "Koop may set up new centre for alternative medicine," *Nature,* vol. 370, no. 6491, p. 591, 1994.

[104] Pandey MM, Rastogi S, Rawat AK. Indian traditional ayurvedic system of medicine and nutritional supplementation. *Evid Based Complement Alternat Med.* 2013;2013:376327.

[105] NIH National Center for Complementary and Integrative Health. NCCIH Policy: *Natural Product Integrity.* Available online: https://nccih.nih.gov/research/policies/naturalproduct.htm.

[106] NIH Office of Extramural Research. Grants & Funcing—Rigor and Reproducibility. Available online: https://grants.nih.gov/reproducibility/index.htm#guidance.

[107] Sebastian, R.S., Wilkinson Enns, C., Goldman, J.D., Moshfegh, A.J. Dietary flavonoid intake is inversely associated with cardiovascular disease risk as assessed by body mass index and waist circumference among adults in the United States. *Nutrients* 2017, *9*, 827.

[108] Dwyer, J.T., Peterson, J. Tea and flavonoids: Where we are, where to go next. *Am. J. Clin. Nutr.* 2013, *98*, 1611s–1618s.

[109] González-Sarrías, A., Combet, E., Pinto, P., Mena, P., Dall'Asta, M., Garcia-Aloy, M., Rodríguez-Mateos, A., Gibney, E.R., Dumont, J., Massaro, M., et al. A systematic review and meta-analysis of the effects of flavanol-containing tea, cocoa and apple products on body composition and blood lipids: Exploring the factors responsible for variability in their efficacy. *Nutrients* 2017, *9*, 746.

[110] Kim, K., Vance, T., Chun, O. Greater total antioxidant capacity from diet and supplements is associated with a less atherogenic blood profile in U.S. adults. *Nutrients* 2016, *8*, 15.

[111] Kuhman, D.J., Joyner, K.J., Bloomer, R.J. Cognitive performance and mood following ingestion of a theacrinecontaining dietary supplement, caffeine, or placebo by young men and women. *Nutrients* 2015, *7*, 9618–9632.

[112] Costello, R.B., Dwyer, J.T., Bailey, R.L. Chromium supplements for glycemic control in type 2 diabetes: Limited evidence of effectiveness. *Nutr. Rev.* 2016, *74*, 455–468.

[113] Delmas, D. *Nutrients Journal Selected Papers from Resveratrol Regional Meeting 2015—Special Issue.* Available online: http://www.mdpi.com/journal/nutrients/special_issues/resveratrol_regional_meeting_2015.

[114] Davis, C.D. The gut microbiome and its role in obesity. *Nutr. Today* 2016, *51*, 167–174.

[115] Perez-Cano, F.J., Castell, M. Flavonoids, inflammation and immune system. *Nutrients* 2016, *8*, 659.

[116] Chamcheu, J.C., Syed, D.N. *Nutrients Journal Special Issue* "Nutraceuticals and the Skin: Roles in Health and Disease." Available online:

[117] Castell, M., Perez Cano, F.J. *Nutrients Journal Special Issue* "Flavonoids, Inflammation and Immune System." Available online: http://www.mdpi.com/journal/nutrients/special_issues/flavonoids-inflammationimmune-system.

[118] Wardenaar, F., Brinkmans, N., Ceelen, I., Van Rooij, B., Mensink, M., Witkamp, R., De Vries, J. Micronutrient intakes in 553 Dutch elite and sub-elite athletes: Prevalence of low and high intakes in users and non-users of nutritional supplements. *Nutrients* 2017, *9*, 142.

[119] Chiba, T., Sato, Y., Suzuki, S., Umegaki, K. Concomitant use of dietary supplements and medicines in patients due to miscommunication with physicians in Japan. *Nutrients* 2015, *7*, 2947–2960.

[120] Chiba, T., Sato, Y., Nakanishi, T., Yokotani, K., Suzuki, S., Umegaki, K. Inappropriate usage of dietary supplements in patients by miscommunication with physicians in Japan. *Nutrients* 2014, *6*, 5392–5404.

[121] Taylor, C.L., Yetley, E.A. Nutrient risk assessment as a tool for providing scientific assessments to regulators. *J. Nutr.* 2008, *138*, 1987s–1991s.

[122] Yetley, E.A. Science in the regulatory setting: A challenging but incompatible mix? *Novartis Found. Symp.* 2007, *282*, 59–68; discussion 69–76, 212–218.

Chapter 8

NATURAL FOODS AND INDIAN HERBS OF CARDIOVASCULAR INTEREST

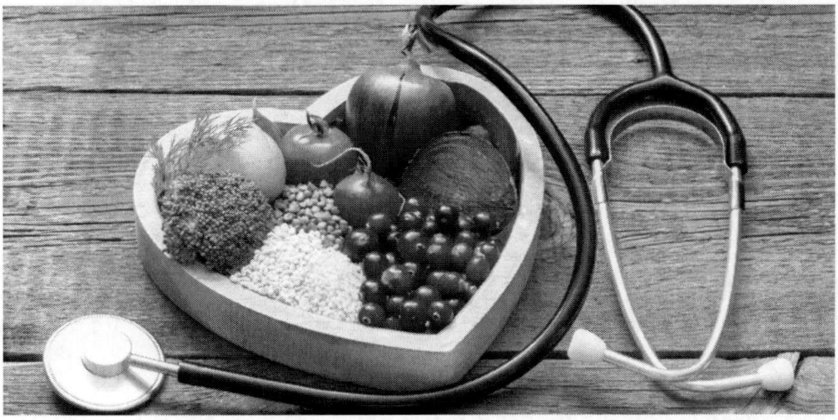

1. ABSTRACT

Since the beginning of human civilization, herbs have been an integral part of society, valued for both their culinary and medicinal properties. Cardiovascular disease is the number one killer in the United States. Diet and lifestyle play an important role in preventing and reversing heart disease, and certain herbs and supplements can help in lowering risk for heart disease and treat heart conditions. Compared with conventional medications, herbal medications do not require clinical studies before their marketing or formal approval from regulatory agencies, and for this reason their efficacy and safety are rarely proven. Herbal treatments have been used in patients with congestive heart failure, systolic hypertension, angina pectoris, atherosclerosis, cerebral insufficiency, venous insufficiency, and arrhythmia, CHF, since centuries. However, many herbal remedies used today have not undergone careful scientific assessment, and some have the potential to cause serious toxic effects and major drug-to-drug interactions. Despite most of these herbs showing an effect on biological mechanisms related to the cardiovascular system, data on their clinical effects are lacking. Potentially relevant side effects, including increased risk of drug interactions, are described, and the possibility of contamination or substitution with other medications represents a concern. Physicians should always assess the use of herbal medications with patients and discuss the possible benefits and side effects with them. Multidisciplinary research is still required to exploit the vast potential of these plants. Potential synergistic and adverse side effects of herb-drug interactions also need to be studied. These approaches will help in establishing them as remedies for cardiovascular diseases and including them in the mainstream of healthcare system. Although it has long been proved that vitamin D, ascorbic acid, and vitamin B12 are the key to treating chronic illnesses, including CVDs. Numerous natural carotenoids are present in fresh fruits and vegetables, and some have been studied extensively in the prevention of coronary heart disease (CHD).

Keywords: anti-oxidant, hypertension, cholesterol, atherosclerosis; cardioprotective; stroke

ABBREVIATIONS

CHF	Congestive Heart Failure
EMNs	Essential Micronutrients
CHD	Coronary Heart Disease
ABI	Ankle-Brachial Index
hsCRP	high-sensitivity C-Reactive Protein
CAC	Coronary Artery Calcium
ACC	American College of Cardiology
AHA	American Heart Association
CVH	Cardiovascular Health
DBH	Diastolic Blood Pressure
SBP	Systolic Blood Pressure
LMICs	Low- and Middle- Income Countries
PURE	Prospective Rural Urban Epidemiology
MD	Mediterranean Diet
CAD	Coronary Artery Disease
MIs	Myocardial infarctions
AMI	Acute Myocardial Infarction
GSPEs	Grape Seed Proanthocyanidin Extracts
GSSE	Grape Seed And Skin Extract
GPE	Grape Pomace Extract
GSE	Grape Seed Extract
HUVECs	Human Umbilical Vein Endothelial Cells
SMA	Small Mesenteric Artery
EPC	Endothelial Progenitor Cells
SHR	Spontaneously Hypertensive Rat

WKY	Wistar-Kyoto
DOCA	Deoxycorticosterone Acetate
DVT	Deep Vein Thrombosis
BKA	Blackberry Anthocyanin Fraction
BCA	Blackcurrant Anthocyanin Fraction
CAIMT	Carotid Artery Intima-Media Thickness
baPWV	brachial–ankle Pulse Wave Velocity
LSS	Laminar Shear Stress
PUFAs	Polyunsaturated Fatty Acids
AIP	Atherogenic Index of the Plasma
SNIR	State of Non-Specifically Increased Resistance
IAYT	Integrated Approach of Yoga Therapy
SREBP	Sterol Regulatory Element-Binding Protein
LXR-α	Liver X receptor-α
ABCA1	ATP-binding cassette transporter
VSMC	Vascular Smooth Muscle Cells
ROS	Reactive Oxygen Species

2. INTRODUCTION

The use of herbal medicine has skyrocketed over the last 10 years, with health expenditure estimated more than 18% of the GDP in US in 2018 (Statista Portal, 2019). In the traditional Indian system of medicine Ayurveda and Siddha various spices and herbs are described to possess medicinal properties, such as being antithrombotic, anti-atherosclerotic, hypolipidemic, hypoglycemic, anti-inflammatory, antiarthritic, etc. It has been believed for some time that dietary factors play a key role in the development of some human diseases, including cardiovascular disease. Several herbs and spices of culinary origin were included in the "approved" monographs, such as caraway oil and seed, cardamom seed, cinnamon bark, cloves, coriander seed, dill seed, fennel oil and seed, garlic, ginger root, licorice root, mint oil, onion, paprika, parsley herb and root, peppermint leaf and oil, rosemary, sage, thyme, turmeric root, and white mustard seed. Spices are rich in antioxidants, and a scientific study suggests they are also potent inhibitors of tissue damage and inflammation caused by high levels of blood sugar and circulating lipids. Apart from the treatment of cardiovascular risk factors with pharmacological agents and the use of antithrombotic drugs, there is growing awareness of the role of dietary factors and herbal medicines in the prevention of CVD and the possibility of their use in treatment. Much of this interest centers on the use of antioxidant vitamins and the antioxidant properties of herbal materials, although some herbal materials may also improve conventional cardiovascular risk factors or have antithrombotic effects. Herb–drug interactions are likely to be more serious with drugs having a narrow therapeutic index, such as warfarin or digoxin. The use of supplements of essential micronutrients (EMNs) in orthodox medical practice remains controversial, although adequate amounts of these substances are known to be necessary for the maintenance of health like Carotenoids, Vitamins B, C, D, E and K, Flavonoids, Magnesium and Iron, L-Carnitine, Omega-3 Polyunsaturated Fatty Acids, Coenzyme Q10. Multiple beneficial cardiovascular effects have been found with garlic, Danshen, Lingzhi, Maidenhair Tree, Foxglove, Ginseng etc. The evidence to support the

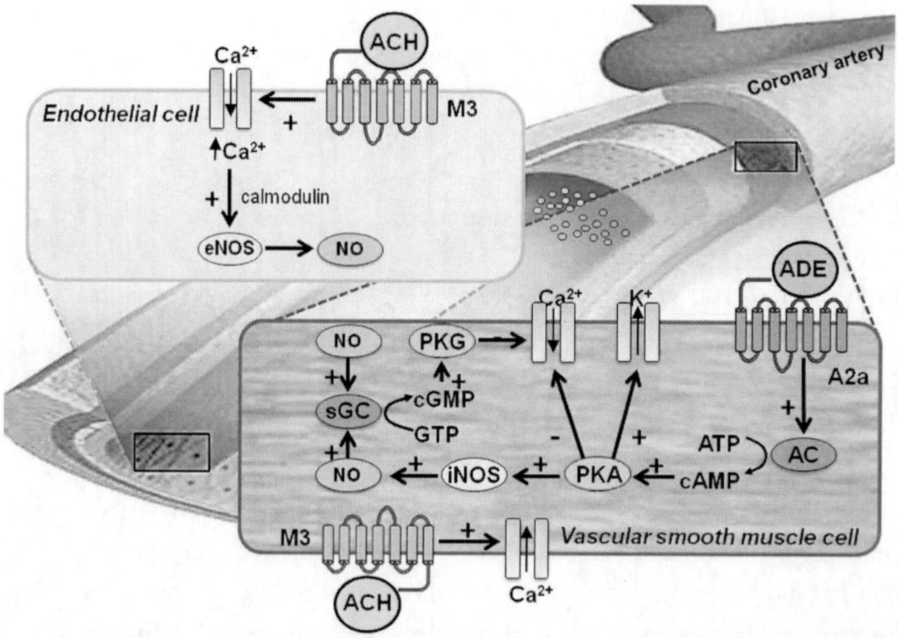

Figure 1. Acetylcholine and Adenosine Coronary Vascular Effects. Acetylcholine and Adenosine Coronary Vascular Effects Acetylcholine (ACH) has dual antithetical effects on the coronary arteries. By binding to muscarinic 3 (M3) receptors on the surface of vascular smooth muscle cells, it elicits (arrow and +) an intracellular release of calcium ions (Ca2+), leading to vasoconstriction, whereas endothelial M3 receptor–mediated Ca2+ release activates the endothelial nitric oxide (NO) synthase (eNOS, NOS III) through a calmodulin-dependent pathway. NO is then released and, in vascular smooth muscle cells, activates soluble guanylate-cyclase (sGC), which converts (curved arrow) guanosine triphosphate (GTP) into cyclic guanosine monophosphate (cGMP). The subsequent activation of GMP-dependent protein kinase (PKG) induces a cascade of intracellular events with the final effect of decreasing (arrow and −) intracellular Ca2+ concentrations, leading to vasodilation. Adenosine (ADE) binds to its receptors (A2a) on the surface of vascular smooth muscle cells, activating adenylate cyclase (AC) and leading to an increase in cyclic adenosine monophosphate (cAMP) concentration and cAMP-dependent protein kinase (PKA) activation. The latter results in potassium (K+) channel opening, resulting in a hyperpolarization of vascular smooth muscle cells, inhibits the entry of Ca2+ and also activates inducible NOS (iNOS) (NOS II), thus producing vasodilation. ATP = adenosine triphosphate. (Source: Radico F, Cicchitti V, Zimarino M, De Caterina R. Angina Pectoris and Myocardial Ischemia in the Absence of Obstructive Coronary Artery Disease: Practical Considerations for Diagnostic Tests. JACC: Cardiovascular Interventions Volume 7, Issue 5, May 2014 DOI: 10.1016/j.jcin.2014.01.157.)

use of these alternative therapies from clinical trials is not yet secure, but custom and practice make it likely that they will continue to be used for the prevention or treatment of CVDs, among other indications. Current trends for obesity management involve multiple pharmacological strategies, including blocking nutrient absorption, modulating fat metabolism, regulating adipose signals, and modulating the satiety center, also lies within the scope of cardiac management. Dietary phytochemicals have recently aroused considerable interest as the potential therapeutic agents for health promotion and to counteract obesity. Due to their chemical diversity and ability to act on various biological targets, plant products have long been a thriving source for the discovery of new drugs, and these find use among the most common complementary and alternative medicine systems.

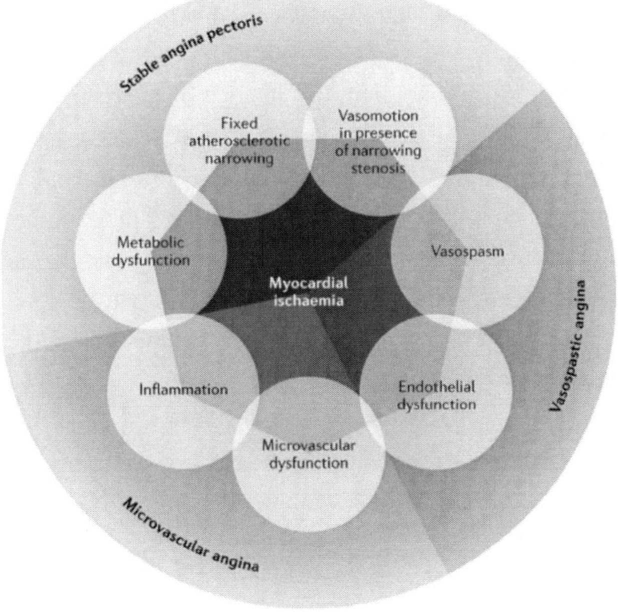

Figure 2. Different manifestations of myocardial ischemia. Stable angina occurs when myocardial ischemia is caused by fixed atherosclerotic narrowing of one or more epicardial coronary arteries. In some circumstances, the angina is associated with a coronary spasm and metabolic dysfunction. Vasospastic angina occurs when myocardial ischemia is caused by a coronary artery spasm with or without endothelial dysfunction. Microvascular angina refers to the absence of an obstructed epicardial coronary artery. Myocardial ischemia in this case can be caused by microvascular and/or endothelial dysfunction and inflammation. (Source: Ferrari R, Camici PG, Crea F, Danchin N, Fox K, Maggioni AP, Manolis AJ, Marzilli M, Rosano GMC, Lopez-Sendon JL. Expert consensus document: A 'diamond' approach to personalized treatment of angina. Nat Rev Cardiol. 2018 Feb;15(2):120-132. doi: 10.1038/nrcardio.2017.131. Epub 2017 Sep 7. Review. PubMed PMID: 28880025.)

2.1. Heart Disease and Significance

Cardiovascular diseases involve the blood vessels, the heart, or both [1]. These include numerous problems, many of which are related to a process called atherosclerosis.

Atherosclerosis is a condition that develops when a substance called plaque builds up in the walls of the arteries [2]. Arrhythmia refers to an abnormal heart rhythm [3]. There are various types of arrhythmias. The heart can beat too slow, too fast or irregularly. When heart valves don't open enough to allow the blood to flow through as it should, a condition called stenosis results. When the heart valves don't close properly and thus allow blood to leak through, it's called regurgitation. If the valve leaflets bulge or prolapse back into the upper chamber, it's a condition called prolapse [4, 5]. Hypertension is another name for high blood pressure. It can lead to severe complications and increases the risk of heart disease, stroke, and death. Blood pressure is the force exerted by the blood against the walls of the blood vessels [6]. Myocardial ischemia occurs when blood flow to heart is reduced, preventing it from receiving enough oxygen. The reduced blood flow is usually the result of a partial or complete blockage of heart's arteries (coronary arteries) [7]. Traditional risk factors for CVD include older age, smoking, high blood pressure, being overweight or obese, diabetes, high cholesterol, and a family history of heart disease [8]. Examples of other "nontraditional" risk factors that are sometimes used for risk assessment include the ankle-brachial index (ABI), high-sensitivity C-reactive protein (hsCRP) level, and the coronary artery calcium (CAC) score. The ABI is calculated by comparing blood pressure values measured at the ankle and the arm (brachial artery). High-sensitivity CRP is a protein involved in inflammation that is measured by its level in a person's blood. The CAC score measures the amount of calcium in the blood vessels of the heart based on a computed tomographic scan of the chest [9-13].

Exhibit 1. Complications of heart disease [14-25]

Heart failure	One of the most common complications of heart disease, heart failure occurs when heart can't pump enough blood to meet body's needs. Heart failure can result from many forms of heart disease, including heart defects, cardiovascular disease, valvular heart disease, heart infections or cardiomyopathy.
Heart attack	A blood clot blocking the blood flow through a blood vessel that feeds the heart causes a heart attack, possibly damaging or destroying a part of the heart muscle. Atherosclerosis can cause a heart attack.
Stroke	The risk factors that lead to cardiovascular disease also can lead to an ischemic stroke, which happens when the arteries to brain are narrowed or blocked so that too little blood reaches brain. A stroke is a medical emergency — brain tissue begins to die within just a few minutes of a stroke.
Aneurysm	A serious complication that can occur anywhere in your body, an aneurysm is a bulge in the wall of your artery. If an aneurysm bursts, you may face life-threatening internal bleeding.
Peripheral artery disease	Atherosclerosis also can lead to peripheral artery disease. When peripheral artery disease is developed in extremities, usually legs don't receive enough blood flow. This causes symptoms, most notably leg pain when walking (claudication).
Sudden cardiac arrest	Sudden cardiac arrest is the sudden, unexpected loss of heart function, breathing and consciousness, often caused by an arrhythmia. Sudden cardiac arrest is a medical emergency. If not treated immediately, it is fatal, resulting in sudden cardiac death.

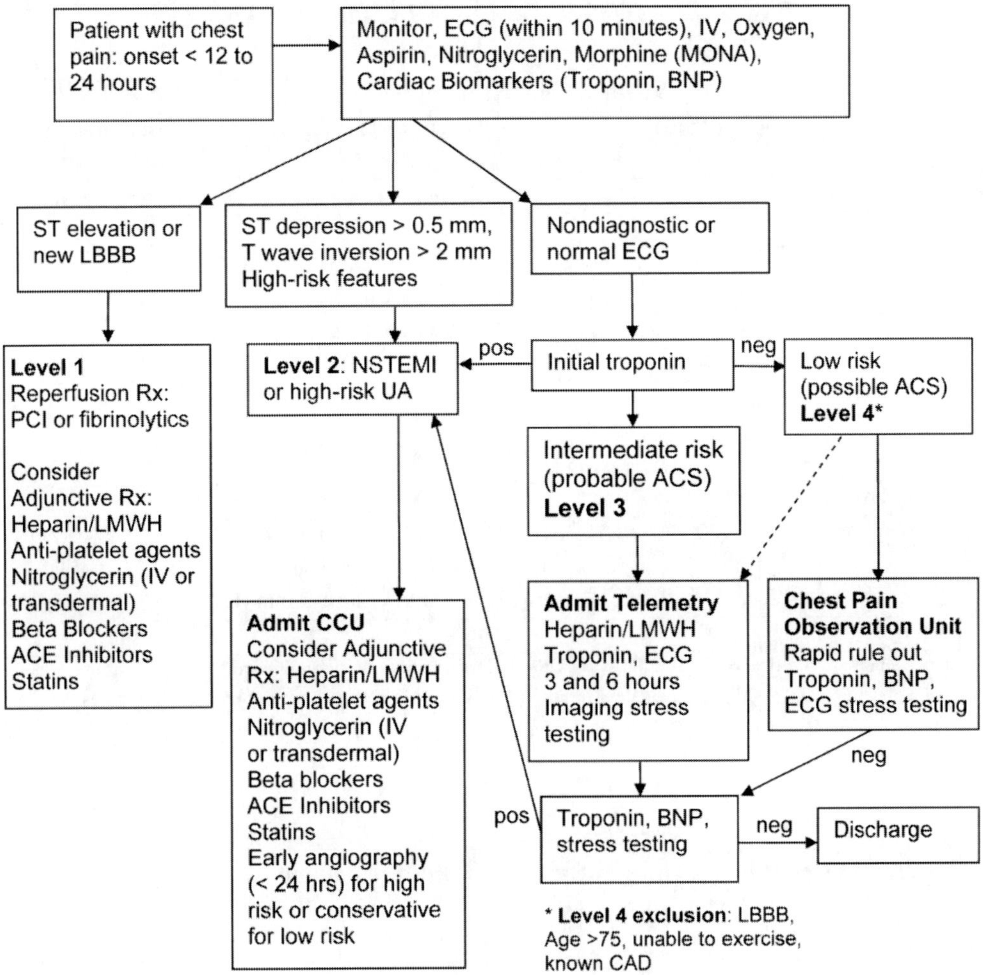

Figure 3. Chest Pain Evaluation Algorithm. An algorithm that integrates information from the above clinical decision rules with ECG findings. Low-risk patients are unlikely to have chest pain resulting from acute or chronic cardiac disease, although other serious causes (e.g., anxiety disorder, reflux disease, peptic ulcer, pulmonary embolism) should be considered. Patients at high risk of CAD require urgent evaluation and, in many cases, hospitalization. For patients at moderate risk, ECG and clinical findings can be used to identify those who are at high or low risk. Cardiac troponin testing can be used for risk stratification if it is available (e.g., in urgent care settings). A normal troponin level at least six hours after the onset of chest pain in combination with normal or near-normal ECG findings is a good prognostic sign; only one in 300 patients with this combination of findings have a cardiovascular event within 30 days.9 Although this algorithm has not been prospectively validated, it is based on prospectively validated diagnostic data. (Source: Ebell MH. Evaluation of Chest Pain in Primary Care Patients. Am Fam Physician. 2011 Mar 1;83(5):603-605. Available From Web American Academy of Family Physicians.)

In 2011, the AHA created a new set of strategic Impact Goals not only to reduce CVD deaths, but also to improve cardiovascular health, composed of 7 metrics (Life's Simple 7). These include 4 health behaviors (diet, physical activity, smoking, and body mass index) and 3 health factors (blood cholesterol, blood pressure, and blood glucose) [36].

Exhibit 2. AHA's life's simple 7 CVH score [36]

CVH Metric	Ideal CVH Definition (2 Points)	Intermediate CVH Definition (1 Point)	Poor CVH Definition (0 Point)
Smoking	**Never smoker**	**Former smoker**	**Current smoker**
Body mass index, kg/m^2	<25	25–29.9	>30
Physical activity	≥150 min/wk moderate or ≥75 min/wk vigorous or ≥150 min/wk moderate+vigorous activity	1–149 min/wk moderate or 1–74 min/wk vigorous or 1–149 min/wk moderate+vigorous activity	None
Diet score, no. of components [a]	4–5	2–3	0–1
Total cholesterol, mg/dL	<200[b]	200–239[b] or treated to goal	≥240
Blood pressure	<120/<80 mm Hg[b]	SBP 120–139 mm Hg[b] and/or DBP 80–89 mm Hg[b] or treated to <120/<80 mm Hg	SBP ≥140 mm Hg and/or DBP ≥90 mm Hg
Fasting glucose, mg/dL[b]	<100	100–125	≥126

[a]Fruits and vegetables: ≥4.5 cups/d; fish: ≥2 3.5-oz servings/wk (preferably oily fish); fiber-rich whole grains (≥1.1 g of fiber per 10 g of carbohydrate): ≥3 1-oz equivalent servings/d; sodium: <1500 mg/d; sugar-sweetened beverages: ≤450 kcal (36 oz)/wk.

[b] Untreated values.

2.2. Prevalence and Economic Burden of Cardiac Diseases

In 2014, US life expectancy ranked 43rd in the world, although the United States spent the most ($3.0 trillion) on health care, exceeding the median amount spent by Organization for Economic Co-operation and Development countries by 35% [39]. CVD was the leading cause of death in the United States in 2016, accounting for more than 900 000 deaths. Most CVD burden in the United States is from atherosclerotic vascular disease, and 80% can be attributed to known causal risk factors [30]. Nearly 1 in 3 (approximately 80 million) adults have some form of CVD, which imparts a heavy economic burden, including estimated direct costs of approximately $444 billion in US. The CVD costs of care are continuing to rise, with the current costs for treatment accounting for nearly $1 of every $6 spent on health care [40]. The evidence on the economic burden of CVD in LMICs remains scarce. The costs per episode for hypertension and generic CVD were fairly homogeneous across studies; ranging between $500 and $1500. In contrast, for CHD and stroke cost estimates were generally higher and more heterogeneous, with several estimates in excess of $5000 per episode. Average monthly treatment costs for stroke and CHD ranged between $300 and $1000 in in China, Brazil, India and Mexico [41]. Prevalence of confirmed hypertension in children to range between 2% and 4% [26]. In some countries, up to 75% of older adults are hypertensive [27]. 87% of the adults in the US who self-reported having hypertension engage in two or more activities to reduce blood pressure, such as taking medication, engaging in physical activity, changing diet, and reducing alcohol consumption [28]. In November 2017, new guidelines from the American College of Cardiology and the American Heart Association (ACC/AHA) expanded the definition of hypertension, extending the label to 46% of adults in the United States [31]. CHD is a major cause of death and disability in developed countries. Although the mortality for this condition has gradually declined over the last decades in western countries, it still causes about one-third of all deaths in people older than 35 years [38]. Atrial fibrillation is the most common sustained arrhythmia, increases with age, and presents with a wide spectrum of symptoms and severity [32]. The most recent studies have confirmed this perception and shown that the prevalence of AF in the general adult population of Europe is more than double that reported just one decade earlier, ranging from 1.9% in Italy, Iceland, and England to 2.3% in Germany and 2.9% in Sweden [33]. The estimated prevalence is lower in women (373 per 100,000) than in men (596 per 100,000). AF incidence has been shown to increase disproportionately with increasing age in both women and men, reaching as high as 30.4 per 1000 person-years in women and 32.9 per 1000 person-years in men by age 85–89 years [34]. Most studies of acute myocardial infarction (AMI) epidemiology and treatment have focused on patients who experience the onset of AMI outside of the hospital. It is increasingly recognized that AMI also occurs among patients already hospitalized for other conditions [35]. Globally, stroke is the second leading cause of death and third leading cause of disability.1 More than 74% of the burden of stroke has been attributed to smoking, poor diet, and low physical activity, while more than 72% has been attributed to metabolic risk factors (high plasma glucose, high cholesterol, high blood pressure, overweight and obesity, and kidney disease) [37]. Myocardial infarctions (MIs) are among the leading causes of morbidity and mortality in the United States and lead to >$11 billion in annual hospitalization costs. Of individuals >45 years of age who have a first MI, incidence of recurrent MI or fatal coronary heart disease within 5 years ranges from 17% to 20%, and heart failure rates are similar, adding further healthcare costs, which are projected to increase by almost 100% by 2030 [36].

3. Nutritional Recommendations for Cardiovascular Disease Prevention

Cardiometabolic diseases are estimated to cause over 700,000 deaths per year in the US and nearly 50% of these deaths are directly related to diet [43]. Lifestyle factors, including nutrition, play an important role in the etiology of CVD. CVD risk in postmenopausal women appears to be sensitive to a change to a low-fat dietary pattern and, among healthy women, includes both CHD benefit and stroke risk [44]. Factors that influence individuals to consume a low-quality diet are myriad and include lack of knowledge, lack of availability, high cost, time scarcity, social and cultural norms, marketing of poor-quality foods, and palatability [42]. The medical literature is still full of articles arguing opposing positions. For example, in 2017, after a review of the evidence, the AHA Presidential Advisory strongly endorsed that "lowering intake of saturated fat and replacing it with unsaturated fats, especially polyunsaturated fats, will lower the incidence of CVD." Three months later, the 18-country observational Prospective Rural Urban Epidemiology (PURE) Study concluded much the opposite: "Total fat and types of fat were not associated with cardiovascular disease, myocardial infarction, or cardiovascular disease mortality" [45]. Today, there continues to be an interest in low-carb approaches such as Atkins, Banting, ketogenic, and South Beach. While diets inducing weight-loss produces a caloric deficit, the mechanism of low-carb diets remains in debate. When lowering carbohydrates from the diet, the macronutrient intake of fat and protein generally increases to compensate for the reduction of carbohydrates. One hypothesis of why low-carb approaches produces rapid weight loss compared to other diets is that fats and protein increase satiety and produce less concomitant hypoglycemia. This increase in satiety and less rebound hypoglycemia then reduces hunger and overall food intake and produces a caloric deficit [46]. Both high and low percentages of carbohydrate diets were associated with increased mortality, with minimal risk observed at 50–55% carbohydrate intake. Plant-derived protein and fat intake, from sources such as vegetables, nuts, peanut butter, and whole-grain breads, were associated with lower mortality, suggesting that the source of food notably modifies the association between carbohydrate intake and mortality [47]. The traditional Mediterranean diet is characterized by the consumption of whole grains, legumes, fruits, vegetables, nuts, fish and olive oil, wine in moderation, and a moderate intake of meat, dairy products, processed foods and sweets [48]. Mediterranean diet reduced cardiovascular disease mortality risk related to long-term exposure to air pollutants in a large prospective U.S cohort. Increased consumption of foods rich in antioxidant compounds may aid in reducing the considerable disease burden associated with ambient air pollution [49]. As shown in a meta-analysis of seven cohort studies; a 2-point increase in adherence to the Mediterranean diet was associated with a significant reduction of overall mortality [50]. In addition, a meta-analysis of 23 prospective cohort studies of 937,665 participants and 18,047 CHD patients showed that fruit consumption was inversely associated with a risk of CHD [51]. Low-grade inflammation, rather than lipids, is likely to be on the pathway of the interaction between MD and statins towards mortality risk. MD lowered the risk of all-cause, cardiovascular and CAD/cerebrovascular mortality CVD patients, net of statins [52].

Exhibit 3. Recommendations of dietary patterns in prevention of CVD [50]

Food Pattern	Recommendations
Low-fat diet	Low-fat diet with restricted calories may present a healthy alternative to the typical Western diet. It may improve quality and life expectancy in healthy people, as well as in patients with overweight, diabetes, and CVD.
Low-carbohydrate Diet	In the short-run, low-carbohydrate diets lead to a greater weight loss compared to low-fat diets. Some studies have shown that this advantage is retained at 2 years but not at longer follow-up periods
	Low-carbohydrate diets are preferable to a low-fat diet in reducing TG levels and increasing HDL-C blood levels. It should be emphasized that carbohydrates should preferably be replaced by unsaturated vegetable fats.
	Low-carbohydrate diets, which include 30%–40% of calories from carbohydrates and are low in saturated fat and high in monounsaturated fat, were found to be safe in healthy and overweight individuals at follow-up up to 4 years.
Mediterranean Diet	A Mediterranean diet with restricted calories may present a healthy alternative to the typical Western diet. It may improve quality and life expectancy in healthy people, as well as in patients with overweight, diabetes, and CVD.
	Mediterranean diets are preferable to a low-fat diet in reducing TG levels, increasing HDL-C blood levels, and improving insulin sensitivity.
DASH Diet	The DASH diet is recommended to prevent hypertension and lower blood pressure. The diet should be accompanied by lifestyle changes such as: weight reduction in overweight people, increased physical activity, sodium restriction, and alcohol avoidance.

4. Natural Foods as Means of Cardio-Preventive Measures

Compared to refined grains, whole grains are higher in fiber, which may help reduce "bad" LDL cholesterol and decrease the risk of heart disease [54. Berries are also rich in antioxidants like anthocyanins, which protect against the oxidative stress and inflammation that contribute to the development of heart disease [55]. Avocados are an excellent source of heart-healthy monounsaturated fats, which have been linked to reduced levels of cholesterol and a lower risk of heart disease [56]. Walnuts are a great source of fiber and micronutrients like magnesium, copper and manganese. Of the fatty acids, oleic and linoleic acids represent more than half of the total fat content in pistachios. Pistachios are also a good source of vegetable protein (about 21% of total weight), with an essential amino acid ratio higher than most other commonly consumed nuts (ie, almonds, walnuts, pecans, and hazelnuts), and they have a high percentage of branched chain amino acids [57]. Dark chocolate is rich in antioxidants like flavonoids, which can help boost heart health [58]. Tomatoes are loaded with lycopene, a natural plant pigment with powerful antioxidant properties [59]. Almonds are also a good source of heart-healthy monounsaturated fats and fiber, two important nutrients that can help protect against heart disease [60].

Exhibit 4. The cardioprotective abilities of fruits [51]

Fruit	Subject	Study Type	Dose	Main Effects
freeze-dried grape powder	SHR and Wistar-Kyoto (WKY) rats	in vivo	600 mg/day	BP↓, arterial relaxation↑, vascular compliance↑, cardiac hypertrophy↓
GSPE	SHR	in vivo	250 mg/kg/day	arterial remodeling↓, ET-1↓, NO↑, SOD↑, CAT↑, MDA↓
GP-EE	rat aorta and small mesenteric artery (SMA) segments	in vitro	0.3 and 10 μM	endothelium- and NO-dependent vasodilatation↑, phenylephrine(Phe)-induced response in aortic rings↓, O_2^-↓, contraction elicited by ET-1↓
red grape skin and seeds polyphenols	human endothelial progenitor cells (EPC)	in vitro	5, 50 and 150 μg/mL	EPC viability and function↑, endothelial dysfunction↓, hyperglycemia effect↓, ROS production↓
GSPE	ouabain induced hypertensive rats model	in vivo	250 mg/kg/day	BP↓, aortic NO production↑
	HUVECs	in vitro	10 μg/mL	eNOS expression↑
GPE	endothelial (EA. hy926) cells	in vitro	0.068 and 0.250 μg/mL	GCS levels↑, GST activity↑, antioxidant activity↑
GSE	HUVECs	in vitro	1 μg/mL	platelet reactivity↓
red grape berry powder	rats with metabolic syndrome	in vivo	200, 400 and 800 mg/kg/day	BP↓, plasma TG↓, insulin↓
	HUVECs	in vitro	20–1400 μg/mL	ET-1↓
			0.011, 0.058, 0.29, 1.46 and 3.66 mg/mL	eNOS level↑
grape seed procyanidin extract	hamster	in vivo	25 mg/kg/day	body weight gain↓, adiposity index↓, weight of white adipose tissue depots↓, plasma phospholipids↓, plasma FFA↓, mesenteric lipid and triglyceride accumulation↓
grape polyphenols from *Vitis vinifera* grapes	24-month-old obese rats	in vivo	90 mg/kg/day	plasma HDL PON activity↑, LCAT activity↑, CETP activity↓
grape seed procyanidin extract	SHR	in vivo	375 mg/kg	SBP↓, DBP↓, GSH activity↑
GSE or black chokeberry (*Aronia melanocarpa*) extract	human platelets incubated with Hcy (100 μM) or HTL (1 μM)	in vitro	2.5, 5, 10 μg/mL	platelet adhesion to collagen and fibrinogen↓, platelet aggregation↓, $O_2^{\bullet-}$ production in platelet↓
malvidin-rich red grape skin extract	isolated and Langendorff perfused rat heart	in vitro	1–1000 ng/mL	I/R damages↓, coronary dilation↑, active PI3K/NO/cGMP/PKG pathway, intracellular cGMP↑, eNOS, PI3K-AKT, ERK1/2, and GSK-3 β phosphorylation↑
GSSE	a rat model of global ischemia	in vivo	2.5 g/kg	brain damage size and histology↓, oxidative stress↓, transition metals associated enzyme activities↑

Fruit	Subject	Study Type	Dose	Main Effects
GSPE	isolated rat hearts	in vitro	NA	RA↓, Na^+/K^+-ATPase activity↑, Na^+/K^+-ATPase α1 subunit↑, free radical↓
GSPE	a rat model of deep vein thrombosis (DVT)	in vivo	400 mg/kg/day	thrombus length and weight↓, protecte endothelium integrity, IL-6, IL-8 and TNF-α↓
blueberry extract (*Vaccinium ashei* Reade)	hypercholesterole mic rat	in vivo	25, 50 mg/kg	aortic lesions↓, oxidative damage to lipids and proteins↓, TC↓, LDL-C↓, TG↓, activity of CAT, SOD and GSH-Px↑
freeze-dried blueberry powder	rats fed a high-fat/cholesterol diet	in vivo	2% (*w*/*w*)	SBP↓, aorta relaxation↑, endothelial dysfunction↓
7 phenolic acids of freeze-dried blueberry	murine macrophage cell line RAW 264.7	in vitro	NA	TNF-α and IL-6 mRNA expression and protein levels↓, MAPK, JNK, p38, and Erk1/2 phosphorylation↓, mRNA expression and protein levels of scavenger receptor CD36↓, foam cell formation↓, expression and protein levels of ABCA1↑
PE	SR-BI/apoE double KO mice	in vivo	307.5 μL/L in water	aortic sinus and coronary artery atherosclerosis↓, oxidative stress and inflammation in the vessel wall↓
PE containing 40% punicalagin	SHR	in vivo	150 mg/kg/day	BP↓, cardiac hypertrophy↓, oxidative stress↓, antioxidant defense system↑, paraventricular nucleus inflammation↓, mitochondrial superoxide anion levels↓, mitochondrial function↑
PE containing 40% punicalagin	heart of a high-fat diet-induced obesity rat model	in vivo	150 mg/kg/day	mitochondrial biogenesis↑, oxidative stress↓, phase II enzymes↑, cardiac metabolic disorders↓
pomegranate seed extract	CHI rat model	in vivo	100, 200, 400, 800 mg/kg/day	motor and cognitive coordination↑
Bravo de Esmolfe apple	male Wistar rats fed a cholesterol-enriched diet (+2% cholesterol)	in vivo	20% (*w*/*w*) = 5g/rat/day (~2–3 apples/perso n/day) for 30 days	serum TG↓, TC↓, LDL-C↓, oxLDL↓
Fuji apple peel Granny Smith apple peel	CF-1 mice with MS $apoE^{-/-}$ mice	in vivo	20% (*w*/*w*) for 43 days 20% (*w*/*w*) for 10 weeks	glycaemia↓, TC↓, HDL-C↓, LDL-C↓, ureic nitrogen↓, TG↓, insulin↓, ADMA↓ atherogenic progression↓, cholesterol accumulation area↓
HFC	$apoE^{-/-}$ atherosclerotic mice with high blood lipid levels fed with a high cholesterol diet	in vivo	0.5 mL/day	TG↓, LDL-C/TC ratio↓
HPPS	the liver of high fat diet induced hyperlipidemic mice	in vivo	150 mg/kg	weight gain↓, TG↓, lipid excretion in feces↑, mRNAs and activities of acyl-CoA oxidase, carnitine palmitoyltransferase I, 3-ketoacyl-CoA thiolase, and 2,4-dienoyl-CoA reductase↑, gene and protein expressions of PPAR-α↑

Exhibit 4. (Continued)

Fruit	Subject	Study Type	Dose	Main Effects
freeze dried hawthorn fruit (*Crataegus pinnatifida)*	apo$E^{-/-}$ mice	in vivo	1% (*w/w*)	atherosclerotic lesions↓, TC↓, TG↓, T-AOC values↑, SOD and GSH-Px activities↑, hepatic FAS and SREBP-1c mRNA levels↓, hepatic SOD1, SOD2, Gpx3 mRNA levels↑
sugar-free aqueous extract of hawthorn fruit (*Crataegus pinnatifida* var. Major)	high fat diet fed rats	in vivo	72 and 288 mg/kg/day	TC, TG and LDL-C↓, HDL-C↑, CRP, IL-1β, IL-8 and IL-18↓, ET, 6-keto-PGF1α and TXB2↑, pathological changes in the arteries↓, IMT↓
avocado pulp (*Persea americana*) extract	male adult CD 1 mice	in vivo	25 mg/kg	thrombus formation↓
	platelet	in vitro	10 μL	platelet aggregation↓
avocado oil	rats ingested with sucrose	in vivo	7.5% (*w/w*)	TG↓, VLDL↓, LDL↓, hs-CRP↓
freeze-dried mango pulp	male C57BL/6J mice fed a high-fat diet	in vivo	1% or 10% (*w/w*)	epididymal fat mass↓, percentage of body fat↓, improve glucose tolerance, insulin resistance↓
methanolic extract of papaya (*Carica papaya*)	SHR	in vivo	100 mg/kg (twice a day)	BP↓, angiotensin converting enzyme(ACE) activity↓, cardiac hypertrophy↓, improve baroreflex sensitivity
sour cherry seed kernel extract	hearts from Sprague-Dawley rats	in vitro	30 mg/kg/day	post ischemic cardiac functions↑, infarct size↓, heme oxygenase-1 (HO-1)↑, Bcl-2↑
total flavonoids of Guangzao (*Choerospondias axillaris*)	I/R male Sprague-Dawley rats	in vivo	75, 150 and 300 mg/kg/day	cardiac function↑, heart pathologic lesion↓, CAT↑, GSH-Px↑, SOD↑, MDA↓, TUNEL-positive nuclear staining↓, Bcl-2-associated X protein (Bax)↓, caspase-3↓, Bcl-2↑, p38 MAPK activity↓, JNK activity↓
hydroalcoholic extract of acai (*Euterpe oleracea* Mart.) seeds	male Wistar rats subjected to myocardial infarction	in vivo	100 mg/kg/day	prevent the development of exercise intolerance, cardiac hypertrophy, fibrosis, and dysfunction
acai pulp	female Fischer rat of dietary-induced hypercholesterole mia	in vivo	2% (*w/w*)	TC↓, LDL-C↓, atherogenic index↓, HDL-C↑, cholesterol excretion in feces↑, expression of the LDL-R, ABCG5, and ABCG8 genes↑
bilberry (*Vaccinium myrtillus* L.) anthocyanin-rich extract	apo$E^{-/-}$ mice	in vivo	0.02% (*w/w*)	improve hypercholesterolemia against atherosclerosis
unrefined black raspberry seed oils	male Syrian hamsters fed high-cholesterol (0.12%), high-fat (9%) diets	in vivo	NA	plasma and liver TG↓, hypertriglyceridemia↓
polyphenols from sea buckthorn berry	rats with hyperlipidemia	in vivo	7–28 mg/kg	serum lipids↓, TNF-α↓, IL-6↓, antioxidant enzymes activity↑, eNOS, ICAM-1, and LOX-1 mRNA expression and proteins in aortas↓
Jujube (*Zizyphus jujuba)* fructus and semen extract	human macrophages	in vitro	NA	the foam cell formation induced by acetylated LDL↓, prevent atherosclerosis

Fruit	Subject	Study Type	Dose	Main Effects
methanol extract of blackberry (*Rubus allegheniensis* Port.)	human monocyte-derived macrophages induced by acetylated LDL	in vitro	50 μM	foam cell formation↓
yellow passion fruit pulp	SHR	in vivo	5, 6 or 8 g/kg/day	SBP↓, GSH↑, thiobarbituric acid-reactive substances (TBARS)↓
proanthocyanidins in boysenberry seed extract	SHR	in vivo	100 and 200 mg/kg	SBP↓
	rat aorta rings	in vitro		vasorelaxant activity↑
methanolic extract of date palm (*Phoenix dactylifera* L.)	cerebral ischemia rats	in vivo	100, 300 mg/kg	SOD↑, CAT↑, GSH↑, glutathione reductase↑, lipid peroxidation↓, oxidative stress↓, neuronal damage↓
black chokeberry (*Aronia melanocarpa*) extract	bovine coronary artery endothelial cells	in vitro	0.1 g/mL	NO↑, eNOS phosphorylation↑
saskatoon berry powder	leptin receptor-deficient diabetic mice	in vivo	5% (*w/w*)	monocyte adhesion to aorta↓, inflammatory, fibrinolytic or stress regulators in aorta or heart apex↓
saskatoon berry powder	leptin receptor-deficient diabetic mice	in vivo	5% (*w/w*)	endoplasmic reticulum stress (ERS)↓, unfolded protein response (UPR)↓
	glycated LDL-treated HUVECs	in vitro		
19 fruits widely consumed in central Chile	NA	in vitro	1 mg/mL	anticoagulant activities: grape, raspberry fibrinolytic activity: raspberry
peach (*Prunus persica*) pulp ethylacetate extract	cultured vascular smooth muscle cells (VSMCs)	in vitro	50, 100, or 200 μg/mL	Angiotensin II (Ang II) induced intracellular Ca^{2+} elevation↓, generation of ROS↓
methanolic extract of Lingonberry (*Vaccinium vitis-idaea* L.)	H9c2 rat myoblasts simulated IR	in vitro	5 and 10 μM	apoptosis↓, markers of nuclei condensation, caspase-3 activation, and MAPK signaling↓
blueberry anthocyanin fraction (BBA), blackberry anthocyanin fraction (BKA), and blackcurrant anthocyanin fraction (BCA)	RAW 264.7 macrophages treated by LPS bone marrow-derived macrophages from $Nrf2^{+/+}$ mice treated by LPS	in vitro	0–20 μg/mL	IL-1 β mRNA levels↓, NF-κB p65 translocation to the nucleus↓, cellular ROS levels↓, IL-1β mRNA levels↓
pomegranate juice, together with date fruit and date seeds extract	$apoE^{-/-}$ mice	in vivo	0.5 μM gallic acid equivalents (GAE)/day	TC↓, TG↓, PON1 activity↑, mouse peritoneal macrophage (MPM) oxidative stress↓, MPM cholesterol content↓, and MPM LDL uptake↓, aortas lipid peroxide content↓, aortas PON lactonase activity↑

5. Herbs as Sources of Cardo-Protective EMNs

Several herbs and supplements may help in fighting atherosclerosis, the underlying cause of most heart disease. In fact, certain herbs can influence blood pressure, triglycerides, cholesterol levels and inflammation, all of which are risk factors for heart disease. They're also high in dietary nitrates, which have been shown to reduce blood pressure, decrease arterial stiffness and improve the function of cells lining the blood vessels [53].

5.1. Carotenoids

Carotenoids are a class of natural, fat-soluble pigments found principally in plants. They have potential antioxidant biological properties because of their chemical structure and interaction with biological membranes. Carotenoids are largely widespread in the vegetable kingdom and are found in high concentrations in algae and microorganisms. Humans and other animals cannot synthesize them, so they are necessary in their diet [61]. The range of applications of microalgae as source of carotenoids is not limited to astaxanthin-based products but also to the manufacture of supplements with biologically active carotenoids like β-carotene, lutein and zeaxanthin with significant contributions to human health that enter in the nutrition and supplement market, which is expected to reach 220 $ billion globally in 2022 [79].

- *Astaxanthin:* Astaxanthin (3,3′-dihydroxy-β,β′-carotene-4,4′-dione), a red carotenoid pigment classified as a xanthophyll, is known to have a powerful antioxidant ability. The highest known level of astaxanthin in nature is in the chlorophyte alga *Haematococcus pluvialis* [62]. Astaxanthin used in nutritional supplements is usually a mixture of configurational isomers produced by Haematococcus pluvialis, a unicellular microalga. Astaxanthin administered orally for five-weeks in stroke prone SHR also resulted in a significant BP reduction. Oral astaxanthin also enhanced nitric oxide induced vascular relaxation in the rat aortas [63]. Astaxanthin limits exercise-induced skeletal and cardiac muscle damage in mice [64]. Astaxanthin effects on blood pressure in spontaneously hypertensive rats (SHR), normotensive Wistar Kyoto rats (NWKR) and stroke prone spontaneously hypertensive rats (SPSHR) were reported. Human umbilical vien endothelial cells and platelets treated with the astaxanthin showed increased nitric oxide levels and decrease in peroxynitrite levels [65].

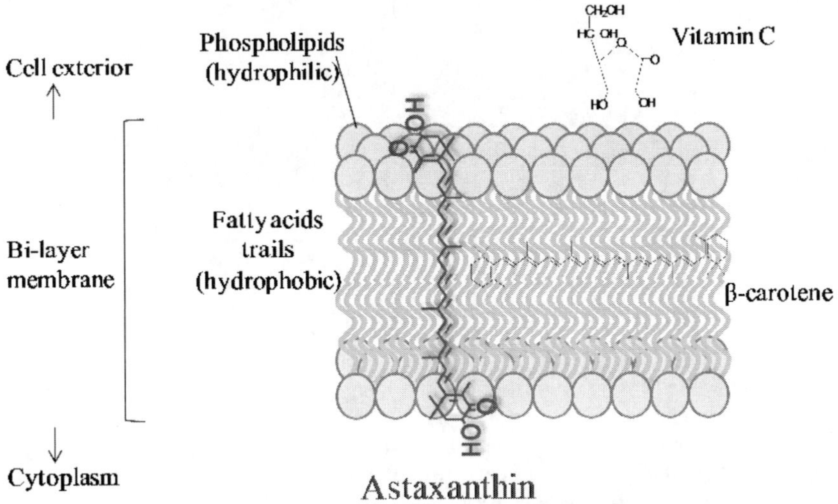

Figure 4. Transmembrane orientation of astaxanthin. The polar end groups overlap the polar boundary zones of the membrane, while the nonpolar middle fits the membrane 's nonpolar interior. The dashed red line speculatively indicates "lightning-rod" conduction of electrons along the astaxanthin molecule, possibly to vitamin C or other antioxidants located outside the membrane. (Source: Pashk ow F J, Watumull DG, Campbell CL. Astaxanthin: a novel potential treatment for oxidative stress and inflammation in cardiovascular disease. Am J Car diol 2008;101(suppl):58D-68D.)

5.2. Fucoxanthin

Fucoxanthin is an orange carotenoid present in edible brown seaweeds, such as *Undaria pinnatifida* (Wakame), *Hijikia fusiformis* (Hijiki), *Laminaria japonica* (Ma-Kombu), and *Sargassum fulvellum* [61]. Fucoxanthin, a carotenoid compound, is found in the chloroplasts of brown seaweed. This phytochemical has highly anti-inflammatory and antioxidant properties [66]. Fucoidan and fucoxanthin in combination can potentially reduce cardiac hypertrophy, cardiac fibrosis, ROS level, and shortened QT interval in aging mice subjects. There were also significant improvements in cardiac morphology and muscular function after the aging mice were fed with fucoidan alone or fucoidan supplemented with fucoxanthin [67]. Moreover, fucoxanthin also showed antiobesity, antidiabetes, anti-inflammatory, anticancer, and hepatoprotective activities as well as cerebrovascular protective effects. Fucoxanthin can improve the lipid profile and prevent the damage in cardiovascular system by promoting the proportion of DHA in the liver [68]. *Laminaria japonica* and *Undaria pinnatifida* are among the most popular food ingredients of Japanese cuisine. Fucoxanthin, and its metabolite fucoxanthinol, attenuate inflammatory changes in the interaction between adipocytes and macrophages. These results suggest that Fucoxanthin contained in edible algae is useful as a food ingredient for controlling obesity-related insulin resistance and for preventing metabolic syndrome [69].

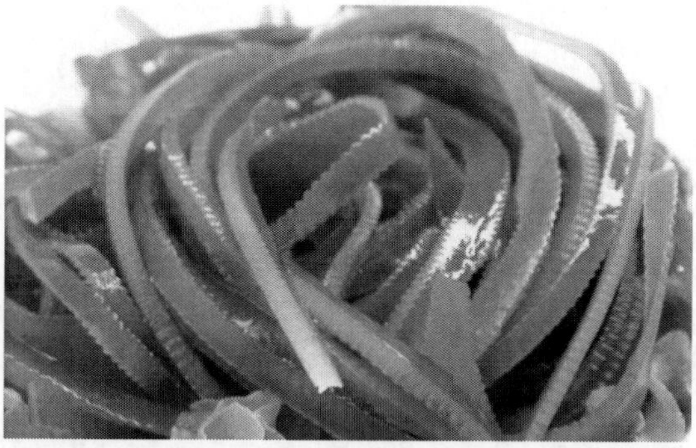

Figure 5. *Laminaria japonica* (Ma-Kombu). Laminaria japonica has frequently been used as a food supplement and drug in traditional oriental medicine. Among the major active constituents responsible for the bioactivities of L. japonica, fucoxanthin (FX) has been considered as a potential antioxidant. A low molecular weight fucoidan (DFPS), obtained from the brown seaweed Laminaria japonica, was separated into three fractions by anion-exchange column chromatography. Available data presented the content of sulfate group, the molar ratio of sulfate/fucose and sulfate/total sugar, and the molecular weight played an important role on antioxidant and anticoagulant activity (Wang J, Zhang Q, Zhang Z, Song H, Li P. Potential antioxidant and anticoagulant capacity of low molecular weight fucoidan fractions extracted from *Laminaria japonica*. Int J Biol Macromol. 2010 Jan 1;46(1):6-12. doi: 10.1016/j.ijbiomac.2009.10.015. Epub 2009 Oct 31. PubMed PMID: 19883681).

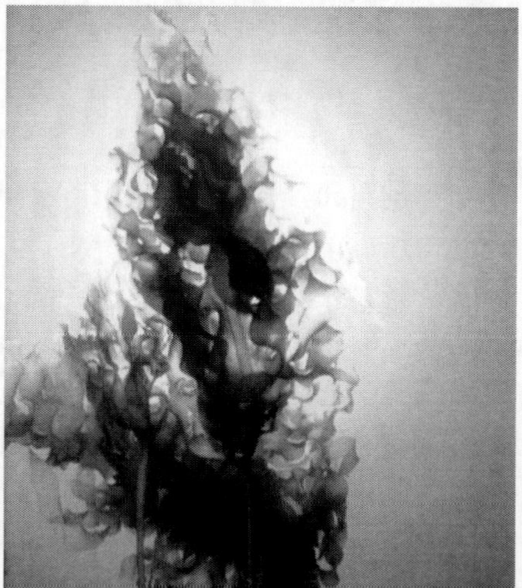

Figure 6. *Undaria pinnatifida* (Wakame). Brown algae and its carotenoids have been shown to have a positive influence on obesity and its comorbidities. Additionally, the treatments, ameliorated adipose tissue accumulation, insulin resistance, blood pressure, cholesterol and triglycerides concentration in serum, and reduced lipogenesis and inflammation by downregulating acetyl-CoA carboxylase (ACC) gene expression, increasing serum concentration and expression of adiponectin as well as downregulating IL-6 expression. (Source: Grasa-López A, Miliar-García Á, Quevedo-Corona L, Paniagua-Castro N, Escalona-Cardoso G, Reyes-Maldonado E, Jaramillo-Flores ME. Undaria pinnatifida and Fucoxanthin Ameliorate Lipogenesis and Markers of Both Inflammation and Cardiovascular Dysfunction in an Animal Model of Diet-Induced Obesity. Mar Drugs. 2016 Aug 3;14(8). pii: E148. doi: 10.3390/md14080148. PubMed PMID: 27527189; PubMed Central PMCID: PMC4999909.)

5.3. Lycopene

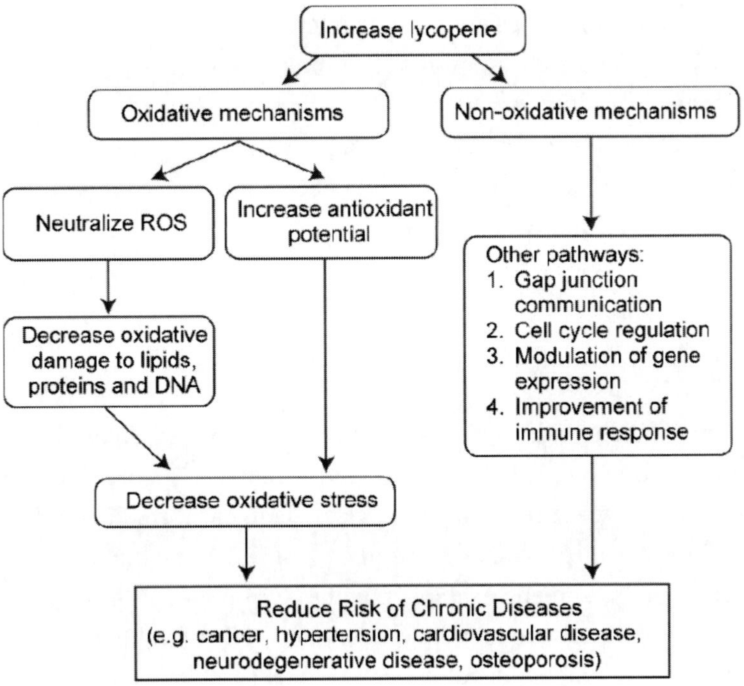

Figure 7. General mechanisms of action of lycopene. The proposed mechanisms of action of lycopene (oxidative and nonoxidative) that decreases the risk of oxidative stress-mediated diseases. Lycopene most likely acts via the oxidative mechanism of action to prevent oxidative stress. Lycopene treatment has been shown to cause a 37% suppression of cellular cholesterol synthesis in J-774A.1 macrophage cell line, and augment the activity of macrophage LDL receptors. Oxidized LDLs are highly atherogenic as they stimulate cholesterol accumulation and foam cell formation, initiating the fatty streaks of atherosclerosis. LDL susceptibility to oxidative modifications is decrease by an acyl analog of platelet-activating (PAF), acyl-PAF, which experts its beneficial role during the initiation and progression of atherosclerosis. Purified lycopene in association with α - tocopherol or tomato lipophilic extracts has been shown to enhance acyl-PAF biosynthesis in endothelial cells during oxidative stress. ROS: reactive oxygen species. (Source: Amany M. M. Basuny (October 3rd 2012). The Anti-Atherogenic Effects of Lycopene, Lipoproteins, Sasa Frank and Gerhard Kostner, IntechOpen, DOI: 10.5772/48134.)

Lycopene is the pigment responsible for the red color in some fruits and vegetables, which can be found in high concentration in tomato products, red grapefruits, and watermelons. It is an unsaturated carotenoid, resulting in an efficient antioxidant, and consumption can prevent both aging and CVD [61]. Overall dietary lycopene intake and high-serum concentration of lycopene, significantly reduced the risk of major cardiovascular events [70]. Lutein and lycopene supplementation significantly increased the serum concentration of lutein and lycopene with a decrease in carotid artery CAIMT [71]. Benefits of lycopene should be especially considered in patients with high cardiovascular risk, statin intolerance, borderline hypertension, aspirin resistance, hyperactive platelets, vascular inflammatory diseases, metabolic syndrome and coronary heart disease, and its inclusion in combination therapies for the mentioned disorders, should be approached [72]. Cholesterol reduction, inhibition of oxidation processes, modulation of inflammatory markers, enhanced intercellular communication, inhibition of tumourigenesis and induction of apoptosis, metabolism to retinoids and antiangiogenic effects was reported in another study [73]. However, the possible inverse associations noted for higher levels of tomato-based products, particularly tomato sauce and pizza, with CVD suggest that dietary lycopene or other phytochemicals consumed as oil-based tomato products confer cardiovascular benefits [74].

5.4. Lutein

It is a pigment (xanthophyll) and a dietary oxygenated carotenoid consisting of 40-carbon hydroxylated compounds found in the human retina in high concentration. It is an isomer of the carotenoid zeaxanthin, with identical chemical formulas [61]. it can just be obtained from yellow corn, egg yolk, orange juice, honeydew melon, and other fruits, but especially occurring in dark green vegetables such as turnip greens, kale, parsley, spinach, and broccoli [75]. Lutein exerts potent antioxidant and anti-inflammatory effects in aortic tissue that may protect against development of atherosclerosis in guinea pigs [76]. Consumption of lutein increases plasma lutein concentrations, and that this increase is associated with increases in activity and reductions in time spent engaged in sedentary activities [77]. Lutein may act as a chemo-preventive agent against atherosclerosis, including oxidative stress and lipid metabolism improvements. Decreased mRNA and protein expression levels of hepatic peroxisome proliferator-activated receptor-α, carnitine palmitoyl-transferase 1A, acyl CoA oxidase 1, low density lipoprotein receptors and scavenger receptor class B type I observed in mice with atherosclerosis were markedly enhanced after treatment with lutein [78].

5.5. Zeaxanthin

Like lutein, zeaxanthin is an oxygenated non-pro-vitamin A carotenoid that consists of a 40-carbon hydroxylated compound and they both are found from same dietary sources [79]. Higher dietary and serum carotenoid levels are associated with lower carotid intima-media thickness in middle-aged and elderly people [80]. Higher levels of plasma oxygenated carotenoids (lutein, zeaxanthin, beta-cryptoxanthin) and alpha-carotene may be protective against early atherosclerosis [81]. Researchers found a relationship between the level of lutein and zeaxanthin in the adipose tissue and diet and the risk for heart attack [82].

5.6. β-Cryptoxanthin

β-cryptoxanthin is a xanthophylls and one of the lesser-known carotenoids, whose best food sources are oranges, peach, tangerines, red peppers and tropical fruits such as papaya and pumpkin. It also has pro-vitamin A activity and seems to have protective health action. The concentrations of β-cryptoxanthin in most mammalian tissues generally are low compared with those of other dietary antioxidants such as vitamins E and C [83]. Acute β-cryptoxanthin treatment exhibits greater cardioprotective efficacy against I/R injury than astaxanthin and vitamin E by reducing infarct sizes and attenuating apoptosis, oxidative stress, and mitochondrial dysfunction in mice [84]. Serum β-cryptoxanthin and lutein plus zeaxanthin were inversely related to the extent of atherosclerosis [85]. β-cryptoxanthin has anti-obesity and antioxidative effects in C. elegans, it is tempting to hypothesize that β-cryptoxanthin may have a protective effect against development of the metabolic syndrome. The metabolic syndrome is a complex disorder clustering obesity, diabetes mellitus, and atherosclerotic cardiovascular diseases. β-cryptoxanthin concentrations in serum are inversely related to indices of oxidative DNA damage and lipid peroxidation [86]. An inverse association of baPWV with β-carotene and β-cryptoxanthin was observed independently of the glycemic state [87].

5.7. Beta-Carotene

Beta-carotene is one of the most widely studied carotenoids for both its pro-vitamin A activity and its abundance in fruits and vegetables, such as carrot, orange, kale, spinach, turnip greens, apricot, and tomato [61]. Low serum carotenoid levels may reflect either increased lipoprotein density or the presence of inflammation, both factors emerging as important novel risk factors for coronary heart disease [88]. In addition to its ability to affect risk and pathogenesis of cancer, beta-carotene has been considered for use in management of heart disease based on its free radical scavenging capacities, with the cautionary note that it may also act as a tissue-damaging prooxidant—depending on the physiologic environment [89, 90]. Apparent cardioprotective effect of beta-carotene at one selected dosage and mitigation or elimination of that protection at a higher dose is speculative based on the outcomes [91]. One-month tobacco-smoke exposure induces functional and morphological cardiac alterations and BC supplementation attenuates this ventricular remodeling process [92]. More information is needed to ascertain the association between the intake of single nutrients, such as carotenoids, and the risk of CVD. Currently, the consumption of carotenoids in pharmaceutical forms for the treatment or prevention of heart diseases cannot be recommended [93].

5.8. Homocysteine Level Maintenance

Homocysteine levels increase in the body when the metabolism to cysteine of methionine to cysteine is impaired. This may be due to dietary deficiencies in vitamin B6, vitamin B12, and folic acid [94]. Elevated homocysteine level has been shown to be associated with the development of atherosclerotic heart disease, stroke, and myocardial ischemia [98]. A rise in serum creatinine also leads to a rise in fasting total homocysteine. The major route of homocysteine clearance from plasma is the kidney, and the rise is due to defective metabolism of homocysteine by the kidney [95]. A 25% reduction in homocysteine levels was associated with an 11% lower ischemic heart disease risk and a 19% lower stroke risk [96]. Trimethylglycine, Folate, Vitamin B12, Vitamin B6, Taurine, Creatine, Choline, N-Acetyl-Cysteine, Omega-3 Fatty Acids keep homocysteine levels in check [97].

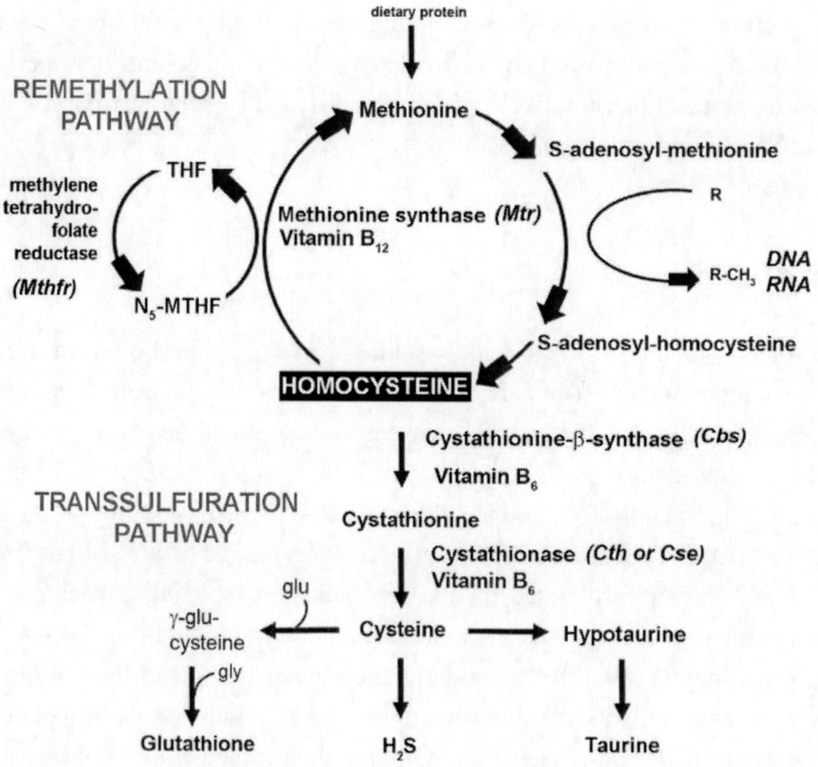

Figure 8. Pathways for the metabolism of homocysteine. Normal trans-sulfuration requires cystathionine β synthase with vitamin B6 as cofactor. Re-methylation requires 5, 10-methylenetetrahydrofolate reductase and methionine synthase. The latter requires folate as co-substrate and vitamin B12 (cobalamin) as cofactor. An alternative re-methylation pathway also exists using the cobalamin independent betaine–homocysteine methyltransferase. For some years, attention focused on the role of heterozygosity for homocystinuria6 as a possible cause of the high homocysteine concentrations that are seen in up to 30–40% of patients with coronary artery disease. (Source: Robinson K. Homocysteine, B vitamins, and risk of cardiovascular disease. Heart 2000;83:127-130.)

5.9. Flavonoids

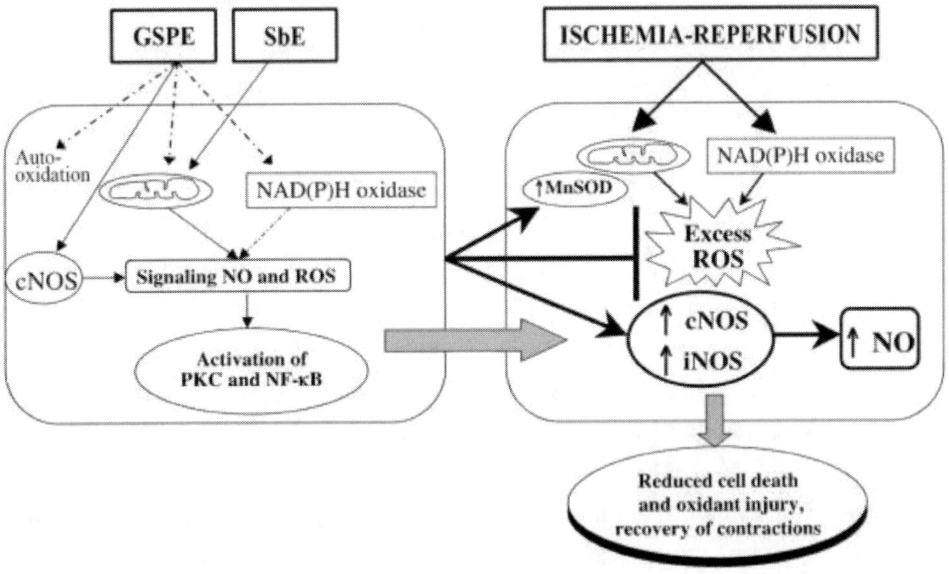

Figure 9. Potential mechanisms of *Scutellaria baicalensis* extract (SbE) and grape seed proanthocyanidin extract (GSPE) in delayed preconditioning in cardiomyocytes. NO-nitric oxide; ROS-reactive oxygen species; PKC-protein kinase C; MnSOD-manganese superoxide dismutase; cNOS-constitutive nitric oxide synthase; iNOS-inducible NOS. With respect to NO, flavonoids in SbE such as wogonin and baicalein, suppress its release by inhibiting NOS/guanylate cyclase. In normal tissue GSPE stimulates NO release via a purinergic pathway. GSPE has shown a reduced NO release, although only in models of inflammation, which could be an indirect effect of suppression of iNOS upregulating cytokines. Data suggest that cardiomyocytes show a non-toxic ROS response to SbE treatment but NO release with GSPE treatment during the induction phase. It appears that the two extracts may induce two distinct preconditioning mechanisms (Wang CZ, Mehendale SR, Calway T, Yuan CS. Botanical flavonoids on coronary heart disease. Am J Chin Med. 2011;39(4):661-71. Review. PubMed PMID: 21721147; PubMed Central PMCID: PMC3277260).

A large body of evidence supports that the dietary intake of polyphenols - particularly of flavonoids and the specific class of flavonoids named flavanols - might be able to exert some beneficial vascular effects and reduce the risk for cardiovascular morbidity and mortality [99]. A number of flavonoids of dietary significance have been shown to impart beneficial impact on parameters associated with atherosclerosis, including lipoprotein oxidation, blood platelet aggregation and cardiovascular reactivity [100]. In a study of approximately 5,000 subjects, the intake of dietary flavonoids and tea was inversely associated with myocardial infarction [101]. Flavonoids' protective effects against ischemic heart disease is based on several clinical studies that positively correlate flavonoid intake to a reduced incidence of the disease. Consuming flavonoids like catechin, which is present in plant seeds and teas, resulted in a 20% reduction in the incidence of the disease [102] (Further details of flavonoids in CVD prevention is discussed in later section).

5.10. Magnesium and Iron

The role of copper, iron, and other metal elements in ischemic heart injury has been well established [103]. Legumes (lentils, beans and peas) pumpkin, sesame, hemp and flaxseeds, cashews, pine nuts and other nuts, tomato, potatoes, mushrooms, palm, prune, olives, mulberries, whole, grains (amaranth, oats), coconut milk, dark chocolate, dried thyme are rich source of iron [105]. Brazil nuts, almonds, pecans, cashews, walnuts, pumpkin seeds, flaxseeds, sunflower seeds, sesame seeds, quinoa seeds, cumin seeds, peach apricots, avocado, banana, blackberries, spinach, okra, broccoli, beetroot, swiss chard, green bell peppers, artichokes, buckwheat are rich sources of magnesium [106]. Iron is a component of hemoglobin and thus plays a key role in tissue oxygenation. It is also a component of myoglobin, which is an oxygen-binding protein found in skeletal muscle and myocytes, allowing oxygen release in hypoxic conditions [107]. The prevalence of iron deficiency in heart failure patients has been reported as being up to 50%, even in patients without anemia. So, IV iron should be considered in symptomatic HF patients with ID [108]. Investigation of the long-term safety of the various intravenous iron supplementation strategies may still be warranted [109].

Exhibit. Summary of studies evaluating the effect of magnesium on cardiovascular-related outcomes in the general population [104]

Study Type	Clinical Setting	No. of Subjects	Outcome	Conclusion
Meta-analysis of prospective studies	General population	>1,000,000	CVD (coronary heart disease, ischemic heart disease, stroke) and all-cause mortality	Increasing dietary Mg is associated with a reduced risk of stroke and heart failure, but not with total CVD, and all-cause mortality.
Observational	Elderly	1400	All-cause and cause-specific mortality	Low plasma Mg levels increase all-cause mortality.
Meta-analysis of prospective studies	General population	532,979	CVD	Inverse association between dietary Mg intake and CVD risk.
		313,041	Incidence of CVD, including IHD	Plasma and dietary Mg are inversely associated with CVD risk.
Prospective	Individuals at high risk of CVD	7216	CVD and all-cause mortality	Mg intake is associated with a lower mortality risk in this population, but not with CV events.
	Women free of disease	86,323	CHD	Dietary Mg intake was inversely associated with fatal CHD.

5.11. Omega-3 Polyunsaturated Fatty Acids

Early secondary prevention trials of fish and omega-3 polyunsaturated fatty acid (PUFA) capsules reported beneficial effects on CVD outcomes, including all-cause mortality and sudden cardiac death [110]. Besides many health benefits, paradoxically, intense exercise can result in oxidative damage to cellular constituents. At rest, muscle receives approximately 20% of the total blood flow, but, during exercise, this can increase to more than 80%. N-3 PUFAs seem to be among the most useful supplements for a huge range of the population (premature infants, elderly with sarcopenia, athletes, and patients with metabolic and inflammatory diseases). N–3 PUFAs has the potential to be an ergogenic aid that enhances training and sport performance at low cost and little risk [111]. Omega-3 fatty acids like EPA only at a pharmacologic dose reduce fasting TG and interfere with mechanisms of atherosclerosis that results in reduced cardiovascular events. Additional mechanistic trials will provide further insights into their role in reducing cardiovascular risk in subjects with well-managed LDL-C but elevated TG levels [112].

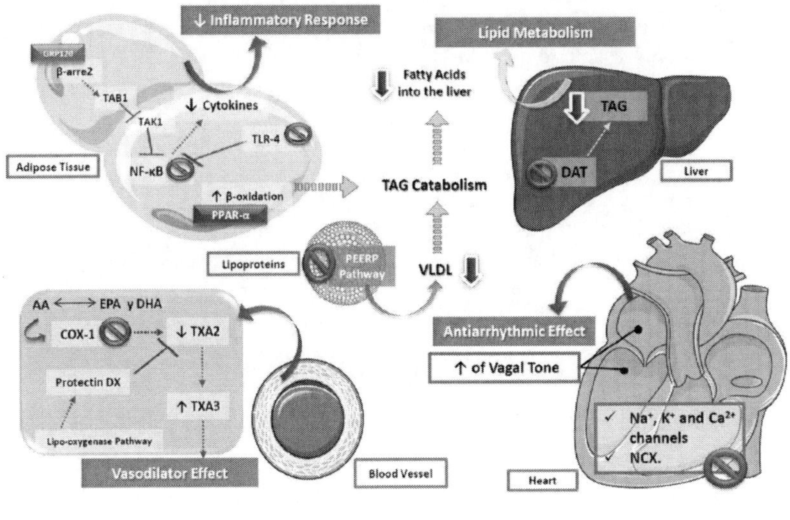

Figure 10. Role of polyunsaturated fatty acids in cardiovascular function. The actions of n3-PUFAs are diverse, including the decrease of the inflammatory response via NF-kB inhibition, as well as an increase of β-oxidation, causing the catabolism of triaclyglycerides and contributing to the decrease of lipids stored both in the liver and vessel walls. In addition, by increasing the production of TXA3 in vessel walls, PUFAs decrease vascular resistance, reducing blood pressure. On the other hand, one of the most described effects of n3-PUFAs is their action on cardiac arrhythmia, by inhibiting voltage-gated ion channels and exchangers, as well as increasing the vagal tone of the atria and ventricles, which leads to a lower heart rate. PUFA: polyunsaturated fatty acids; TXA2: thromboxane A2; TXA3: thromboxane A3; COX-1: cyclooxygenase 1; DAT: 1,2 diglyceride acyltransferase; TAG: triacylglycerides; NF-kB: nuclear factor kappa B; TLR-4: toll-like receptor 4; VLDL: very low-density lipoproteins (María José Calvo1, María Sofía Martínez1 et al. Omega-3 polyunsaturated fatty acids and cardiovascular health: a molecular view into structure and function. Vessel Plus 2017;1:116-28.10.20517/2574-1209.2017.14© 2017).

5.12. Co-Enzyme 10 (Q10)

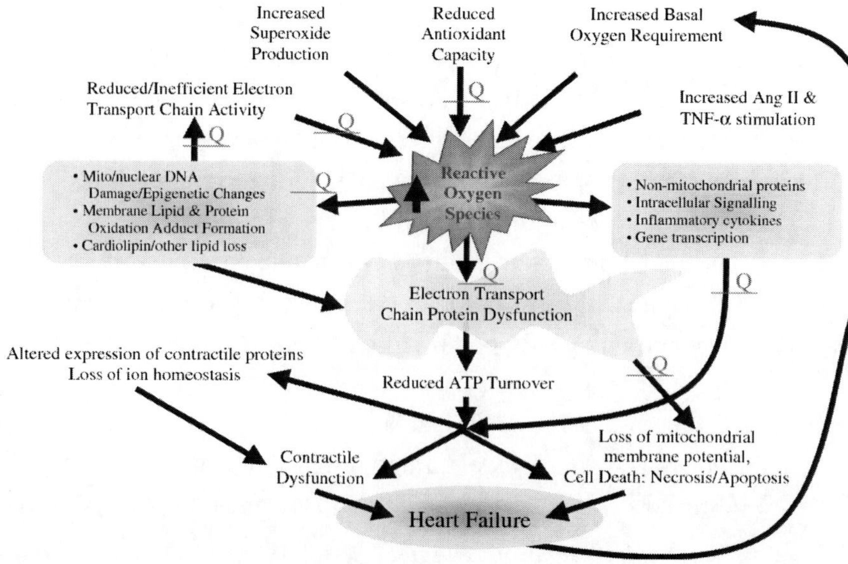

Figure 11. Q10 treatment may intervene in the scheme where augmented ROS production contributes to post-ischemic injury and progression to heart failure. Reactive oxygen species (ROS) Increased myocardial levels of oxidative stress markers have been demonstrated in animal models of heart failure produced by coronary ligation (Hill and Singal, 1996), pressure overload (Dhalla and Singal, 1994) and rapid car- diac pacing (Ide et al., 2000). ROS are key pathophysiolog- ical mediators in myocardial remodelling in heart failure (Singal et al., 1993). In human heart failure, there is also evidence of increased levels of oxidative stress markers such as malondialdehyde (MDA) in serum (Belch et al., 1991), and isoprostanes in urine (Cracowski et al., 2000). Further- more the levels of these markers correlate with the severity of heart failure. (Source: Pepe S, Marasco SF, Haas SJ, Sheeran FL, Krum H, Rosenfeldt FL. Coenzyme Q10 in cardiovascular disease. Mitochondrion. 2007 Jun;7 Suppl:S154-67. Epub 2007 Mar 16. Review. PubMed PMID: 17485243.)

CoQ10 is not FDA-approved to treat any medical condition although it is widely available over-the-counter as a dietary supplement and recommended by primary care physicians and specialists alike [113]. Q10 can increase the production of key antioxidants such as superoxide dismutase, an enzyme capable of reducing vascular oxidative stress in hypertensive patients. Q10 reduces levels of lipid peroxidation via the reduction of pro-oxidative compounds. Q10 can enhance blood flow and protect blood vessels via the preservation of nitric oxide [114]. There's a strong role of CoQ10 in hypertension, ischemic heart disease, myocardial infarction, heart failure, viral myocarditis, cardiomyopathies, cardiac toxicity, dyslipidemia, obesity, type 2 diabetes mellitus, metabolic syndrome, cardiac procedures and resuscitation [115]. Q10 has the potential in hypertensive patients to lower systolic blood pressure by up to 17 mm Hg and diastolic blood pressure by up to 10 mm Hg without significant side effects [116]. Evidence suggests that the CoQ10 supplement may be a useful tool for managing patients with heart failure [117]. Despite positive findings, a larger prospective trial is warranted to support routine use of CoQ10 [118].

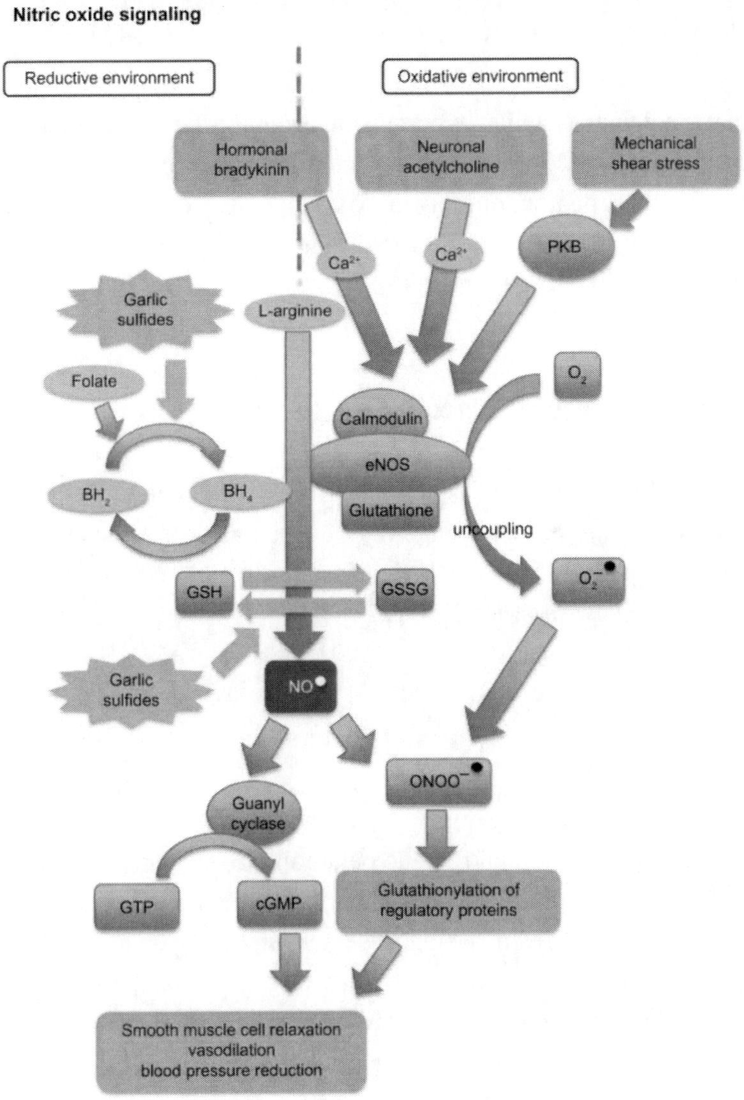

Figure 12. Effect of garlic on blood pressure via the NO pathway. N.B. Blue rectangles illustrate metabolites, blue circles represent enzymes, orange circles are dietary cofactors, green star shapes are garlic and other organosulfur-containing nutrients, red rectangle represents NO, and purple rectangles denote direct and indirect influence of NO on vasodilation and blood pressure. NO pathway: in the presence of BH4, eNOS produces NO, which triggers pathways leading to smooth muscle cell relaxation and vasodilation. eNOS uncoupling leads to the formation of O2−. NO and O2− combine to form OONO−, which rapidly reacts with thiols and tyrosine residues of proteins, which in turn, leads to vasodilation and BP reduction independent of cGMP. Garlic and other dietary organosulfides may play a role in the regulation of the NO signaling pathway by creating a more reductive environment and therefore supporting NO production. Abbreviations: BH2, dihypdrobiopterin; BH4, tetrahydrobiopterin; Ca2+, calcium ion; cGMP, cyclic-guanosyl-monophosphate; GSSG, oxidized glutathione; eNOS, endothelial-nitric-oxide-synthase; GSH, reduced free glutathione; GTP, guanosyl-tri-phosphate; NO, nitric oxide (radical); ONOO, peroxynitrite; O2, oxygen; O2−, superoxide anion radical; PKB, protein kinase-B. (Source: Ried K, Fakler P. Potential of garlic (Allium sativum) in lowering high blood pressure: mechanisms of action and clinical relevance. Integr Blood Press Control. 2014 Dec 9;7:71-82. doi: 10.2147/IBPC.S51434. eCollection 2014. Review. PubMed PMID: 25525386; PubMed Central PMCID: PMC4266250.)

6. Indian Herbs for the CVD Management

In traditional medicinal systems, hypertension is diagnosed by its apparent symptoms. The traditional healing also describes other symptoms such as severe headache, fatigue, chest pain, irregular heart beat among others for a diagnosis of cardiac ailments. A 2009 study showed that 25% of modern drug and 75% of new medicines against virulent diseases are obtained from natural plant resources [120].

6.1. *Allium sativum* (Family: Alliaceae or Liliaceae)

The protective mechanisms of the beneficial effects of garlic in CVDs may be achieved by suppressing LDL oxidation, increasing HDL, as well as decreasing TC and TG [121]. While garlic supplementation reduced BP significantly in hypertensive patients, it did not appreciably affect patients with normal BP [122].

6.2. *Terminalia arjuna* (Family: Combretaceae)

Bark of T. arjuna contains a very high level of flavonoids, namely arjunolone, flavones, luteolin, baicaleiin, quercetin, kempferol, and pelargonidin evaluated with other medicinal plants particularly having favorable effects on cardiovascular diseases [123]. *T. arjuna* is widely used for treatment of cardiovascular diseases, including heart diseases and related chest pain, high blood pressure and high cholesterol. A number of clinical studies have also reported its beneficial effects in patients of chronic stable angina, endothelial dysfunction, heart failure and even ischemic mitral regurgitation [124]. Its bark decoction is being used in the Indian subcontinent for anginal pain, hypertension, congestive heart failure, and dyslipidemia, based on the observations of ancient physicians for centuries [125]. No systematic review has been conducted for Terminalia arjuna in patients of chronic stable angina [126]. It nourishes and strengthens the heart muscle and promotes cardiac functioning by regulating blood pressure and cholesterol [127]. T. arjuna significantly decreases TC, LDL and TG levels and increases HDL and lessens atherosclerotic lesion in aorta of hypercholesterolemic rabbits [128]. The effectiveness of T. arjuna stem bark as a cardioprotective and potent antioxidant has been sufficiently demonstrated in different experimental and clinical studies. However, continuous research progress on T. arjuna stem bark is very much needed in the regard of exact molecular mechanism, drug administration, drug-drug interactions, and toxicological studies [129].

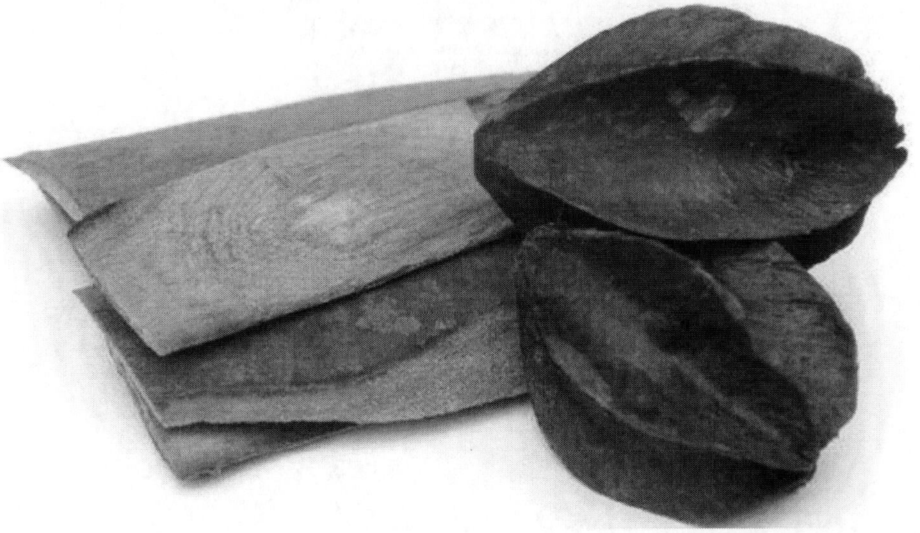

Figure 13. Medicine Grade *Terminalia arjuna* Bark and Dried Fruits. (Source: Indiamart.)

6.3. *Allium cepa* (Onion)

Onion peel extract supplementation for 2 weeks is beneficial as it reduces the possibility of developing key risk factors for cardiovascular disease by altering the lipid profiles in healthy young women [130]. Garlic oil and onion oil have anti-obesity properties that can counteract the effects of an HFD on body weight, adipose tissue weight, and serum lipid profiles [131]. HPLC analysis of onion peel extract revealed that it contains quercetin, one of the major flavonoids, which has anti-platelet effect (an effective inhibitor of collagen-stimulated platelet aggregation in vitro), therefore, it can be a promising and safe strategy for anti-cardiovascular diseases [132]. Hyperglycemia has been identified as a major risk factor for cardiovascular complications linked to T2DM, and thereby known as an effective therapeutic target in the treatment of T2DM. Heat-processed onion extract can be a significant source of arginyl-fructose, a major bioactive Amadori rearrangement compounds in heat-processed onion, and phenolic compounds that exert postprandial blood glucose-lowering and antioxidant effects, respectively [133]. Administration of garlic plus lemon juice resulted in an improvement in lipid levels, fibrinogen and blood pressure of patients with hyperlipidemia [134]. Onion bulbs (*Allium cepa* L.) are among the richest sources of dietary flavonoids and contribute to a large extent to the overall intake of flavonoids [135-137].

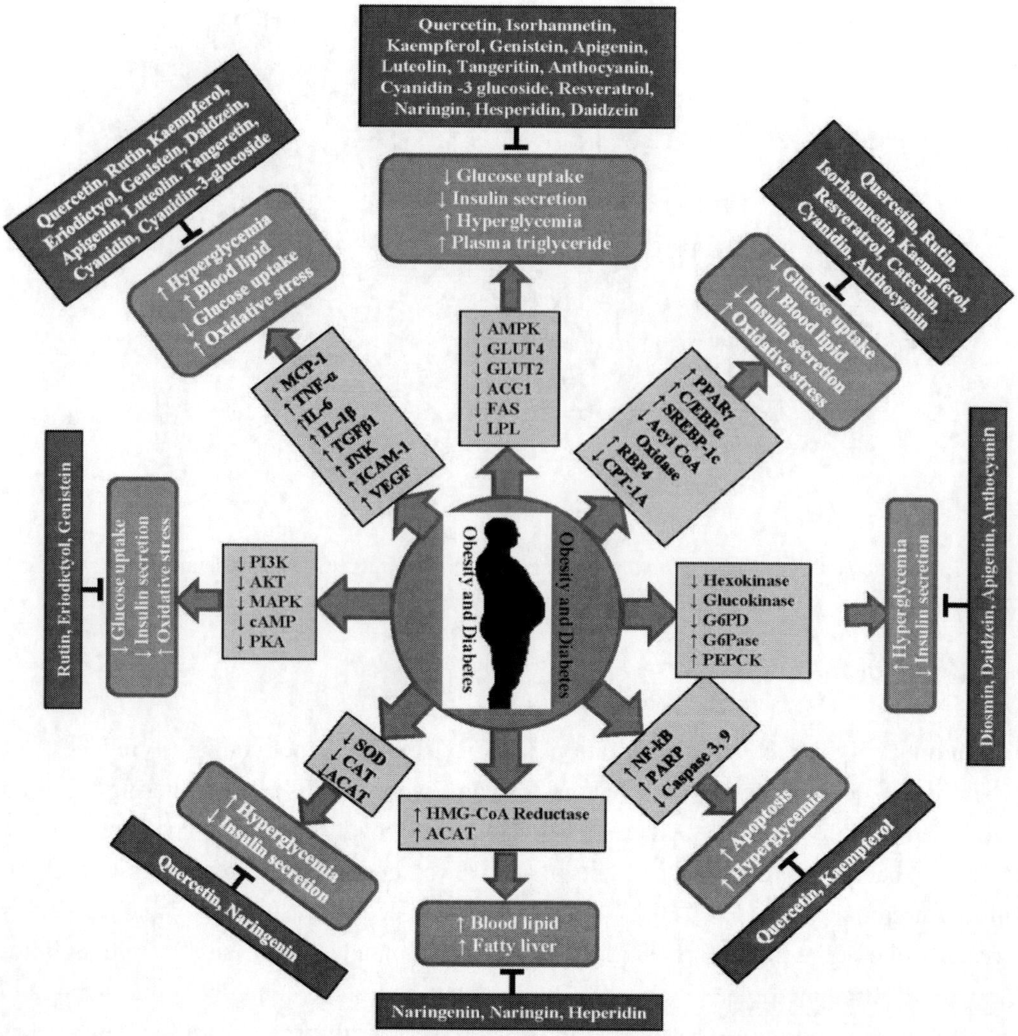

Figure 14. Schematic presentation of molecular functions of different flavonoids with anti-obesity and anti-diabetic effects. Flavonoids showed anti-obesity and anti-diabetic effects by activating or inhibiting different cytokines, enzymes, and metabolites to prevent inflammation, oxidative stress, and metabolism to protect against obesity and diabetes. MCP-1: monocyte-chemo-attractant protein-1; TNF-α: tumor necrosis factor alpha; IL-6: interleukin-6; IL-1β: interleukin 1 beta; FFA: free fatty acid, IRS1: insulin receptor substrate 1; PI3K: phosphatidylinositol 3-kinase; AKT: serine/threonine kinase; FA: fatty acid; IGT: impaired glucose tolerance; PARP: poly(ADP-ribose) polymerase; BCl-2: B-cell lymphoma 2; Bax: Bcl-2-associated X protein; Bak: Bcl-2 homologous antagonist/killer; Caspase 3: cysteine-dependent aspartate-directed proteases 3; PPAR γ: peroxisomal proliferator-activated receptor gamma; SREBP1c: sterol regulatory element binding protein-1c; LPL: lipo protein lipase; AMPK: 5′ adenosine monophosphate-activated protein kinase; HOMA-IR: homeostatic model assessment for insulin resistance; HbA1c: hemoglobin A1c; GLUT4: glucose transporter 4; G6PDH: glucose-6-phosphate dehydrogenase; HMG-CoA: 3-hydroxy-3-methylglutaryl-coenzyme; ACAT: acyl CoA: cholesterol acyltransferase; G6pase: glucose-6-phosphatase; cAMP: cyclic adenosine monophosphate; PKA: protein kinase A. (Source: Kawser Hossain M, Abdal Dayem A, Han J, Yin Y, Kim K, Kumar Saha S, Yang GM, Choi HY, Cho SG. Molecular Mechanisms of the Anti-Obesity and Anti-Diabetic Properties of Flavonoids. Int J Mol Sci. 2016 Apr 15;17(4):569. doi: 10.3390/ijms17040569. Review. PubMed PMID: 27092490; PubMed Central PMCID: PMC4849025.)

6.4. Amla (*Emblica officinalis*)

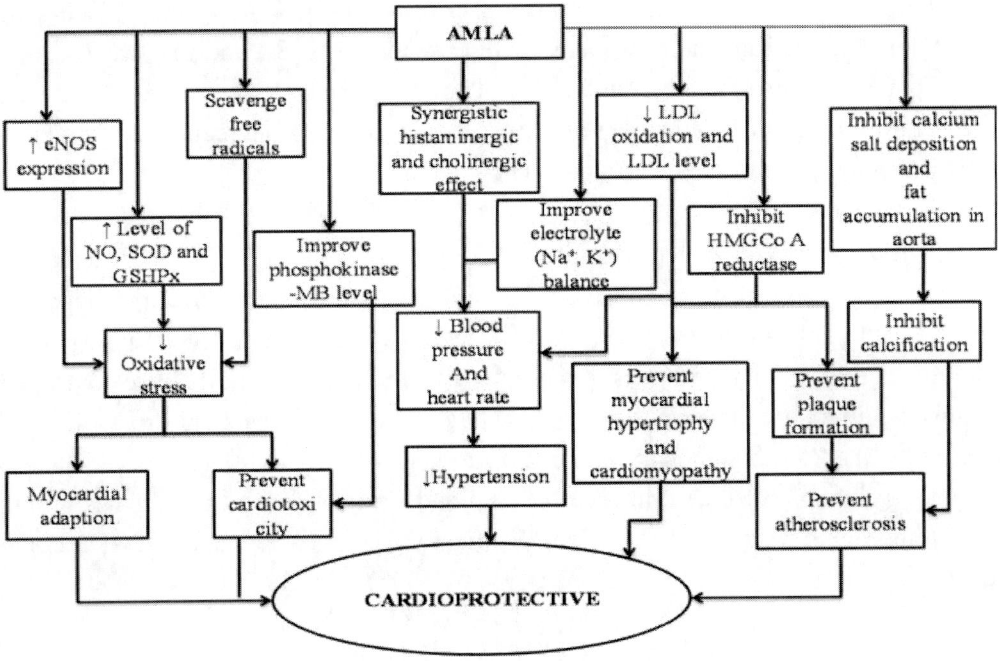

Figure 15. Mechanism of Amla as cardioprotective agent. (1) Reduction in hypertension and oxidative stress by increasing the expression of eNOS, by ameliorating the levels of nitric oxide (NO), SOD, GSHPx and electrolytes like Na+ and K+. (2) Aqueous extract of amla lowers the mean arterial blood pressure, heart rate and respiratory rate by showing synergistic histaminergic and cholinergic effect. (3) Cardioprotective potential in isoproterenol-induced cardiotoxicity through ameliorating the levels of antioxidant enzymes and creatinine phosphokinase-MB and LDH by its antioxidant free radical scavenging activity. (4) Amla fruit juice at dose of 1 ml/kg p.o for 8 weeks in diabetes-induced MI showed preventive action in myocardial hypertrophy, cardiomyopathy and hypertension by increasing heart rate, lowering blood pressure through its antioxidant potential and by maintaining the lipid profile and enzyme levels. (5) Methanolic extract and fruit powder of amla has been known to attenuate the induction and progression of atherosclerosis by preventing the formation of plaque in blood vessels and aorta via inhibiting HMG CoA reductase and LDL oxidation; and by reducing LDL cholesterol levels and subsequently increasing HDL levels [Source: Kaur J, Kaur D, Singh H, Khan MU. Emblica Officinalis: A Meritocratic Drug for Treating Various Disorders. Indo American Journal of Pharm Research.2013:3(6).]

Amla produced significant hypolipidemic effect along with a reduction in blood pressure. Addition of Amla to the currently available hypolipidemic therapy would offer significant protection against atherosclerosis and coronary artery disease, with reduction in the dose and adverse effects of the hypolipidemic agents [138]. It has beneficial role on dyslipidemia and cardiac autonomic functions in rats treated with high fat diet [139]. A potent inhibition of collagen-induced platelet aggregation in response to oral supplementation of a standardized extract of Phyllanthus emblica. Additionally, the extract significantly inhibited hypercholesterolemia and hs-CRP in overweight/Class-1 obese adults from the US population [140]. In a 2019 study, Amla extract has shown significant potential in reducing TC and TG levels as well as lipid ratios, AIP and apoB/apo A-I in dyslipidemic persons (apo B, apo A-I is a major apolipoprotein of HDL particles which helps the reversal transport of cholesterol from peripheral tissue to liver, thus reducing the risk of developing inflammatory response and growth of plaques) and thus has scope to treat general as well as diabetic dyslipidemia. A single agent to reduce cholesterol as well as TG is rare. Cholesterol reduction is achieved without concomitant reduction of Co Q10, in contrast to what is observed with statins [141, 142].

6.5. *Withania somnifera* (Ashwagandha)

Ashwagandha root extract enhances the cardiorespiratory endurance and improves QOL in healthy athletic adults [143]. Ashwagandha is shown in the literature to be an anxiolytic, antidepressant, and antistress adaptogen. A number of studies have confirmed the antistress effect of ashwagandha [144-147]. It also appears to exert a positive influence on the endocrine, cardiopulmonary, and central nervous systems [148]. prevented increase in adrenal weight and decrease in ascorbic acid and Cortisol content of adrenals during stress. It appears to induce a state of non-specifically increased resistance (SNIR) during stress [149].

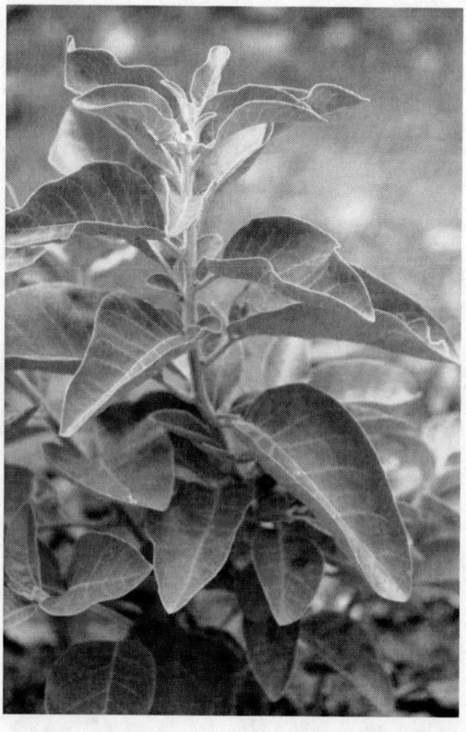

Figure 16. Ashwagandha (Withania somnifera). (Source: Red Moon Herbs.)

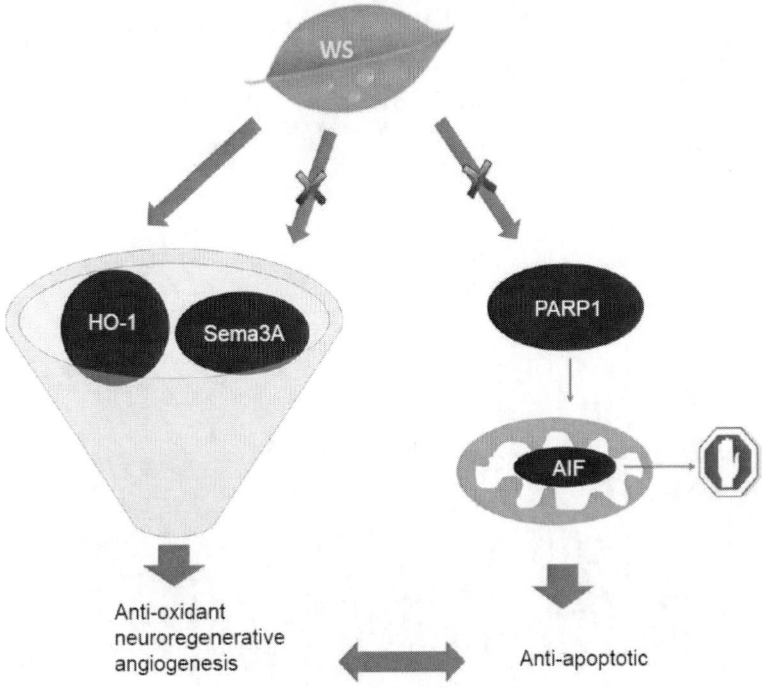

Figure 17. Probable mechanisms of action of an aqueous extract of *Withania somnifera* (WS) in ischemic stroke. WS-mediated attenuation of the expression of Semaphorin 3A (Sema3A) could promote neuronal regeneration. Moreover, HO-1 mediated vascular endothelial growth factor (VEGF) induction and the antagonistic effects of Sema3A and VEGF could have the combined result of higher VEGF levels and a resulting pro-angiogenic effect. WS was also found to reduce levels of poly (ADP-ribose) polymerase 1 (PARP1), which prevents translocation of anti-apoptotic factor (AIF) from the mitochondria to the nucleus. The PARP1-AIF pathway is a prime mediator of caspase-independent apoptosis, which is prevented by WS in this model of stroke. (Source: Raghavan A, Shah ZA. Withania somnifera: a pre-clinical study on neuroregenerative therapy for stroke. Neural Regen Res. 2015 Feb;10(2):183-5. doi: 10.4103/1673-5374.152362. PubMed PMID: 25883607; PubMed Central PMCID: PMC4392656.)

*6.6. Nardostachys jatamansi (*Valerianaceae)

Possesses significant anti-stress activity, which may be due to its antioxidant activity [150]. In vitro antioxidant activity of hydroethanolic extract (70%) of N. jatamansi was studied by measuring the free radical scavenging activity. Rakatchap Har (Each 500 mg cap contains Sarpgandha 150 mg, Shankhpushpi 75 mg, Jatamansi 75 mg, Jahar Mohra Khatai Pishti 75 mg, Moti Pishti 75 mg, Ras Sindoor 50 mg) along with life style modification and psychotherapy is a safe and efficacious remedy for the treatment of all grades of hypertension in all age groups with no limitation to its use [151]. Brahmyadi Churna (Brahmi, Shankhapushpi, Jatamansi, Jyotishmati, Vacha, Ashwagandha Churna 1 part each) caused marked reduction in the levels of total BP. Symptoms such as headache, insomnia, and giddiness showed marked improvement while not much reduction was observed in other symptoms such as chest pain, fatigue, and palpitation. SBP reduced considerably than DBP.reduction in BP was observed markedly with $P < 0.000$ [152]. The aqueous extracts also exhibited protective effects against 2K1C-induced cardiac hypertrophy in a rat model [153].

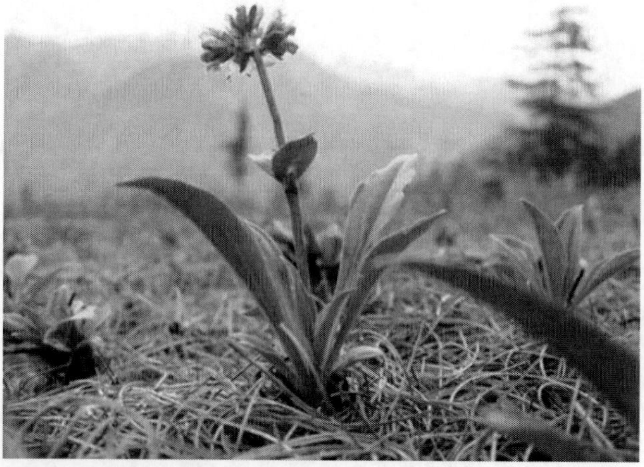

Figure 18. Nardostachys jatamansi or spikenard. (Source: fragnatica.com.)

6.7. Triphala (Combination Drug)

a well-recognized, polyherbal Ayurvedic medicine consisting of fruits of the plant species *Emblica officinalis* (Amalaki), *Terminalia bellerica* (Bibhitaki), and *Terminalia chebula* (Haritaki) in equal proportion 1:1:1 [154, 158]. Potentially effective for several clinical uses such as appetite stimulation, reduction of hyperacidity, antioxidant, anti-inflammatory, immunomodulating, antibacterial, antimutagenic, adaptogenic, hypo-glycemic, antineoplastic, chemoprotective, and radioprotective effects, and prevention of dental caries [155]. Laghu shankha prakshalana kriya (LSP), a yogic bowel cleansing technique, integrated approach of yoga therapy (IAYT) is a safe and useful procedure for patients with essential hypertension. LSP with triphala is more useful [156]. Plays an important role in blood pressure control and balances cholesterol [157]. Triphala and its constituents can counter the effects of an environment (ie, high dietary intake of fats) and have the potential for use as antiobesity agents with desirable lipid-profile modulating properties [159]. *Terminalia bellerica* may influence cholesterol level i.e., increase the level of HDL and decrease LDL, and simultaneously be useful in the treatment of coronary artery disease [160]. β-sitosterol, which is the main constituent of *T. chebula,* is an organic compound belonging to the family of phytosterols, whose chemical structure resembles cholesterol. β-sitosterol and phytosterols may affect lipid metabolism by inhibiting the absorption of cholesterol from the digestive tract. β-sitosterol has also been studied for its potential in lowering high levels of blood-cholesterol [161]. Triphala formulation was associated with hypolipidemic effects on the experimentally induced hypercholesteremic rats [162]. Triphala tablets help helps to improve the circulation and is a very effective formula for hypercholesterolemia [163].

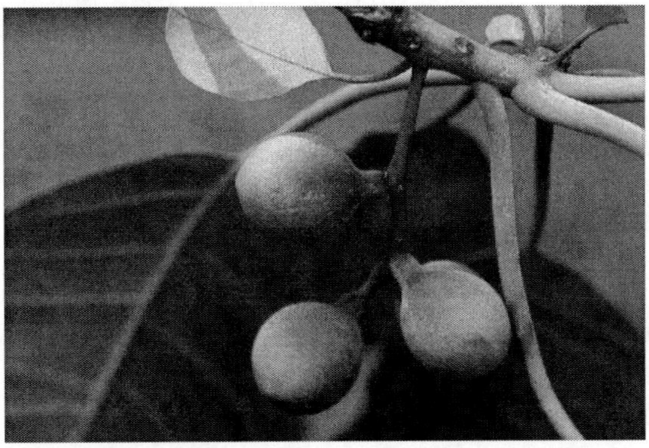

Figure 19. *Terminalia bellerica* (Bahera). (Source: Alibaba.com.)

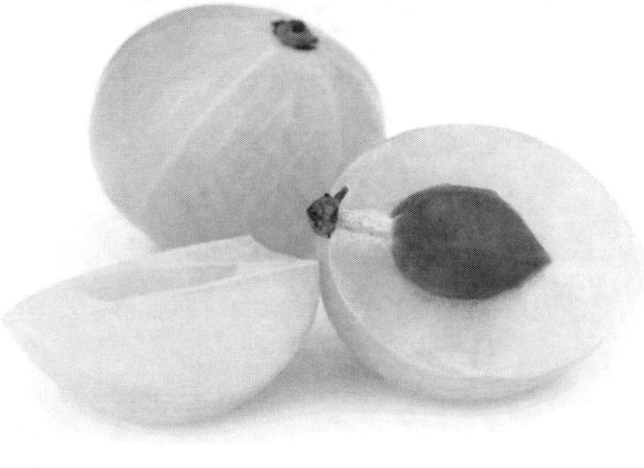

Figure 20. *Phyllanthus Emblica* (Amla). (Source: Ayurtimes.com.)

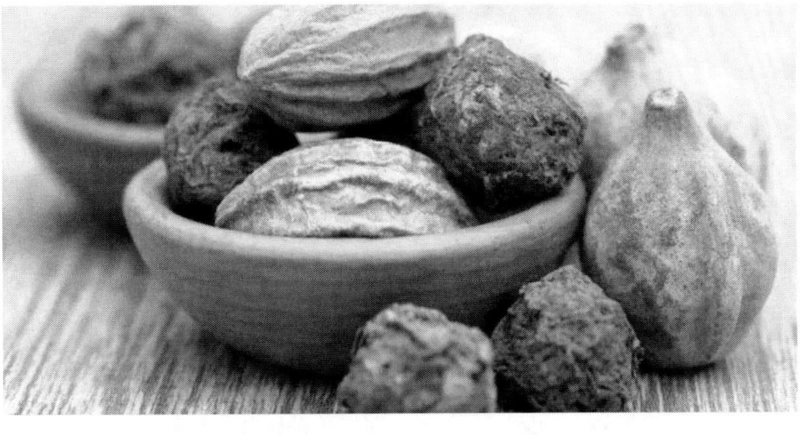

Figure 21. *Terminalia chebula* (Haritaki). (Source: AliExpress.com.)

6.8. *Boerhavia diffusa* (Nyctaginaceae)

Punarnava, a well-known cardiotonic edible medicinal plant against apoptosis in Angiotensin II (Ang II)-stimulated hypertrophic cardiac cells (H9c2), effective in attenuating apoptosis in cardiac cells, which is a major contributor to sudden cardiac death in addition to its nutraceutical properties [164]. Various active compounds in B. diffusa include punarnavine, ursolic acid, punarnavoside, liriodendrin, eupalitin, eupalitin-3-O-â-D-galactopyranoside, rotenoids like boeravinones A, B, C, D, E, F and G, quercetin, kaempferol, etc [165, 166]. Among these, quercetin exhibits antioxidant, antihypertrophic and antihypertensive potential in in vitro and in vivo experimental models [167,168]. Ursolic acid is reported to possess cardioprotective potential via inducing uncoupling of mitochondrial oxidative phosphorylation and reducing mitochondrial H2O2 production [169]. Kaempferol is also reported to possess cardioprotective potential and boeravinone G is another antioxidant and genoprotective compound in B.diffusa [170, 171]. Liriodendrin isolated from B.diffusa is reported to possess Ca2+ channel antagonistic properties in heart [172]. Presence of these active constituents might be responsible for its protective activity against Ang II induced hypertrophy. Cell organelles are also the targets of Arsenic trioxide (ATO)-induced cardiotoxicity in addition to other reported targets like ion channels, and ethanolic extract of *Boerhavia diffusa* has the potential to protect the cardiotoxicity induced by ATO [173].

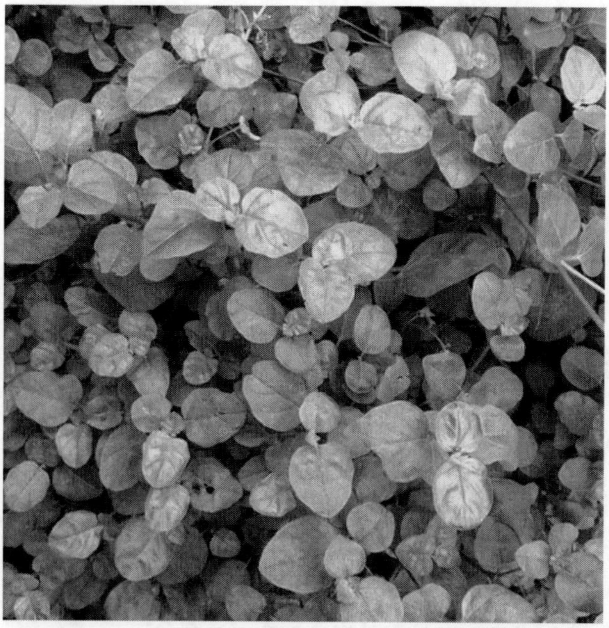

Figure 22. *Boerhavia diffusa* (Nyctaginaceae), Punarnava. (Source: Indiamart.)

6.9. Cruciferous Vegetables

These include broccoli, Brussel sprouts, cabbage, cauliflower, kale, radish, rutabaga, turnip and even arugula. cruciferous vegetables contain isothiocyanates, which can produce the redox-regulated cardioprotective protein, thioredoxin, it was reasoned that consumption of broccoli could be beneficial to the heart. Sulforaphane is by far the most widely studied and best characterized isothiocyanates [174, 175]. Research is showing that sulforaphane helps with inflammation of the arterial walls, inhibits obesity, relieves hypertension, and other conditions that are part of or lead to CVD [176]. Oxidative stress caused by reduced production of nitric oxide and/or increased production of ROS (mainly superoxide) may promote endothelial dysfunction. Therefore, increased oxidative stress represents one possible driver of the increased prevalence of hypertension. A diet containing broccoli sprouts high in Grn (Grn+) decreased oxidative stress and associated problems in male spontaneously hypertensive stroke-prone rats (SHRsp) [177]. As one of Grn key metabolites, SFN was also found to improve blood pressure. Obesity is associated with metabolic disorder, which is another risk factor for atherosclerosis and CVD. Choi et al. investigated whether SFN prevented high-fat diet- (HFD-) induced obesity in C57BL/6N mice. SFN may induce anti-obesity effects by inhibiting adipogenesis [178]. 75% of the sulforaphane will be absorbed into the bloodstream after eaten and taken up by cells. Once inside sulforaphane can damage important intracellular structures like mitochondria and enzymes. This depletes glutathione (most potent human antioxidant) leaving cells vulnerable to further oxidative damage. Sulforaphane can even disrupt epithelial barriers providing yet another plant chemical that can contribute to "leaky gut" [179].

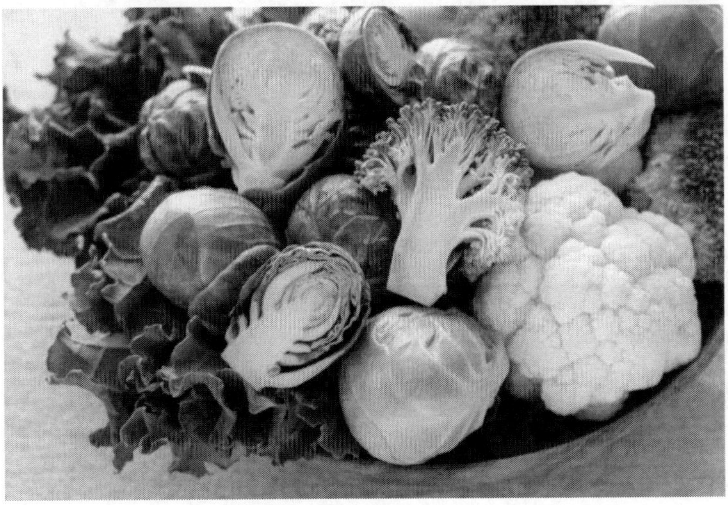

Figure 23. Cruciferous vegetables. (Source: roswellpark.org.)

6.10. *Nigella sativa* (Ranunculaceae)

It has been used in traditional medicine and several studies have been performed in the last decades to reveal the effects of it on different medical disorders such as diabetes, dyslipidemia, hypertension, and obesity [180]. N. sativa oil at a dose of 2.5 mg/kg attenuates the Nω-nitro-L-arginine methyl ester (L-NAME)-induced increase in BP and was associated with a reduction in cardiac redox status and angiotensin-converting enzyme activity and an increase in heme oxygenase (HO-1) activity. N. sativa oil also prevented plasma NO loss. Notably, the BP-lowering effect was comparable to that of nicardipine in hypertensive rats [181]. N. sativa and its component thymoquinone have the beneficial effect on hypertension probably due to attenuation cardiovascular effects of angiotensin II [182]. Thymoquinone (the main constituent *Nigella sativa*) supplementation attenuates cyclophosphamide -induced cardiotoxicity, at least in part, by its ability to decrease oxidative and nitrosative stress and to preserve the activity of antioxidant enzymes as well as its ability to improve the mitochondrial function and energy production [183]. A similar study was found with cyclosporine A and Doxorubicin. N. sativa oil reduced the subsequent cyclosporine A injury in rat heart, demonstrated by normalized cardiac histopathology, decrease in lipid peroxidation, improvement in antioxidant enzyme status and cellular protein oxidation [184]. Thymoquinone as a potentially selective cytoprotective agent, which may ameliorate cardiotoxicity without decreasing DOX antitumor activity [185].

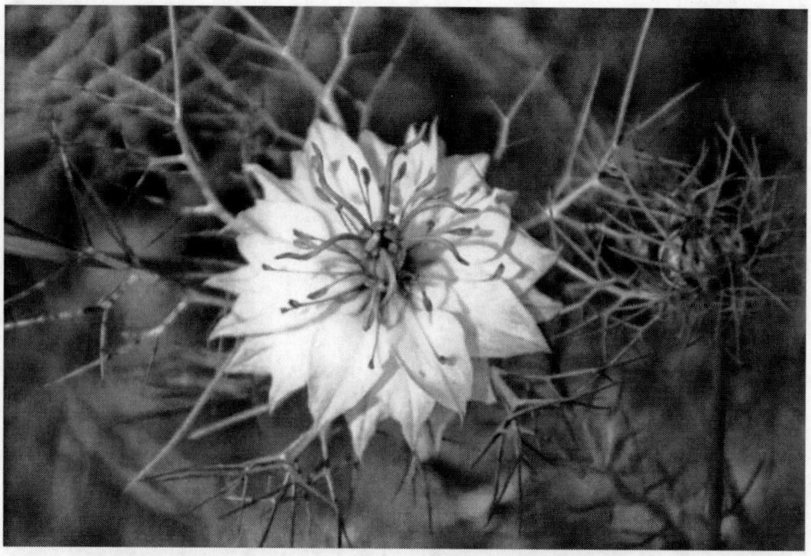

Figure 24. Nigella sativa (black cumin). (Source: Healthy Buddha Magazine.)

6.11. *Zingiber officinale* (Zingiberaceae)

The pharmacological activities of ginger were mainly attributed to its active phytocompounds 6-gingerol, 6-shogaol, zingerone beside other phenolics and flavonoids. 6-gingerol was reported as the most abundant bioactive compound in ginger with various pharmacological effects including antioxidant, analgesic, anti-inflammatory and antipyretic properties. Also, other studies showed that 6-shogaol with lowest concentration in ginger represent more biologically actives compared to 6-gingerol [191]. According to animal studies ginger has the potential to offer a natural alternative dietary supplementation to conventional anti-hypertensive agents, but more human trials of ginger on hypertensive patients using different dosage of a standardized extract are needed [186]. The antihyperlipidemic effect of ginger was supported by animal studies, gingerol prevents HFD-induced hyperlipidemia by modulating the expression of enzymes important to cholesterol metabolism [187]. In addition, the lowering effect of ginger on serum cholesterol may be due to the inhibitory effect of cholesterol biosynthesis and the transformation of cholesterol into bile acids by elevating the activity of hepatic cholesterol 7 alpha-hydroxylase. Furthermore, niacin, a nutrient in ginger, may be a potential active ingredient in lowering serum triglyceride level, increasing clearance of VLDL, enhancing hepatic uptake of LDL-c, and inhibiting cholesterol synthesis [188]. Recent study shows, 6-gingerol could decrease cellular total cholesterol and free cholesterol levels via up-regulation of LDLR through activation of SREBP2 as well as up-regulation of cholesterol efflux-related genes LXRα and ABCA1 (member 1 of human transporter sub-family ABCA) [189]. Daily administration of 1g ginger reduces serum triglyceride concentration, which is a risk factor for cardiovascular disease, in peritoneal dialysis patients [190].

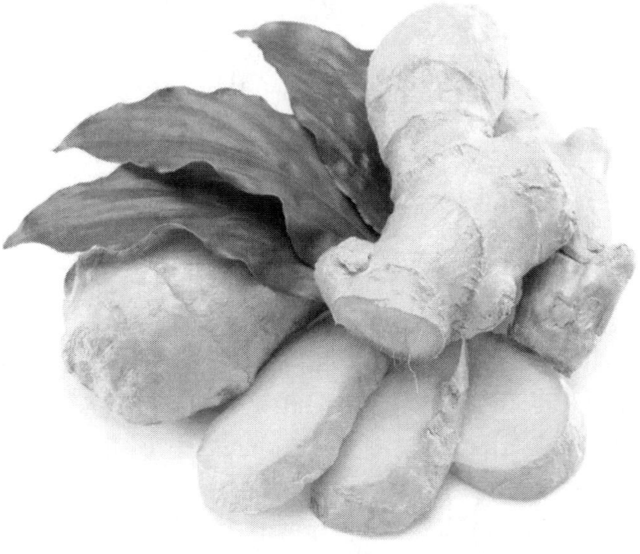

Figure 25. Zingiber officinale (Zingiberaceae) Rhizome. (Source: WordPress.com.)

Conclusion

The pharmacological actions of herbs or herbal isolates appear to favorably modulate several parameters implicated in the pathogenesis of blood pressure, including but not limited to ROS production, VSMC phenotype, endothelial function, platelet activation, pro-inflammatory signaling, and gene expression. With such a broad spectrum of actions, one may predict that herbal remedies will receive even more attention in the coming years, perhaps accentuating the need for further experimentations and clinical trials. Indeed, the lack of sufficient clinical trials constitutes a significant limitation on the ir use at the present time. Of equal importance, it may be advisable that patients be appropriately educated, particularly in relation to herbs whose consumption has been considered safe for thousands of years (black cumin, Chinese sage, coriander, garlic, ginger, ginseng, and tea), and has been supported by sound scientific evidence such as one based on clinical trials with large population groups. The renewed interest in the search for new drugs from natural sources, especially from plant sources, has gained global attention during the last two decades. The tropical rain forests have become an important point of this activity, primarily due to the rich biodiversity they harbor, which promises a high diversity of chemicals with the potential novel structures. However, of this rich biodiversity, only a small portion has been studied for its medicinal potential. The evidence presented is strongly indicative of the notion that herbs and plants are becoming part of evidence-based medicine in the prevention and/or treatment of CVD.

References

[1] Jin J. Screening for Cardiovascular Disease Risk With ECG. *JAMA*. 2018;319(22):2346. doi:10.1001/jama.2018.7311.

[2] Cholesterol and Atherosclerosis. *JAMA*. 2001;285(19):2536. doi:10.1001/jama.285.19.2536.

[3] Kronhaus KD. Dysrhythmia vs Arrhythmia. *JAMA*. 1979;241(1):28. doi:10.1001/jama.1979.03290270020009.

[4] White Pd. An Unusual Type Of Gross Cardiac Arrhythmia. *JAMA*. 1915;LXV(15):1276. doi:10.1001/jama.1915.02580150050016.

[5] Cardiac Arrhythmias: Diagnosis and Treatment. *Arch Intern Med*. 1977;137(11):1643. doi:10.1001/archinte.1977.03630230109039.

[6] Stefano Caselli, Andrea Serdoz, Federica Mango, Erika Lemme, Antonia Vaquer Seguì, Alberto Milan, Christine Attenhofer Jost, Christian Schmied, Antonio Spataro, Antonio Pelliccia; High blood pressure response to exercise predicts future

development of hypertension in young athletes, *European Heart Journal,* Volume 40, Issue 1, 1 January 2019, Pages 62–68, https://doi.org/10.1093/eurheartj/ehy810.

[7] Kristian Thygesen, Joseph S Alpert, Allan S Jaffe, Bernard R Chaitman, Jeroen J Bax, David A Morrow, Harvey D White, ESC Scientific Document Group; Fourth universal definition of myocardial infarction (2018), *European Heart Journal,* Volume 40, Issue 3, 14 January 2019, Pages 237–269, https://doi.org/10.1093/eurheartj/ehy462.

[8] Zhao-Jun Yang, China National Diabetes and Metabolic Disorders Study Group, Jie Liu, China National Diabetes and Metabolic Disorders Study Group, Jia-Pu Ge, China National Diabetes and Metabolic Disorders Study Group, Li Chen, China National Diabetes and Metabolic Disorders Study Group, Zhi-Gang Zhao, China National Diabetes and Metabolic Disorders Study Group, Wen-Ying Yang, China National Diabetes and Metabolic Disorders Study Group; Prevalence of cardiovascular disease risk factor in the Chinese population: the 2007–2008 China National Diabetes and Metabolic Disorders Study, *European Heart Journal,* Volume 33, Issue 2, 1 January 2012, Pages 213–220, https://doi.org/10.1093/eurheartj/ehr205.

[9] Jin J. Risk Assessment for Cardiovascular Disease with Nontraditional Risk Factors. *JAMA.* 2018;320(3):316. doi:10.1001/jama.2018.9122.

[10] Joanne M. Murabito, Chao-Yu Guo, Caroline S. Fox, Ralph B. D'Agostino; Heritability of the Ankle-Brachial Index: The Framingham Offspring Study, *American Journal of Epidemiology,* Volume 164, Issue 10, 15 November 2006, Pages 963–968, https://doi.org/10.1093/aje/kwj295.

[11] Kimio Satoh, Hiroaki Shimokawa; High-sensitivity C-reactive protein: still need for next-generation biomarkers for remote future cardiovascular events, *European Heart Journal,* Volume 35, Issue 27, 14 July 2014, Pages 1776–1778, https://doi.org/10.1093/eurheartj/ehu115.

[12] Rajesh Tota-Maharaj, Michael J. Blaha, John W. McEvoy, Roger S. Blumenthal, Evan D. Muse, Matthew J. Budoff, Leslee J. Shaw, Daniel S. Berman, Jamal S. Rana, John Rumberger, Tracy Callister, Juan Rivera, Arthur Agatston, Khurram Nasir; Coronary artery calcium for the prediction of mortality in young adults <45 years old and elderly adults >75 years old, *European Heart Journal,* Volume 33, Issue 23, 1 December 2012, Pages 2955–2962, https://doi.org/10.1093/eurheartj/ehs230.

[13] M S J R Shahi, M Dey, A K Chowdhury; 20P A study on possibility of high sensitivity C - reactive protein (hs-CRP) and circulating interluekin-6 (IL-6) as biomarker in breast cancer patients, *Annals of Oncology*, Volume 29, Issue suppl_9, 1 November 2018, mdy426.018, https://doi.org/10.1093/annonc/mdy426.018.

[14] Dipak Kotecha, Jonathan P. Piccini; Atrial fibrillation in heart failure: what should we do?, *European Heart Journal,* Volume 36, Issue 46, 7 December 2015, Pages 3250–3257, https://doi.org/10.1093/eurheartj/ehv513.

[15] Aidan P Bolger, Andrew J.S Coats, Michael A Gatzoulis; Congenital heart disease: the original heart failure syndrome, *European Heart Journal,* Volume 24, Issue 10, 1 May 2003, Pages 970–976, https://doi.org/10.1016/S0195-668X(03)00005-8.

[16] Thomas F Lüscher; Outcome of congenital heart disease with modern cardiac care, *European Heart Journal,* Volume 39, Issue 12, 21 March 2018, Pages 969–971, https://doi.org/10.1093/eurheartj/ehy166.

[17] Fukui M, Gupta A, Abdelkarim I, et al. Association of Structural and Functional Cardiac Changes With Transcatheter Aortic Valve Replacement Outcomes in Patients With Aortic Stenosis. *JAMA Cardiol.* Published online February 06, 2019. doi:10.1001/jamacardio.2018.4830.

[18] Maron BJ, Lesser JR, Schiller NB, Harris KM, Brown C, Rehm HL. Implications of Hypertrophic Cardiomyopathy Transmitted by Sperm Donation. *JAMA.* 2009;302(15):1681–1684. doi:10.1001/jama.2009.1507.

[19] Angus DC. Successful Resuscitation From In-Hospital Cardiac Arrest—What Happens Next? *JAMA.* 2015;314(12):1238–1239. doi:10.1001/jama.2015.11735.

[20] Myerburg RJ, Goldberger JJ. Sudden Cardiac Arrest Risk Assessment: Population Science and the Individual Risk Mandate. *JAMA Cardiol.* 2017;2(6):689–694. doi:10.1001/jamacardio.2017.0266.

[21] Hess CN, Hiatt WR. Antithrombotic Therapy for Peripheral Artery Disease in 2018. *JAMA.* 2018;319(22):2329–2330. doi:10.1001/jama.2018.5422.

[22] Voelker R. Aneurysm Guidelines. JAMA. 2000;284(20):2585. doi:10.1001/jama.284.20.2585-JQU00009-2-1.

[23] Dan Laukka, Emily Pan, Terhi Fordell, Kemal Alpay, Melissa Rahi, Jussi Hirvonen, Jaakko Rinne, Jarmo Gunn; *317 Prevalence of Thoracic Aneurysms or Dilatations in Patients With the Intracranial Aneurysms, Neurosurgery,* Volume 65, Issue CN_suppl_1, 1 September 2018, Pages 128, https://doi.org/10.1093/neuros/nyy303.317.

[24] Mehmet Kanbay, Laura-Gabriela Sánchez-Lozada, Martha Franco, Magdalena Madero, Yalcin Solak, Bernardo Rodriguez-Iturbe, Adrian Covic, Richard J. Johnson; Microvascular disease and its role in the brain and cardiovascular system: a potential role for uric acid as a cardiorenal toxin, *Nephrology Dialysis Transplantation,* Volume 26, Issue 2, 1 February 2011, Pages 430–437, https://doi.org/10.1093/ndt/gfq635.

[25] S Coccheri, G Palareti; The cardiovascular risk burden of intermittent claudication, *European Heart Journal Supplements,* Volume 4, Issue suppl_B, 1 March 2002, Pages B46–B49, https://doi.org/10.1016/S1520-765X(02)90017-9.

[26] Bell CS, Samuel JP, Samuels JA. Prevalence of Hypertension in Children. *Hypertension.* 2019 Jan;73(1):148-152. doi: 10.1161/hypertensionaha.118.11673. PubMed PMID: 30571555; PubMed Central PMCID: PMC6291260.

[27] Anker D, Santos-Eggimann B, Santschi V, Del Giovane C, Wolfson C, Streit S, Rodondi N, Chiolero A. Screening and treatment of hypertension in older adults: less is more? *Public Health Rev.* 2018 Sep 3;39:26. doi: 10.1186/s40985-018-0101-z. eCollection 2018. Review. PubMed PMID: 30186660; PubMed Central PMCID: PMC6120092.

[28] Kim H, Andrade FCD. Diagnostic status and age at diagnosis of hypertension on adherence to lifestyle recommendations. *Prev Med Rep.* 2018 Nov 13;13:52-56. doi: 10.1016/j.pmedr.2018.11.005. eCollection 2019 Mar. PubMed PMID: 30510893; PubMed Central PMCID: PMC6260446.

[29] Moynihan RN, Clark J, Albarqouni L. Media Coverage of the Benefits and Harms of the 2017 Expanded Definition of High Blood Pressure. *JAMA Intern Med.* 2019;179(2):272–273. doi:10.1001/jamainternmed.2018.6201.

[30] Global Burden of Cardiovascular Diseases Collaboration. The Burden of Cardiovascular Diseases Among US States, 1990-2016. *JAMA Cardiol.* 2018;3(5):375–389. doi:10.1001/jamacardio.2018.0385.

[31] Khera R, Lu Y, Lu J, Saxena A, Nasir K, Jiang L, Krumholz HM. Impact of 2017 ACC/AHA guidelines on prevalence of hypertension and eligibility for antihypertensive treatment in United States and China: nationally representative cross sectional study. *BMJ.* 2018 Jul 11;362:k2357. doi: 10.1136/bmj.k2357. PubMed PMID: 29997129; PubMed Central PMCID: PMC6039831.

[32] Wyndham CR. Atrial fibrillation: the most common arrhythmia. *Tex Heart Inst J.* 2000;27(3):257-67. Review. PubMed PMID: 11093410; PubMed Central PMCID: PMC101077.

[33] Zoni-Berisso M, Lercari F, Carazza T, Domenicucci S. Epidemiology of atrial fibrillation: European perspective. *Clin Epidemiol.* 2014 Jun 16;6:213-20. doi: 10.2147/CLEP.S47385. eCollection 2014. Review. PubMed PMID: 24966695; PubMed Central PMCID: PMC4064952.

[34] Ko D, Rahman F, Schnabel RB, Yin X, Benjamin EJ, Christophersen IE. Atrial fibrillation in women: epidemiology, pathophysiology, presentation, and prognosis. *Nat Rev Cardiol.* 2016 Jun;13(6):321-32. doi: 10.1038/nrcardio.2016.45. Epub 2016 Apr 7. Review. PubMed PMID: 27053455; PubMed Central PMCID: PMC5579870.

[35] Bradley SM, Borgerding JA, Wood GB, Maynard C, Fihn SD. Incidence, Risk Factors, and Outcomes Associated With In-Hospital Acute Myocardial Infarction. *JAMA Netw Open.* 2019;2(1):e187348. doi:10.1001/jamanetworkopen.2018.7348.

[36] Kayani WT, Ballantyne CM. Improving Outcomes After Myocardial Infarction in the US Population. *J Am Heart Assoc.* 2018 Feb 17;7(4). pii: e008407. doi: 10.1161/JAHA.117.008407. PubMed PMID: 29455157; PubMed Central PMCID: PMC5850209.

[37] Kim J, Thrift AG. A Promising Skills-Based Intervention to Reduce Blood Pressure in Individuals with Stroke and Transient Ischemic Attack. *JAMA Neurol.* 2019;76(1):13–14. doi:10.1001/jamaneurol.2018.2935.

[38] Sanchis-Gomar F, Perez-Quilis C, Leischik R, Lucia A. Epidemiology of coronary heart disease and acute coronary syndrome. *Ann Transl Med.* 2016 Jul;4(13):256. doi: 10.21037/atm.2016.06.33. Review. PubMed PMID: 27500157; PubMed Central PMCID: PMC4958723.

[39] The US Burden of Disease Collaborators. The State of US Health, 1990-2016: Burden of Diseases, Injuries, and Risk Factors Among US States. *JAMA.* 2018;319(14):1444–1472. doi:10.1001/jama.2018.0158.

[40] Shaw LJ, Goyal A, Mehta C, Xie J, Phillips L, Kelkar A, Knapper J, Berman DS, Nasir K, Veledar E, Blaha MJ, Blumenthal R, Min JK, Fazel R, Wilson PWF, Budoff MJ. 10-Year Resource Utilization and Costs for Cardiovascular Care. *J Am Coll Cardiol.* 2018 Mar 13;71(10):1078-1089. doi: 10.1016/j.jacc.2017.12.064. PubMed PMID: 29519347; PubMed Central PMCID: PMC5846485.

[41] Gheorghe A, Griffiths U, Murphy A, Legido-Quigley H, Lamptey P, Perel P. The economic burden of cardiovascular disease and hypertension in low- and middle-income countries: a systematic review. *BMC Public Health.* 2018 Aug 6;18(1):975. doi: 10.1186/s12889-018-5806-x. PubMed PMID: 30081871; PubMed Central PMCID: PMC6090747.

[42] Yu E, Malik VS, Hu FB. Cardiovascular Disease Prevention by Diet Modification: JACC Health Promotion Series. *J Am Coll Cardiol.* 2018 Aug 21;72(8):914-926. doi: 10.1016/j.jacc.2018.02.085. Review. PubMed PMID: 30115231; PubMed Central PMCID: PMC6100800.

[43] Billingsley HE, Carbone S, Lavie CJ. Dietary Fats and Chronic Noncommunicable Diseases. *Nutrients.* 2018 Sep 30;10(10). pii: E1385. doi: 10.3390/nu10101385. Review. PubMed PMID: 30274325; PubMed Central PMCID: PMC6213917.

[44] Prentice RL, Aragaki AK, Van Horn L, Thomson CA, Beresford SA, Robinson J, Snetselaar L, Anderson GL, Manson JE, Allison MA, Rossouw JE, Howard BV. Low-fat dietary pattern and cardiovascular disease: results from the Women's Health Initiative randomized controlled trial. *Am J Clin Nutr.* 2017 Jul;106(1):35-43. doi: 10.3945/ajcn.117.153270. Epub 2017 May 17. PubMed PMID: 28515068; PubMed Central PMCID: PMC5486201.

[45] Forouhi NG, Krauss RM, Taubes G, Willett W. Dietary fat and cardiometabolic health: evidence, controversies, and consensus for guidance. *BMJ.* 2018 Jun 13;361:k2139. doi: 10.1136/bmj.k2139. PubMed PMID: 29898882; PubMed Central PMCID: PMC6053258.

[46] Oh R, Uppaluri KR. Low Carbohydrate Diet. 2019 Jan 28. *StatPearls [Internet].* Treasure Island (FL): StatPearls Publishing; 2018 Jan-. Available from http://www.ncbi.nlm.nih.gov/books/NBK537084/ PubMed PMID: 30725769.

[47] Seidelmann SB, Claggett B, Cheng S, Henglin M, Shah A, Steffen LM, Folsom AR, Rimm EB, Willett WC, Solomon SD. Dietary carbohydrate intake and mortality: a prospective cohort study and meta-analysis. *Lancet Public Health.* 2018 Sep;3(9):e419-e428. doi: 10.1016/S2468-2667(18)30135-X. Epub 2018 Aug 17. PubMed PMID: 30122560; PubMed Central PMCID: PMC6339822.

[48] Vitale M, Masulli M, Calabrese I, Rivellese AA, Bonora E, Signorini S, Perriello G, Squatrito S, Buzzetti R, Sartore G, Babini AC, Gregori G, Giordano C, Clemente G, Grioni S, Dolce P, Riccardi G, Vaccaro O; TOSCA.IT Study Group. Impact of a Mediterranean Dietary Pattern and Its Components on Cardiovascular Risk Factors, Glucose Control, and Body Weight in People with Type 2 Diabetes: A Real-Life Study. *Nutrients.* 2018 Aug 10;10(8). pii: E1067. doi: 10.3390/nu10081067. PubMed PMID: 30103444; PubMed Central PMCID: PMC6115857.

[49] Lim CC, Hayes RB, Ahn J, Shao Y, Silverman DT, Jones RR, Thurston GD. Mediterranean Diet and the Association Between Air Pollution and Cardiovascular Disease Mortality Risk. *Circulation.* 2019 Jan 31. doi: 10.1161/CIRCULATIONAHA.118.035742. [Epub ahead of print] PubMed PMID: 30700142.

[50] Eilat-Adar S, Sinai T, Yosefy C, Henkin Y. Nutritional recommendations for cardiovascular disease prevention. *Nutrients.* 2013 Sep 17;5(9):3646-83. doi: 10.3390/nu5093646. Review. PubMed PMID: 24067391; PubMed Central PMCID: PMC3798927.

[51] Zhao CN, Meng X, Li Y, Li S, Liu Q, Tang GY, Li HB. Fruits for Prevention and Treatment of Cardiovascular Diseases. *Nutrients.* 2017 Jun 13;9(6). pii: E598. doi: 10.3390/nu9060598. Review. PubMed PMID: 28608832; PubMed Central PMCID: PMC5490577.

[52] Bonaccio M, Di Castelnuovo A, Costanzo S, Persichillo M, De Curtis A, Cerletti C, Donati MB, de Gaetano G, Iacoviello L; Moli-sani Study Investigators. Interaction between Mediterranean diet and statins on mortality risk in patients with cardiovascular disease: Findings from the Moli-sani Study. *Int J Cardiol.* 2019 Feb 1;276:248-254. doi: 10.1016/j.ijcard.2018.11.117. Epub 2018 Nov 24. PubMed PMID: 30527993.

[53] Kapil V, Khambata RS, Robertson A, Caulfield MJ, Ahluwalia A. Dietary nitrate provides sustained blood pressure lowering in hypertensive patients: a randomized, phase 2, double-blind, placebo-controlled study. *Hypertension.* 2015 Feb;65(2):320-7. doi: 10.1161/HYPERTENSIONAHA.114.04675. Epub 2014 Nov 24. PubMed PMID: 25421976; PubMed Central PMCID: PMC4288952.

[54] Bazzano LA. Effects of soluble dietary fiber on low-density lipoprotein cholesterol and coronary heart disease risk. *Curr Atheroscler Rep.* 2008 Dec;10(6):473-7. Review. PubMed PMID: 18937894.

[55] Zafra-Stone S, Yasmin T, Bagchi M, Chatterjee A, Vinson JA, Bagchi D. Berry anthocyanins as novel antioxidants in human health and disease prevention. *Mol Nutr Food Res.* 2007 Jun;51(6):675-83. Review. PubMed PMID: 17533652.

[56] Wang L, Bordi PL, Fleming JA, Hill AM, Kris-Etherton PM. Effect of a moderate fat diet with and without avocados on lipoprotein particle number, size and subclasses in overweight and obese adults: a randomized, controlled trial. *J Am Heart Assoc.* 2015 Jan 7;4(1):e001355. doi: 10.1161/JAHA.114.001355. PubMed PMID: 25567051; PubMed Central PMCID: PMC4330060.

[57] Hernández-Alonso P, Bulló M, Salas-Salvadó J. Pistachios for Health: What Do We Know About This Multifaceted Nut? *Nutr Today.* 2016 May;51(3):133-138. Epub 2016 May 19. PubMed PMID: 27340302; PubMed Central PMCID: PMC4890834.

[58] Galleano M, Oteiza PI, Fraga CG. Cocoa, chocolate, and cardiovascular disease. *J Cardiovasc Pharmacol.* 2009 Dec; 54(6):483-90. doi: 10.1097/FJC. 0b013e3181b76787. Review. PubMed PMID: 19701098; PubMed Central PMCID: PMC2797556.

[59] Story EN, Kopec RE, Schwartz SJ, Harris GK. An update on the health effects of tomato lycopene. *Annu Rev Food Sci Technol.* 2010;1:189-210. doi: 10.1146/annurev.food.102308.124120. Review. PubMed PMID: 22129335; PubMed Central PMCID: PMC3850026.

[60] Ros E. Health benefits of nut consumption. Nutrients. 2010 Jul;2(7):652-82. doi: 10.3390/nu2070683. Epub 2010 Jun 24. Review. PubMed PMID: 22254047; PubMed Central PMCID: PMC3257681.

[61] Gammone MA, Riccioni G, D'Orazio N. Carotenoids: potential allies of cardiovascular health? *Food Nutr Res.* 2015 Feb 6;59:26762. doi: 10.3402/fnr.v59.26762. eCollection 2015. PubMed PMID: 25660385; PubMed Central PMCID: PMC4321000.

[62] Kishimoto Y, Yoshida H, Kondo K. Potential Anti-Atherosclerotic Properties of Astaxanthin. *Mar Drugs.* 2016 Feb 5;14(2). pii: E35. doi: 10.3390/md14020035. Review. PubMed PMID: 26861359; PubMed Central PMCID: PMC4771988.

[63] Fassett RG, Coombes JS. Astaxanthin: a potential therapeutic agent in cardiovascular disease. *Mar Drugs.* 2011 Mar 21;9(3):447-65. doi: 10.3390/md9030447. Review. PubMed PMID: 21556169; PubMed Central PMCID: PMC3083660.

[64] Aoi W, Naito Y, Sakuma K, Kuchide M, Tokuda H, Maoka T, Toyokuni S, Oka S, Yasuhara M, Yoshikawa T. Astaxanthin limits exercise-induced skeletal and cardiac muscle damage in mice. *Antioxid Redox Signal.* 2003 Feb;5(1):139-44. PubMed PMID: 12626126.

[65] Ambati RR, Phang SM, Ravi S, Aswathanarayana RG. Astaxanthin: sources, extraction, stability, biological activities and its commercial applications--a review. *Mar Drugs.* 2014 Jan 7;12(1):128-52. doi: 10.3390/md12010128. Review. PubMed PMID: 24402174; PubMed Central PMCID: PMC3917265.

[66] Heo S.J., Yoon W.J., Kim K.N., Ahn G.N., Kang S.M., Kang D.H., Affan A., Oh C., Jung W.K., Jeon Y.J. Evaluation of anti-inflammatory effect of fucoxanthin isolated from brown algae in lipopolysaccharide-stimulated RAW 264.7 macrophages. *Food Chem. Toxicol.* 2010;48:2045–2451. doi: 10.1016/j.fct.2010.05.003.

[67] Chang PM, Li KL, Lin YC. Fucoidan¯Fucoxanthin Ameliorated Cardiac Function via IRS1/GRB2/ SOS1, GSK3β/CREB Pathways and Metabolic Pathways in Senescent Mice. *Mar Drugs.* 2019 Jan 21;17(1). pii: E69. doi: 10.3390/md17010069. PubMed PMID: 30669571; PubMed Central PMCID: PMC6356397.

[68] Zhang H, Tang Y, Zhang Y, Zhang S, Qu J, Wang X, Kong R, Han C, Liu Z. Fucoxanthin: A Promising Medicinal and Nutritional Ingredient. *Evid Based Complement Alternat Med.* 2015;2015:723515. doi: 10.1155/2015/723515. Epub 2015 May 27. Review. PubMed PMID: 26106437; PubMed Central PMCID: PMC4461761.

[69] Maeda H, Kanno S, Kodate M, Hosokawa M, Miyashita K. Fucoxanthinol, Metabolite of Fucoxanthin, Improves Obesity-Induced Inflammation in Adipocyte Cells. *Mar Drugs.* 2015 Aug 4;13(8):4799-813. doi: 10.3390/md13084799. PubMed PMID: 26248075; PubMed Central PMCID: PMC4557005.

[70] Cheng HM, Koutsidis G, Lodge JK, Ashor AW, Siervo M, Lara J. Lycopene and tomato and risk of cardiovascular diseases: A systematic review and meta-analysis of epidemiological evidence. *Crit Rev Food Sci Nutr.* 2017 Aug 11:1-18. doi: 10.1080/10408398.2017.1362630. [Epub ahead of print] PubMed PMID: 28799780.

[71] Zou ZY, Xu XR, Lin XM, Zhang HB, Xiao X, Ouyang L, Huang YM, Wang X, Liu YQ. Effects of lutein and lycopene on carotid intima-media thickness in Chinese subjects with subclinical atherosclerosis: a randomised, double-blind, placebo-controlled trial. *Br J Nutr.* 2014 Feb;111(3):474-80. doi: 10.1017/S0007114513002730. Epub 2013 Sep 19. PubMed PMID: 24047757.

[72] Mozos I, Stoian D, Caraba A, Malainer C, Horbańczuk JO, Atanasov AG. Lycopene and Vascular Health. *Front Pharmacol.* 2018 May 23;9:521. doi: 10.3389/fphar.2018.00521. eCollection 2018. Review. PubMed PMID: 29875663; PubMed Central PMCID: PMC5974099.

[73] Thies F, Mills LM, Moir S, Masson LF. Cardiovascular benefits of lycopene: fantasy or reality? *Proc Nutr Soc.* 2017 May;76(2):122-129. doi: 10.1017/S0029665116000744. Epub 2016 Sep 9. PubMed PMID: 27609297.

[74] Howard D. Sesso, Simin Liu, J. Michael Gaziano, Julie E. Buring; Dietary Lycopene, Tomato-Based Food Products and Cardiovascular Disease in Women, *The Journal of Nutrition,* Volume 133, Issue 7, 1 July 2003, Pages 2336–2341, https://doi.org/10.1093/jn/133.7.2336

[75] Sommerburg O, Keunen JE, Bird AC, van Kuijk FJ. Fruits and vegetables that are sources for lutein and zeaxanthin: the macular pigment in human eyes. *Br J*

Ophthalmol. 1998 Aug;82(8):907-10. PubMed PMID: 9828775; PubMed Central PMCID: PMC1722697.

[76] Kim JE, Leite JO, DeOgburn R, Smyth JA, Clark RM, Fernandez ML. A lutein-enriched diet prevents cholesterol accumulation and decreases oxidized LDL and inflammatory cytokines in the aorta of guinea pigs. *J Nutr.* 2011 Aug;141(8):1458-63. doi: 10.3945/jn.111.141630. Epub 2011 Jun 22. Erratum in: *J Nutr.* 2013 Jun;143(6):934. PubMed PMID: 21697302.

[77] Thomson RL, Coates AM, Howe PR, Bryan J, Matsumoto M, Buckley JD. Increases in plasma lutein through supplementation are correlated with increases in physical activity and reductions in sedentary time in older adults. *Nutrients.* 2014 Mar 3;6(3):974-84. doi: 10.3390/nu6030974. PubMed PMID: 24594505; PubMed Central PMCID: PMC3967172.

[78] Han H, Cui W, Wang L, Xiong Y, Liu L, Sun X, Hao L. Lutein prevents high fat diet-induced atherosclerosis in ApoE-deficient mice by inhibiting NADPH oxidase and increasing PPAR expression. *Lipids.* 2015 Mar;50(3):261-73. doi: 10.1007/s11745-015-3992-1. Epub 2015 Feb 7. PubMed PMID: 25663235.

[79] Viera I, Pérez-Gálvez A, Roca M. Bioaccessibility of Marine Carotenoids. *Mar Drugs.* 2018 Oct 22;16(10). pii: E397. doi: 10.3390/md16100397. Review. PubMed PMID: 30360450; PubMed Central PMCID: PMC6213429.

[80] Wang C, Qiu R, Cao Y, Ouyang WF, Li HB, Ling WH, Chen YM. Higher dietary and serum carotenoid levels are associated with lower carotid intima-media thickness in middle-aged and elderly people. *Br J Nutr.* 2018 Mar;119(5):590-598. doi: 10.1017/S0007114517003932. PubMed PMID: 29508696.

[81] Dwyer JH, Paul-Labrador MJ, Fan J, Shircore AM, Merz CN, Dwyer KM. Progression of carotid intima-media thickness and plasma antioxidants: the Los Angeles Atherosclerosis Study. *Arterioscler Thromb Vasc Biol.* 2004 Feb;24(2):313-9. Epub 2003 Dec 1. PubMed PMID: 14656738.

[82] Lutein and Zeaxanthin Linked to Higher Heart Attack Risk. *Web Jobson Medical Information LLC,* August 15, 2005. Available From: https://www.reviewofoptometry.com/article/lutein-and-zeaxanthin-linked-to-higher-heart-attack-risk.

[83] Burri BJ, La Frano MR, Zhu C. Absorption, metabolism, and functions of β-cryptoxanthin. *Nutr Rev.* 2016 Feb;74(2):69-82. doi: 10.1093/nutrit/nuv064. Epub 2016 Jan 7. Review. PubMed PMID: 26747887; PubMed Central PMCID: PMC4892306.

[84] Pongkan W, Takatori O, Ni Y, Xu L, Nagata N, Chattipakorn SC, Usui S, Kaneko S, Takamura M, Sugiura M, Chattipakorn N, Ota T. β-Cryptoxanthin exerts greater cardioprotective effects on cardiac ischemia-reperfusion injury than astaxanthin by attenuating mitochondrial dysfunction in mice. *Mol Nutr Food Res.* 2017 Oct;61(10). doi: 10.1002/mnfr.201601077. Epub 2017 Jul 18. PubMed PMID: 28544535.

[85] Iribarren C, Folsom AR, Jacobs DR Jr, Gross MD, Belcher JD, Eckfeldt JH. Association of serum vitamin levels, LDL susceptibility to oxida-tion, and autoantibodies against MDA-LDL with carotid atherosclerosis. A case-control study. The ARIC Study Investigators Atherosclerosis Risk in Communities. *Arterioscler Thromb Vasc Biol* 1997; 17:1171 –7.

[86] Llopis S, Rodrigo MJ, González N, Genovés S, Zacarías L, Ramón D, Martorell P. *Nutrients.* 2019 Jan 22;11(2). pii: E232. doi: 10.3390/nu11020232.

[87] Nakamura M, Sugiura M, Aoki N. High beta-carotene and beta-cryptoxanthin are associated with low pulse wave velocity. *Atherosclerosis.* 2006 Feb;184(2):363-9. Epub 2005 Jun 4. PubMed PMID: 15936762.

[88] Stephen B. Kritchevsky; β-Carotene, Carotenoids and the Prevention of Coronary Heart Disease, *The Journal of Nutrition,* Volume 129, Issue 1, 1 January 1999, Pages 5–8, https://doi.org/10.1093/jn/129.1.5

[89] A.J. Alija, N. Bresgen, O. Sommerburg, C.D. Langhans, W. Siems, P.M. Eckl Cyto- and genotoxic potential of beta-carotene and cleavage products under oxidative stress. *Biofactors,* 24 (2005), pp. 159-163.

[90] W. Siems, C. Salerno, C. Crifo, O. Sommerburg, I. Wiswedel Beta-carotene degradation products—formation: toxicity and prevention of toxicity Forum. *Nutr.,* 61 (2009), pp. 75-86.

[91] Csepanyi E, Czompa A, Haines D, Lekli I, Bakondi E, Balla G, Tosaki A, Bak I. Cardiovascular effects of low versus high-dose beta-carotene in a rat model. *Pharmacol Res.* 2015 Oct;100:148-56. doi: 10.1016/j.phrs.2015.07.021. Epub 2015 Jul 28. PubMed PMID: 26225824.

[92] Leonardo A. M. Zornoff, Luiz S. Matsubara, Beatriz B. Matsubara, Marina P. Okoshi, Katashi Okoshi, Maeli Dal Pai-Silva, Robson F. Carvalho, Antonio C. Cicogna, Carlos R. Padovani, Ethel L. Novelli, Rosangela Novo, Álvaro O. Campana, Sergio A. R. Paiva; Beta-Carotene Supplementation Attenuates Cardiac Remodeling Induced by One-Month Tobacco-Smoke Exposure in Rats, *Toxicological Sciences,* Volume 90, Issue 1, 1 March 2006, Pages 259–266, https://doi.org/10.1093/toxsci/kfj080.

[93] Sari Voutilainen, Tarja Nurmi, Jaakko Mursu, Tiina H Rissanen; Carotenoids and cardiovascular health, *The American Journal of Clinical Nutrition,* Volume 83, Issue 6, 1 June 2006, Pages 1265–1271, https://doi.org/10.1093/ajcn/83.6.1265.

[94] Ganguly P, Alam SF. Role of homocysteine in the development of cardiovascular disease. *Nutr J.* 2015 Jan 10;14:6. doi: 10.1186/1475-2891-14-6. Review. PubMed PMID: 25577237; PubMed Central PMCID: PMC4326479.

[95] Hankey GJ, Eikelboom JW. Homocysteine and vascular disease. *Lancet.* 1999 Jul 31;354(9176):407-13. Review. PubMed PMID: 10437885.

[96] Marcus J, Sarnak MJ, Menon V. Homocysteine lowering and cardiovascular disease risk: lost in translation. *Can J Cardiol.* 2007 Jul;23(9):707-10. Review. PubMed PMID: 17622392; PubMed Central PMCID: PMC2651913.

[97] Fallis J. 16 Powerful Ways to Effectively Lower Homocysteine. *Web Optimal Living Dynamics,* August 19, 2017. Available From: https://www.optimallivingdynamics.com/blog/16-proven-ways-to-effectively-lower-homocysteine

[98] Nieva R, Safavynia SA, Lee Bishop K, Laurence S. Herbal, vitamin, and mineral supplement use in patients enrolled in a cardiac rehabilitation program. *J Cardiopulm Rehabil Prev.* 2012 Sep-Oct;32(5):270-7. doi: 10.1097/HCR. 0b013e31825f78f0. PubMed PMID: 22878561; PubMed Central PMCID: PMC4317371.

[99] Grassi D, Desideri G, Croce G, Tiberti S, Aggio A, Ferri C. Flavonoids, vascular function and cardiovascular protection. *Curr Pharm Des.* 2009;15(10):1072-84. Review. PubMed PMID: 19355949.

[100] Panche AN, Diwan AD, Chandra SR. Flavonoids: an overview. *J Nutr Sci.* 2016 Dec 29;5:e47. doi: 10.1017/jns.2016.41. eCollection 2016. Review. PubMed PMID: 28620474; PubMed Central PMCID: PMC5465813.

[101] Geleijnse JM, Launer LJ, Van der Kuip DA, Hofman A, Witteman JC. Inverse association of tea and flavonoid intakes with incident myocardial infarction: the Rotterdam Study. *Am J Clin Nutr.* 2002 May;75(5):880-6. PubMed PMID: 11976162.

[102] Arts IC, Hollman PC, Feskens EJ, Bueno de Mesquita HB, Kromhout D. Catechin intake might explain the inverse relation between tea consumption and ischemic heart disease: the Zutphen Elderly Study. *Am J Clin Nutr.* 2001 Aug;74(2):227-32. PubMed PMID: 11470725.

[103] Kurian, Gino A and Jose Paddikkala. "Effect of IntraOperative Magnesium Supplementation in Plasma Antioxidant Levels Trace Elements and Electrolyte Balance in Serum of Coronary Artery Bypass Graft Patients." (2016). *J Clin Basic Cardiol* 2007; 10 (online): 11.

[104] Muñoz-Castañeda JR, Pendón-Ruiz de Mier MV, Rodríguez M, Rodríguez-Ortiz ME. Magnesium Replacement to Protect Cardiovascular and Kidney Damage? Lack of Prospective Clinical Trials. *Int J Mol Sci.* 2018 Feb 27;19(3). pii: E664. doi: 10.3390/ijms19030664. Review. PubMed PMID: 29495444; PubMed Central PMCID: PMC5877525.

[105] Petre A. *21 Vegetarian Foods That Are Loaded With Iron.* Web HealthLine, May 4, 2017. Available From: https://www.healthline.com/nutrition/iron-rich-plant-foods.

[106] Tadimalla RT. Top 39 Magnesium-Rich Foods You Should Include In Your Diet. Reviewed By Registered Dietitian Staci Gulbin, MS, MEd, RD. Web Stylecraze, January 28, 2019. Available From: https://www.stylecraze.com/articles/magnesium-rich-foods-you-should-include-in-your-diet/#gref.

[107] Ordway GA, Garry DJ. Myoglobin: an essential hemoprotein in striated muscle. *J Exp Biol.* 2004 Sep; 207(Pt 20):3441-6.

[108] Mordi IR, Tee A, Lang CC. Iron Therapy in Heart Failure: Ready for Primetime? *Card Fail Rev.* 2018 May;4(1):28-32. doi: 10.15420/cfr.2018:6:2. Review. PubMed PMID: 29892473; PubMed Central PMCID: PMC5971676.

[109] Kshirsagar AV, Freburger JK, Ellis AR, Wang L, Winkelmayer WC, Brookhart MA. Intravenous iron supplementation practices and short-term risk of cardiovascular events in hemodialysis patients. *PLoS One.* 2013 Nov 1;8(11):e78930. doi: 10.1371/journal.pone.0078930. eCollection 2013. PubMed PMID: 24223866; PubMed Central PMCID: PMC3815308.

[110] Bowen KJ, Harris WS, Kris-Etherton PM. Omega-3 Fatty Acids and Cardiovascular Disease: Are There Benefits? *Curr Treat Options Cardiovasc Med.* 2016 Nov;18(11):69. Review. PubMed PMID: 27747477; PubMed Central PMCID: PMC5067287.

[111] Gammone MA, Riccioni G, Parrinello G, D'Orazio N. Omega-3 Polyunsaturated Fatty Acids: Benefits and Endpoints in Sport. *Nutrients.* 2018 Dec 27;11(1). pii: E46. doi: 10.3390/nu11010046. Review. PubMed PMID: 30591639; PubMed Central PMCID: PMC6357022.

[112] Preston Mason R. New Insights into Mechanisms of Action for Omega-3 Fatty Acids in Atherothrombotic Cardiovascular Disease. *Curr Atheroscler Rep.* 2019 Jan 12;21(1):2. doi: 10.1007/s11883-019-0762-1. Review. PubMed PMID: 30637567; PubMed Central PMCID: PMC6330561.

[113] Du J, Wang T, Huang P, Cui S, Gao C, Lin Y, Fu R, Shen J, He Y, Tan Y, Chen S. Clinical correlates of decreased plasma coenzyme Q10 levels in patients with multiple system atrophy. *Parkinsonism Relat Disord.* 2018 Dec;57:58-62. doi: 10.1016/j.parkreldis.2018.07.017. Epub 2018 Jul 26. PubMed PMID: 30093363.

[114] Sood B, Keenaghan M. Coenzyme Q10. [Updated 2018 Oct 27]. In: *StatPearls [Internet].* Treasure Island (FL): StatPearls Publishing; 2018 Jan-. Available from: https://www.ncbi.nlm.nih.gov/books/NBK531491/

[115] Zozina VI, Covantev S, Goroshko OA, Krasnykh LM, Kukes VG. Coenzyme Q10 in Cardiovascular and Metabolic Diseases: Current State of the Problem. *Curr Cardiol Rev.* 2018;14(3):164-174. doi: 10.2174/1573403X14666180416115428. Review. PubMed PMID: 29663894; PubMed Central PMCID: PMC6131403.

[116] Database of Abstracts of Reviews of Effects (DARE): Quality-assessed Reviews [Internet]. York (UK): *Centre for Reviews and Dissemination (UK); 1995-. Coenzyme Q10 in the treatment of hypertension: a meta-analysis of the clinical trials.* 2007. Available from: https://www.ncbi.nlm.nih.gov/books/NBK74275/

[117] Jafari M, Mousavi SM, Asgharzadeh A, Yazdani N. Coenzyme Q10 in the treatment of heart failure: A systematic review of systematic reviews. *Indian Heart J.* 2018

Jul;70 Suppl 1:S111-S117. doi: 10.1016/j.ihj.2018.01.031. Epub 2018 Jan 31. Review. PubMed PMID: 30122240; PubMed Central PMCID: PMC6097169.

[118] Ayers J, Cook J, Koenig RA, Sisson EM, Dixon DL. Recent Developments in the Role of Coenzyme Q10 for Coronary Heart Disease: a Systematic Review. *Curr Atheroscler Rep.* 2018 May 16;20(6):29. doi: 10.1007/s11883-018-0730-1. Review. PubMed PMID: 29766349.

[119] Bedoya LM, Bermejo P, Abad MJ. Anti-infectious activity in the Cistaceae family in the Iberian Peninsula. *Mini Rev Med Chem.* 2009 May; 9(5):519-25.

[120] Bedoya LM, Bermejo P, Abad MJ. Anti-infectious activity in the Cistaceae family in the Iberian Peninsula. *Mini Rev Med Chem.* 2009 May;9(5):519-25. Review. PubMed PMID: 19456283.

[121] Yue-E S, Weidong W, Jie Q. Anti-hyperlipidemia of garlic by reducing the level of total cholesterol and low-density lipoprotein. *Medicine:* May 2018 - Volume 97 - Issue 18 - p e0255 doi: 10.1097/MD.0000000000010255.

[122] Ried K, Fakler P. Potential of garlic (Allium sativum) in lowering high blood pressure: mechanisms of action and clinical relevance. *Integr Blood Press Control.* 2014 Dec 9;7:71-82. doi: 10.2147/IBPC.S51434. eCollection 2014. Review. PubMed PMID: 25525386; PubMed Central PMCID: PMC4266250.

[123] Maulik SK, Katiyar CK. Terminalia arjuna in cardiovascular diseases: making the transition from traditional to modern medicine in India. *Curr Pharm Biotechnol.* 2010 Dec;11(8):855-60. Review. PubMed PMID: 20874682.

[124] Dwivedi S, Chopra D. Revisiting Terminalia arjuna - An Ancient Cardiovascular Drug. *J Tradit Complement Med.* 2014 Oct;4(4):224-31. doi: 10.4103/2225-4110.139103. Review. PubMed PMID: 25379463; PubMed Central PMCID: PMC4220499.

[125] Kaur N, Shafiq N, Negi H, Pandey A et al. Terminalia arjuna in Chronic Stable Angina: Systematic Review and Meta-Analysis. *Cardiology Research and Practice* Volume 2014, Article ID 281483, 7 pages. http://dx.doi.org/10.1155/2014/281483

[126] Ragini H., Amita P., Jain A.K. An approach to standardize Arjunarishta: a well known ayurvedic formulation using UV and Colorimetric method. *J Med Pharm Allied Sci.* 2012;01:77–84.

[127] Shengule SA, Mishra S, Joshi K, Apte K, Patil D, Kale P, Shah T, Deshpande M, Puranik A. Anti-hyperglycemic and anti-hyperlipidaemic effect of Arjunarishta in high-fat fed animals. *J Ayurveda Integr Med.* 2018 Jan - Mar;9(1):45-52. doi: 10.1016/j.jaim.2017.07.004. Epub 2017 Dec 15. PubMed PMID: 29249636; PubMed Central PMCID: PMC5884182.

[128] Subramaniam S, Subramaniam R, Rajapandian S, Uthrapathi S, Gnanamanickam VR, Dubey GP. Anti-Atherogenic Activity of Ethanolic Fraction of Terminalia arjuna Bark on Hypercholesterolemic Rabbits. *Evid Based Complement Alternat*

Med. 2011;2011:487916. doi: 10.1093/ecam/neq003. Epub 2011 Mar 20. PubMed PMID: 21785628; PubMed Central PMCID: PMC3136348.

[129] Gaikwad D, Jadhav N. A Review On Biogenic Properties Of Stem Bark Of Terminalia Arjuna: AN UPDATE. *Asian J Pharm Clin Res,* Vol 11, Issue 8, 2018, 35-39.

[130] Kim J, Cha YJ, Lee KH, Park E. Effect of onion peel extract supplementation on the lipid profile and antioxidative status of healthy young women: a randomized, placebo-controlled, double-blind, crossover trial. *Nutr Res Pract.* 2013 Oct;7(5):373-9. doi: 10.4162/nrp.2013.7.5.373. Epub 2013 Oct 1. PubMed PMID: 24133616; PubMed Central PMCID: PMC3796662.

[131] Yang C, Li L, Yang L, Lǚ H, Wang S, Sun G. Anti-obesity and Hypolipidemic effects of garlic oil and onion oil in rats fed a high-fat diet. *Nutr Metab* (Lond). 2018 Jun 20;15:43. doi: 10.1186/s12986-018-0275-x. eCollection 2018. PubMed PMID: 29951108; PubMed Central PMCID: PMC6011244.

[132] Ro JY, Ryu JH, Park HJ, Cho HJ. Onion (Allium cepa L.) peel extract has anti-platelet effects in rat platelets. *Springerplus.* 2015 Jan 13;4:17. doi: 10.1186/s40064-015-0786-0. eCollection 2015. PubMed PMID: 25628983; PubMed Central PMCID: PMC4303602.

[133] Kang YR, Choi HY, Lee JY, Jang SI, Kang H, Oh JB, Jang HD, Kwon YI. Calorie Restriction Effect of Heat-Processed Onion Extract (ONI) Using In Vitro and In Vivo Animal Models. *Int J Mol Sci.* 2018 Mar 15;19(3). pii: E874. doi: 10.3390/ijms19030874. PubMed PMID: 29543768; PubMed Central PMCID: PMC5877735.

[134] Aslani N, Entezari MH, Askari G, Maghsoudi Z, Maracy MR. Effect of garlic and lemon juice mixture on lipid profile and some cardiovascular risk factors in people 30-60 years old with moderate hyperlipidaemia: A randomized clinical trial. *Int J Prev Med* 2016;7:95.

[135] Slimestad R, Fossen T, Vågen IM. Onions: a source of unique dietary flavonoids. *J Agric Food Chem.* 2007 Dec 12;55(25):10067-80. Epub 2007 Nov 13. Review. PubMed PMID: 17997520.

[136] Khiari Z, Makris DP. Stability and transformation of major flavonols in onion (Allium cepa) solid wastes. *J Food Sci Technol.* 2012 Aug;49(4):489-94. doi: 10.1007/s13197-010-0201-3. Epub 2010 Dec 22. PubMed PMID: 23904658; PubMed Central PMCID: PMC3550896.

[137] Kawser Hossain M, Abdal Dayem A, Han J, Yin Y, Kim K, Kumar Saha S, Yang GM, Choi HY, Cho SG. Molecular Mechanisms of the Anti-Obesity and Anti-Diabetic Properties of Flavonoids. *Int J Mol Sci.* 2016 Apr 15;17(4):569. doi: 10.3390/ijms17040569. Review. PubMed PMID: 27092490; PubMed Central PMCID: PMC4849025.

[138] Gopa B, Bhatt J, Hemavathi KG. A comparative clinical study of hypolipidemic efficacy of Amla (Emblica officinalis) with 3-hydroxy-3-methylglutaryl-coenzyme-A reductase inhibitor simvastatin. *Indian J Pharmacol.* 2012 Mar;44(2):238-42. doi: 10.4103/0253-7613.93857. PubMed PMID: 22529483; PubMed Central PMCID: PMC3326920.

[139] Kanthe PS, Patil BS, Bagali SC, Reddy RC, Aithala MR, Das KK. Protective effects of Ethanolic Extract of Emblica officinalis (amla) on Cardiovascular Pathophysiology of Rats, Fed with High Fat Diet. *J Clin Diagn Res.* 2017 Sep;11(9):CC05-CC09. doi: 10.7860/JCDR/2017/28474.10628. Epub 2017 Sep 1. PubMed PMID: 29207698; PubMed Central PMCID: PMC5713720.

[140] Khanna S, Das A, Spieldenner J, Rink C, Roy S. Supplementation of a standardized extract from Phyllanthus emblica improves cardiovascular risk factors and platelet aggregation in overweight/class-1 obese adults. *J Med Food.* 2015 Apr;18(4):415-20. doi: 10.1089/jmf.2014.0178. Epub 2015 Mar 10. PubMed PMID: 25756303; PubMed Central PMCID: PMC4390209.

[141] Tamang HK, Timilsina U, Singh KP, Shrestha S, Raman RK, Panta P, Karna P, Khadka L, Dahal C. Apo B/Apo A-I Ratio is Statistically A Better Predictor of Cardiovascular Disease (CVD) than Conventional Lipid Profile: A Study from Kathmandu Valley, Nepal. *J Clin Diagn Res.* 2014 Feb;8(2):34-6. doi: 10.7860/JCDR/2014/7588.4000. Epub 2014 Feb 3. PubMed PMID: 24701475; PubMed Central PMCID: PMC3972591.

[142] Feingold KR, Grunfeld C. *Introduction to Lipids and Lipoproteins.* [Updated 2018 Feb 2]. In: Feingold KR, Anawalt B, Boyce A, et al., editors. Endotext [Internet]. South Dartmouth (MA): MDText.com, Inc.; 2000-. Available from: https://www.ncbi.nlm.nih.gov/books/NBK305896/

[143] Choudhary B, Shetty A, Langade DG. Efficacy of Ashwagandha (Withania somnifera [L.] Dunal) in improving cardiorespiratory endurance in healthy athletic adults. *Ayu.* 2015 Jan-Mar;36(1):63-8. doi: 10.4103/0974-8520.169002. PubMed PMID: 26730141; PubMed Central PMCID: PMC4687242.

[144] Chandrasekhar K, Kapoor J, Anishetty S. A prospective, randomized double-blind, placebo-controlled study of safety and efficacy of a high-concentration full-spectrum extract of ashwagandha root in reducing stress and anxiety in adults. *Indian J Psychol Med.* 2012 Jul;34(3):255-62. doi: 10.4103/0253-7176.106022. PubMed PMID: 23439798; PubMed Central PMCID: PMC3573577.

[145] Auddy B., Hazra J., Mitra A., Abedon B., Ghosal S., City S. L. A standardized Withania somnifera extract significantly reduces stress-related parameters in chronically stressed humans. *Journal of the American Nutraceutical Association.* 2008;11:51–57.

[146] Cooley K, Szczurko O, Perri D, Mills EJ, Bernhardt B, Zhou Q, Seely D. Naturopathic care for anxiety: a randomized controlled trial ISRCTN78958974.

PLoS One. 2009 Aug 31;4(8):e6628. doi: 10.1371/journal.pone.0006628. PubMed PMID: 19718255; PubMed Central PMCID: PMC2729375.

[147] Deshpande A, Irani N, Balakrishnan R. Study protocol and rationale for a prospective, randomized, double-blind, placebo-controlled study to evaluate the effects of Ashwagandha (Withania somnifera) extract on nonrestorative sleep. *Medicine (Baltimore).* 2018 Jun;97(26):e11299. doi: 10.1097/MD.0000000000011299. PubMed PMID: 29953014; PubMed Central PMCID: PMC6039614.

[148] Mishra LC, Singh BB, Dagenais S. Scientific basis for the therapeutic use of Withania somnifera (ashwagandha): a review. *Altern Med Rev.* 2000 Aug;5(4):334-46. Review. PubMed PMID: 10956379.

[149] Singh N, Nath R, Lata A, Singh S, Kohli R, Bhargava K. Withania somnifera (ashwagandha), a rejuvenating herbal drug which enhances survival during stress (an adaptogen). *Int J Crude Drug Res.* 1982;20(1):29–35. doi: 10.3109/13880208209083282.

[150] Lyle N, Bhattacharyya D, Sur TK, Munshi S, Paul S, Chatterjee S, Gomes A. Stress modulating antioxidant effect of Nardostachys jatamansi. *Indian J Biochem Biophys.* 2009 Feb;46(1):93-8. PubMed PMID: 19374260.

[151] Nandha R, Singh H, Moudgill P, Kular G. A pilot study to clinically evaluate the role of herbomineral compound "Rakatchap Har" in the management of essential hypertension. *Ayu.* 2011 Jul;32(3):329-32. doi: 10.4103/0974-8520.93908. PubMed PMID: 22529645; PubMed Central PMCID: PMC3326876.

[152] Ali A, Umar D, Farhan M, Basheer B, Baroudi K. Effect of Brahmyadi Churna (Brahmi, Shankhapushpi, Jatamansi, Jyotishmati, Vacha, Ashwagandha) and tablet Shilajatu in essential hypertension: An observational study. *J Adv Pharm Technol Res.* 2015 Oct-Dec;6(4):148-53. doi: 10.4103/2231-4040.165015. PubMed PMID: 26605154; PubMed Central PMCID: PMC4630720.

[153] Aisa R, Yu Z, Zhang X, Maimaitiyiming D, Huang L, Hasim A, Jiang T, Duan M. The Effects of Aqueous Extract from Nardostachys chinensis Batalin on Blood Pressure and Cardiac Hypertrophy in Two-Kidney One-Clip Hypertensive Rats. *Evid Based Complement Alternat Med.* 2017;2017:4031950. doi: 10.1155/2017/4031950. Epub 2017 Oct 11. PubMed PMID: 29234388; PubMed Central PMCID: PMC5660807.

[154] Peterson CT, Denniston K, Chopra D. Therapeutic Uses of Triphala in Ayurvedic Medicine. *J Altern Complement Med.* 2017 Aug;23(8):607-614. doi: 10.1089/acm.2017.0083. Epub 2017 Jul 11. Review. PubMed PMID: 28696777; PubMed Central PMCID: PMC5567597.

[155] Aggarwal BB, Prasad S, Reuter S, Kannappan R, Yadev VR, Park B, Kim JH, Gupta SC, Phromnoi K, Sundaram C, Prasad S, Chaturvedi MM, Sung B. Identification of novel anti-inflammatory agents from Ayurvedic medicine for prevention of chronic

diseases: "reverse pharmacology" and "bedside to bench" approach. *Curr Drug Targets.* 2011 Oct;12(11):1595-653. PubMed PMID: 21561421; PubMed Central PMCID: PMC3170500.

[156] Mashyal P, Bhargav H, Raghuram N. Safety and usefulness of Laghu shankha prakshalana in patients with essential hypertension: A self controlled clinical study. *J Ayurveda Integr Med.* 2014 Oct-Dec;5(4):227-35. doi: 10.4103/0975-9476.131724. PubMed PMID: 25624697; PubMed Central PMCID: PMC4296435.

[157] Mukherjee PK, Rai S, Bhattacharyya S, Debnath PK, Biswas TK, Jana U, et al. Clinical study of 'Triphala'--A well knownphytomedicine from India. *Ir J Pharmacol and Ther.* 2006;5:51–4.

[158] Singh DP, Mani D. Protective effect of Triphala Rasayana against paracetamol-induced hepato-renal toxicity in mice. *J Ayurveda Integr Med.* 2015 Jul-Sep;6(3):181-6. doi: 10.4103/0975-9476.146553. PubMed PMID: 26604553; PubMed Central PMCID: PMC4630692.

[159] Gurjar S, Pal A, Kapur S. Triphala and its constituents ameliorate visceral adiposity from a high-fat diet in mice with diet-induced obesity. *Altern Ther Health Med.* 2012 Nov-Dec;18(6):38-45. PubMed PMID: 23251942.

[160] Walden R, Tomlinson B. Cardiovascular disease. In: Benzie IFF, Wachtel-Galor S, editors. *Herbal Medicine: Biomolecular and Clinical Aspects,* Chapter 16. 2. Boca Raton: CRC Press/Taylor & Francis; 2011.

[161] Tarasiuk A, Mosińska P, Fichna J. Triphala: current applications and new perspectives on the treatment of functional gastrointestinal disorders. *Chin Med.* 2018 Jul 18;13:39. doi: 10.1186/s13020-018-0197-6. eCollection 2018. Review. PubMed PMID: 30034512; PubMed Central PMCID: PMC6052535.

[162] Saravanan S, Srikumar R, Manikandan S, Jeya Parthasarathy N, Sheela Devi R. Hypolipidemic effect of triphala in experimentally induced hypercholesteremic rats. *Yakugaku Zasshi.* 2007 Feb;127(2):385-8. PubMed PMID: 17268159.

[163] Vinayakumar A. *Ayurvedic Clinical Medicine,* 1st ed. Delhi: Sri Satguru publication, 1997.

[164] A P, P SR, M PR, K G R. Apoptosis in angiotensin II-stimulated hypertrophic cardiac cells -modulation by phenolics rich extract of Boerhavia diffusa L. *Biomed Pharmacother.* 2018 Dec;108:1097-1104. doi: 10.1016/j.biopha.2018.09.114. Epub 2018 Sep 28. PubMed PMID: 30372810.

[165] Prathapan A, Vineetha VP, Abhilash PA, Raghu KG. Boerhaavia diffusa L. attenuates angiotensin II-induced hypertrophy in H9c2 cardiac myoblast cells via modulating oxidative stress and down-regulating NF-κβ and transforming growth factor β1. *Br J Nutr.* 2013 Oct;110(7):1201-10. doi: 10.1017/S0007114513000561. Epub 2013 Apr 16. PubMed PMID: 23591029.

[166] Ferreres F, Sousa C, Justin M, Valentão P, Andrade PB, Llorach R, Rodrigues A, Seabra RM, Leitão A. Characterisation of the phenolic profile of Boerhaavia diffusa

L. by HPLC-PAD-MS/MS as a tool for quality control. *Phytochem Anal.* 2005 Nov-Dec;16(6):451-8. PubMed PMID: 16315490.

[167] Yan L, Zhang JD, Wang B, Lv YJ, Jiang H, Liu GL, Qiao Y, Ren M, Guo XF. Quercetin inhibits left ventricular hypertrophy in spontaneously hypertensive rats and inhibits angiotensin II-induced H9C2 cells hypertrophy by enhancing PPAR-γ expression and suppressing AP-1 activity. *PLoS One.* 2013 Sep 10;8(9):e72548. doi: 10.1371/journal.pone.0072548. eCollection 2013. PubMed PMID: 24039778; PubMed Central PMCID: PMC3769399.

[168] Larson AJ, Symons JD, Jalili T. Therapeutic potential of quercetin to decrease blood pressure: review of efficacy and mechanisms. *Adv Nutr.* 2012 Jan;3(1):39-46. doi: 10.3945/an.111.001271. Epub 2012 Jan 5. Review. PubMed PMID: 22332099; PubMed Central PMCID: PMC3262612.

[169] Liobikas J, Majiene D, Trumbeckaite S, Kursvietiene L, Masteikova R, Kopustinskiene DM, Savickas A, Bernatoniene J. Uncoupling and antioxidant effects of ursolic acid in isolated rat heart mitochondria. *J Nat Prod.* 2011 Jul 22;74(7):1640-4. doi: 10.1021/np200060p. Epub 2011 Jun 7. PubMed PMID: 21648406.

[170] Calderón-Montaño JM, Burgos-Morón E, Pérez-Guerrero C, López-Lázaro M. A review on the dietary flavonoid kaempferol. *Mini Rev Med Chem.* 2011 Apr;11(4):298-344. Review. PubMed PMID: 21428901.

[171] Aviello G, Canadanovic-Brunet JM, Milic N, Capasso R, Fattorusso E, Taglialatela-Scafati O, Fasolino I, Izzo AA, Borrelli F. Potent antioxidant and genoprotective effects of boeravinone G, a rotenoid isolated from Boerhaavia diffusa. *PLoS One.* 2011;6(5):e19628. doi: 10.1371/journal.pone.0019628. Epub 2011 May 20. PubMed PMID: 21625488; PubMed Central PMCID: PMC3098844.

[172] Lami N, Kadota S, Kikuchi T, Momose Y. Constituents of the roots of Boerhaavia diffusa L. III. Identification of Ca2+ channel antagonistic compound from the methanol extract. *Chem Pharm Bull (Tokyo).* 1991 Jun;39(6):1551-5. PubMed PMID: 1934177.

[173] Vineetha VP, Prathapan A, Soumya RS, Raghu KG. Arsenic trioxide toxicity in H9c2 myoblasts--damage to cell organelles and possible amelioration with Boerhavia diffusa. *Cardiovasc Toxicol.* 2013 Jun;13(2):123-37. doi: 10.1007/s12012-012-9191-x. PubMed PMID: 23161055.

[174] Hung, H.C., et al., Fruit and vegetable intake and risk of major chronic disease. *J Natl Cancer Inst,* 2004. 96(21): p. 1577-84.

[175] Wiseman, M., The second World Cancer Research Fund/American Institute for Cancer Research expert report. Food, nutrition, physical activity, and the prevention of cancer: a global perspective. *Proc Nutr Soc,* 2008. 67(3): p. 253-6.

[176] 10 Incredible Reasons to Eat Cruciferous Vegetables Regularly. *Web Food Revolution Network,* February 8, 2017. Available From: https://foodrevolution.org/blog/food-and-health/cruciferous-vegetables-cancer-health-benefits/

[177] Bai Y, Wang X, Zhao S, Ma C, Cui J, Zheng Y. Sulforaphane Protects against Cardiovascular Disease via Nrf2 Activation. *Oxid Med Cell Longev.* 2015;2015:407580. doi: 10.1155/2015/407580. Epub 2015 Oct 25. Review. PubMed PMID: 26583056; PubMed Central PMCID: PMC4637098.

[178] Choi KM, Lee YS, Kim W, Kim SJ, Shin KO, Yu JY, Lee MK, Lee YM, Hong JT, Yun YP, Yoo HS. Sulforaphane attenuates obesity by inhibiting adipogenesis and activating the AMPK pathway in obese mice. *J Nutr Biochem.* 2014 Feb;25(2):201-7. doi: 10.1016/j.jnutbio.2013.10.007. Epub 2013 Nov 14. PubMed PMID: 24445045.

[179] Health Dangers of Cruciferous Vegetables. *Web Kevin Stock,* September 18, 2018. Available From: https://www.kevinstock.io/health/health-dangers-of-cruciferous-vegetables/

[180] Mohtashami A, Entezari MH. Effects of Nigella sativa supplementation on blood parameters and anthropometric indices in adults: A systematic review on clinical trials. *J Res Med Sci.* 2016 Jan 28;21:3. eCollection 2016. Review. PubMed PMID: 27904549; PubMed Central PMCID: PMC5122217.

[181] Jaarin K, Foong WD, Yeoh MH, Kamarul ZY, Qodriyah HM, Azman A, Zuhair JS, Juliana AH, Kamisah Y. Mechanisms of the antihypertensive effects of Nigella sativa oil in L-NAME-induced hypertensive rats. *Clinics (Sao Paulo).* 2015 Nov;70(11):751-7. doi: 10.6061/clinics/2015(11)07. PubMed PMID: 26602523; PubMed Central PMCID: PMC4642492.

[182] Enayatfard L, Mohebbati R, Niazmand S, Hosseini M, Shafei MN. The standardized extract of Nigella sativa and its major ingredient, thymoquinone, ameliorates angiotensin II-induced hypertension in rats. *J Basic Clin Physiol Pharmacol.* 2018 Oct 1. pii: /j/jbcpp.ahead-of-print/jbcpp-2018-0074/jbcpp-2018-0074.xml. doi: 10.1515/jbcpp-2018-0074. [Epub ahead of print] PubMed PMID: 30269105.

[183] Nagi MN, Al-Shabanah OA, Hafez MM, Sayed-Ahmed MM. Thymoquinone supplementation attenuates cyclophosphamide-induced cardiotoxicity in rats. *J Biochem Mol Toxicol.* 2011 May-Jun;25(3):135-42. doi: 10.1002/jbt.20369. Epub 2010 Oct 18. PubMed PMID: 20957680.

[184] Ebru U, Burak U, Yusuf S, Reyhan B, Arif K, Faruk TH, Emin M, Aydin K, Atilla II, Semsettin S, Kemal E. Cardioprotective effects of Nigella sativa oil on cyclosporine A-induced cardiotoxicity in rats. *Basic Clin Pharmacol Toxicol.* 2008 Dec;103(6):574-80. doi: 10.1111/j.1742-7843.2008.00313.x. PubMed PMID: 18801029.

[185] al-Shabanah OA, Badary OA, Nagi MN, al-Gharably NM, al-Rikabi AC, al-Bekairi AM. Thymoquinone protects against doxorubicin-induced cardiotoxicity without

compromising its antitumor activity. *J Exp Clin Cancer Res.* 1998 Jun;17(2):193-8. PubMed PMID: 9700580.

[186] Torabi M, Naeemzadeh F, Ebrahimi V, Taleschian-Tabrizi N, Pashazadeh F, Nazemie H. 133: The Effect Of Zingiber Officinale (Ginger) On Hypertension; A Systematic Review Of Randomised Controlled Trials. *BMJ Open.* 2017;7(Suppl 1):bmjopen-2016-015415.133. Published 2017 Feb 8. doi:10.1136/bmjopen-2016-015415.133.

[187] Brahma Naidu P, Uddandrao VV, Ravindar Naik R, Suresh P, Meriga B, Begum MS, Pandiyan R, Saravanan G. Ameliorative potential of gingerol: Promising modulation of inflammatory factors and lipid marker enzymes expressions in HFD induced obesity in rats. *Mol Cell Endocrinol.* 2016 Jan 5;419:139-47. doi: 10.1016/j.mce.2015.10.007. Epub 2015 Oct 19. PubMed PMID: 26493465.

[188] Zhu J, Chen H, Song Z, Wang X, Sun Z. Effects of Ginger (Zingiber officinale Roscoe) on Type 2 Diabetes Mellitus and Components of the Metabolic Syndrome: A Systematic Review and Meta-Analysis of Randomized Controlled Trials. *Evid Based Complement Alternat Med.* 2018 Jan 9;2018:5692962. doi: 10.1155/2018/5692962. eCollection 2018. Review. PubMed PMID: 29541142; PubMed Central PMCID: PMC5818945.

[189] Li X, Guo J, Liang N, Jiang X, Song Y, Ou S, Hu Y, Jiao R, Bai W. 6-Gingerol Regulates Hepatic Cholesterol Metabolism by Up-regulation of LDLR and Cholesterol Efflux-Related Genes in HepG2 Cells. *Front Pharmacol.* 2018 Feb 27;9:159. doi: 10.3389/fphar.2018.00159. eCollection 2018. PubMed PMID: 29535632; PubMed Central PMCID: PMC5835308.

[190] Tabibi H, Imani H, Atabak S, Najafi I, Hedayati M, Rahmani L. Effects of Ginger on Serum Lipids and Lipoproteins in Peritoneal Dialysis Patients: A Randomized Controlled Trial. *Perit Dial Int.* 2016 Mar-Apr;36(2):140-5. doi: 10.3747/pdi.2015.00006. Epub 2015 Oct 16. PubMed PMID: 26475844; PubMed Central PMCID: PMC4803358.

[191] Ali AMA, El-Nour MEM, Yagi SM. Total phenolic and flavonoid contents and antioxidant activity of ginger (Zingiber officinale Rosc.) rhizome, callus and callus treated with some elicitors. *J Genet Eng Biotechnol.* 2018 Dec;16(2):677-682. doi: 10.1016/j.jgeb.2018.03.003. Epub 2018 Mar 21. PubMed PMID: 30733788; PubMed Central PMCID: PMC6353720.

AUTHOR'S CONTACT INFORMATION

A. K. Mohiuddin
Assistant Professor
World University of Bangladesh
Email: mohiuddin3@pharmacy.wub.edu.bd

INDEX

A

B

C

D

I

J

K

L

M

N

O

T

U

V

W

X

Y

Z

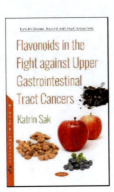